HEALTH POWER
Health by Choice
Not Chance

Aileen Ludington, MD
Hans Diehl, DrHSc, MPH, FACN, CNS

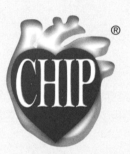

Lifestyle Medicine Institute, LLC
Loma Linda, CA 92354

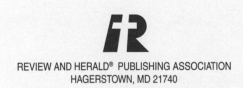

REVIEW AND HERALD® PUBLISHING ASSOCIATION
HAGERSTOWN, MD 21740

This book was
Edited by Aileen Ludington and Hans Diehl
Copyedited by James Cavil
Designed by Darryl Ludington
Cover design by Darryl Ludington
Typeset: 11/14 Helvetica

PRINTED IN U.S.A.

R&H Cataloging Service
Ludington, Aileen, & Diehl, Hans
   p. cm. Health Power: Health by Choice, Not Chance / Aileen Ludington, Hans Diehl.
   Includes index.

   1. Health. 2. Popular Medicine. I. Diehl, Hans, 1946. II. Ludington, Aileen, 1926.

613
ISBN 0-8280-1865-0 Caucasian
ISBN 0-8280-1576-7 African American
ISBN 0-8280-1698-4 Native American

What Others Have Said

Clarity, Charm, and Thoroughness

"The greatest challenge of Western medicine is to educate and motivate patients to adopt a healthier lifestyle. This book is doing exactly that—with clarity, charm, and thoroughness."

—William Castelli, M.D.
Former Director, Framingham Heart Study

A Solid Book

"A solid book, clearly written, providing a sensible introduction to the basis of natural health management."

—John Robbins
Author, Diet for a New America

Extend Your Life

"These are important concepts that, when internalized, will do more to improve your health and extend your life than all the technological wonders of modern medicine."

—Caldwell Esselstyn, Jr., M.D.
Cleveland Clinic

No One Can Read and Remain the Same

"The authors have been in the forefront of preventive medicine since long before it was fashionable. They confront health questions and anxieties with compelling evidence and grace. No one can read even a few of these chapters and remain the same."

—Herbert E. Douglass, Th.D., former president
Weimar Institute

Most Practical Key

"This may be the most practical key to a better lifestyle that many of us have ever found."

—Dan Matthews, executive producer/host
Christian Lifestyle Magazine

Habits Count

"[Most people] suffer because of their own wrong course of action. They disregard the principles of health by their habits of eating, drinking, dressing, and working."

—E. G. White
Pioneer health reformer/educator

The Blame Game

"God is not responsible for the suffering that follows disregard of natural law."

—E. G. White
Pioneer health reformer/educator

Nature's Way

"In nature there are neither rewards nor punishments; there are only consequences."

—Robert B. Ingersoll

Can't Buy Them

"There are four things in life which money cannot buy: friends, time, peace of mind, and good health."

—William F. Kenney

Number One

"The most important things in life aren't things."

Look It Up

"The only place where success comes before work is in a dictionary."

—Vidal Sassoon

3

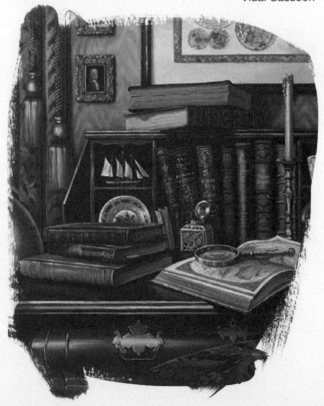

CONTENTS

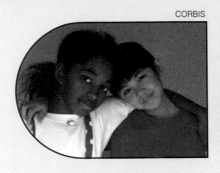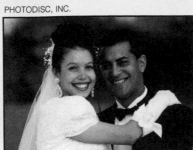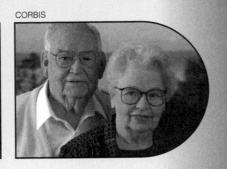

Weight Control

Natural Remedies

Mind-Body Connection

Coda

CAUTION

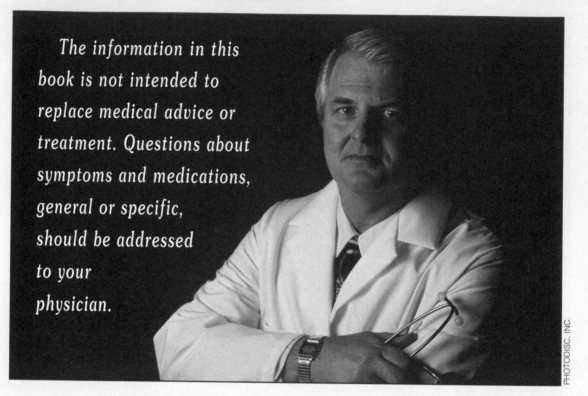

The information in this book is not intended to replace medical advice or treatment. Questions about symptoms and medications, general or specific, should be addressed to your physician.

PHOTODISC, INC.

Acknowledgements

We are indebted to the wholistic (personal health) vision of *The Quiet Hour* broadcast ministries, to their president, Bill Tucker, and to his staff, for believing in this project enough to extend considerable financial support and resources to see it through to completion.

In addition, we wish to give special recognition to Lawson Dumbeck, author of the *Dynamic Living Workbook,* from which the Application pages of this book are abstracted. Mr. Dumbeck is an educator and freelance writer based in Olympia, Washington. He holds graduate degrees in adult education and law.

And lastly, the faithful participants of our CHIP health outreach programs who continue to validate in their daily lives the principles presented in this book.

—Drs. Aileen Ludington and Hans Diehl

PREFACE

Consciously or unconsciously, most people make sacrifices of some sort. Unfortunately, they often sacrifice health, family, religion, or other priceless possessions in order to gain the transitory pleasures of wealth, power, status, or fame.

Imagine life as a game in which you are juggling five balls—work, family, health, friends and religion—in the air, and you are trying to keep all of them off the ground. You will soon realize that work is a rubber ball. If you drop it, it will bounce back. But the other four balls—your family, health, friends, and spiritual life—are much more fragile. If you drop one of these, it will be scuffed, marked, nicked, damaged, or even shattered. It will never be the same again. You must understand that, and strive to balance all parts of your life.

This book will help you realize that all these aspects are largely under your control.

- Learn how you can prevent and even reverse many of today's major killer diseases.

- Learn how to make sense out of confusing and often contradictory health information, and to understand why today's breakthroughs often become tomorrow's embarrassments.

- Learn how to strengthen your social and family relationships, and cultivate a more meaningful spiritual life.

This book will help you discover—day by day and step by step—not a better life, but the *best life!*

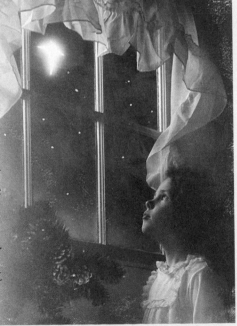

CORBIS

7

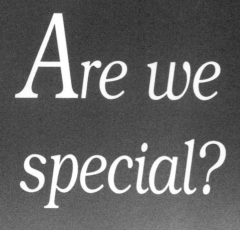

Are we special?

"Sons are a heritage from the Lord, children a reward from him." Psalm 127:3

HEALTH OUTLOOK
FOR THE NEW CENTURY

- **Medical Overview**

- **The Western Diet**

- **Modern Nutrition**

- **Children at Risk**

- **Aging**

WITH THE KNOWLEDGE WE HAVE NOW, WE COULD AND SHOULD LIVE A HEALTHY, HAPPY 100 YEARS.

MEDICAL OVERVIEW

Myths and Miracles

The achievements of science, medicine, and public health in the twentieth century have been enormous. America is now an undisputed leader of quality medical care. There is much to be proud of, and more to come.

That's especially incredible considering that germs were discovered only around 150 years ago.

It has been a big jump from Louis Pasteur's discovery of the germ theory to the place we are now. His findings opened the door to antiseptic surgery, improved sanitation, cleaner water, safer food, and vaccines. All of these impacted infectious diseases such as typhoid, cholera, poliomyelitis and smallpox. Once a leading cause of death in developed countries, infectious diseases have now been upstaged by the noninfectious degenerative-type diseases, increasingly referred to as Western or lifestyle diseases.

What do you consider the medical landmarks of the twentieth century?

There are many. Improved surgical techniques, better anesthesia, and safer blood transfusions, for starters. Antibiotics have saved millions of lives, although their overuse is producing a frightening backlash—resistant strains of bacteria that are often unaffected by present treatments.

Advances in diagnostic technology are prodigious. The inside workings of various bodily organs can now be visualized, measured, and studied, and even thought patterns and emotions can be traced as they travel in the brain.

Molecular biology and genetics are opening doors to more new worlds.

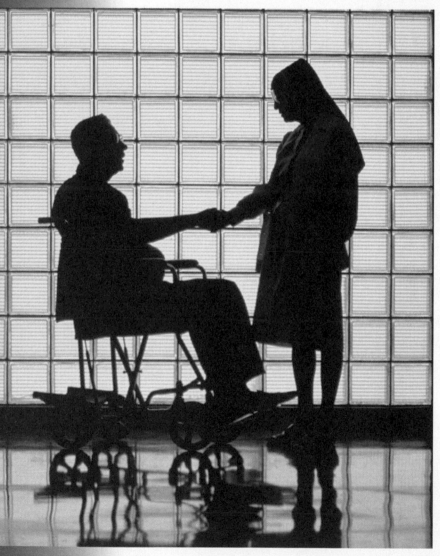

"Dear friend, I pray that you may enjoy good health and that all may go well with you, even as your soul is getting along well." 3 John 2

Many birth defects can now be detected in advance, and some can be corrected in the uterus, before birth. Geneticists are learning to pinpoint predispositions to certain diseases in the DNA, and are looking for ways to affect the outcome.

For medical technology in the years ahead, there is no end in sight. As scientists seek to clone spare body parts from people's own cells, the limiting factors may well be cost and affordability.

No wonder people live so much longer today!

Actually that belief is largely a myth. For years people believed that the miracles of modern medicine were mainly responsible for extending our current life span by some 27 years, when compared to those who were born 100 years ago.

The fact is that around 1900 every sixth baby died before reaching the first year of life, mainly because of infectious diseases. This, then, greatly shortened the average life span of their society.

Today, however, a person age 65 has very nearly the same life expectancy as a person back then who survived that critical first year of life, with perhaps an average gain of around five or six years at most (see graph).

Then why do we see so much more "degenerative disease"? Isn't it because most of our ancestors died while they were still too young to experience the diseases of "old age"?

The term "degenerative disease" is really a misnomer. For years people fatalistically accepted the idea that atherosclerosis-related diseases (such as coronary heart diseases and stroke), cancer, diabetes, diverticulosis, arthritis, and other ailments were diseases of old age and therefore to

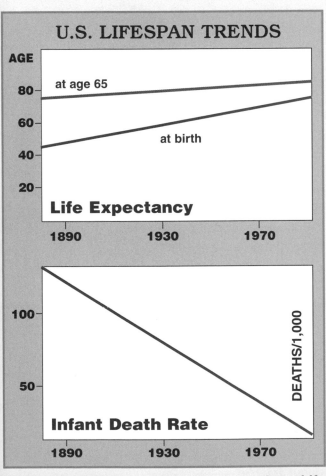

U.S. LIFESPAN TRENDS

Life Expectancy

AGE — at age 65 — at birth

80, 60, 40, 20

1890   1930   1970

Infant Death Rate

DEATHS/1,000

100

50

1890   1930   1970

Life expectancy at birth is increasing. Life expectancy for 65-year-olds, however, has only marginally increased during the past 100 years.

Without health, life is not life; it is only a state of languor and suffering—an image of death.

—Rabelais

be expected.

Nothing could be further from the truth, because in Western society 100 years ago:

● Atherosclerosis-related diseases were virtually unknown. The first description of coronary artery disease and "heart attacks" appeared in medical literature in 1910. Today these diseases are responsible for almost every second death.

● Cancers of the breast, colon, prostate, and lungs were virtually unknown. These cancers are now claiming one out of every four American lives.

● Similarly, very few diabetics were known then. Yet today, diabetes rates are increasing with frightening speed. *(See chart on page 53.)* Diabetes and its complications now represent one of the most frequent causes of death.

In light of the advances in medical science, that is truly amazing. Shouldn't these diseases be decreasing?

It's important to understand that these diseases are actually

Dropping the Ball

THE GOVERNMENT
What They're Doing:
The federal government shells out a mere $2 million on health and on fitness-related initiatives—some policy recommendations here, a public service campaign there.

THE MEDICAL PROFESSION
What They're Doing:
Precious little. Nearly half the people surveyed in a Gallup poll said they'd never heard a word about fitness or wellness from their doctors.

THE FITNESS INDUSTRY
What They're Doing:
Marketing the quick hit ("Thinner Thighs in 30 Days"), exercise that's painful rather than fun ("Go for the Burn"), and sexiness over health.

The Stereotypical Businessman—

over-weight, exhausted, living on cigarettes and three-martini lunches—is out of date. In today's business world, sweat is status, and trimness is success. More and more modern executives are apt to be in prime condition; neither they nor their companies can afford otherwise.

Depending on expensive, high-tech medical facilities and equipment for health is not the solution.

not "degenerative"—they are not necessarily the result of growing older. The fact that an increasing number of younger people are suffering from them refutes this, as does their increase to near epidemic proportions despite everything medical science can do.

Modern epidemiology (the study of disease differences in world populations) is unraveling the mystery—that most of these modern killer diseases are lifestyle-related. They are basically diseases of affluence—too much eating and drinking, too much smoking, and too little exercise. Medical science is treating the symptoms, but it's time to attack the causes.

You mean people create their own diseases? You can't be serious!

Yes, I am serious. The solution to most of our health problems today does not depend on physicians, technological advances, or on the quality of our hospitals. Our health today is determined largely by our lifestyle choices, our physiological inheritance, and our physical environment. Good health in today's world mainly depends on what we're willing to do for ourselves—how we choose to live, especially how we eat, drink, exercise, and whether or not we smoke.

That's pretty scary. Yet it's good to know there are things I can do to improve my own health.

That's the bottom line. People are increasingly waking up to the fact that they must take charge—take responsibility—for their own health. That's what this book is about. How to do it. How to live a quality life, and how to avoid the most common causes of premature disease, disability, suffering, and death. If we take advantage of the knowledge we have right now, most of us could live to be 100 in good health.

"Advances in high-tech medicine have not altered the advances of the killer diseases."

"Before I got into med school, I knew what I was going to do—help people get healthy. But instead of becoming expert in health, I became an expert in disease."

Application

"The concept that Western diseases are lifestyle-related and therefore potentially preventable and reversible is the most important medical discovery of the twentieth century."

—Denis Burkitt, M.D., England
Discoverer of Burkitt's Lymphoma

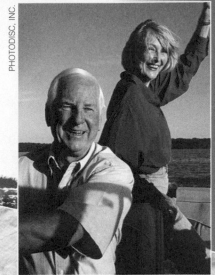

The Future Shape of Healthy Living

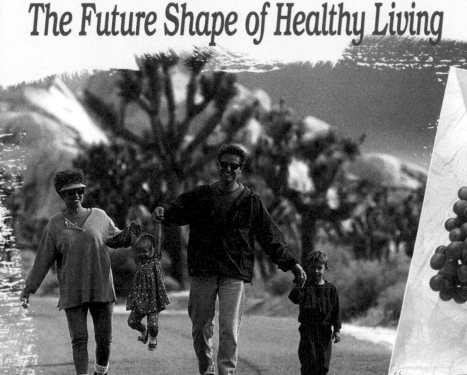

PHOTODISC, INC.

PHOTODISC, INC.

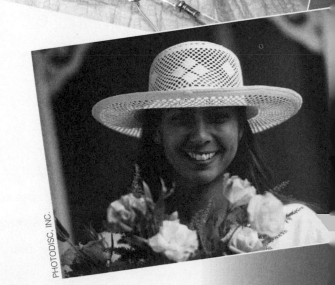

PHOTODISC, INC.

How about you? What are some health habits you would like to work on?

Write them down in this space:

1) _____

2) _____

3) _____

4) _____

5) _____

6) _____

THE WESTERN DIET

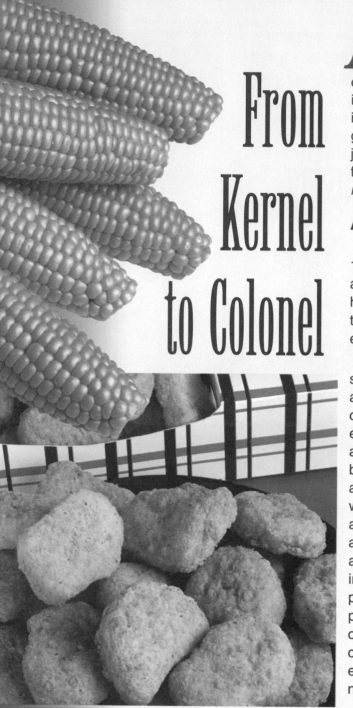

From Kernel to Colonel

Americans are spending 40 percent of their food dollars eating out. Our food is processed, refined, concentrated, sugared, salted, and chemically engineered to produce taste sensations high in calories and low in nutrients. Our cattle are fattened in feedlots without exercise and with antibiotics and growth enhancers. The result: bigger cattle producing juicier steaks containing nearly twice the fat as range-fed cattle. And we are paying dearly for these *advancements.* While we eat to live, what we eat is killing us.

Are you saying that food can cause disease?

The statistics are pretty convincing. In 1900, about 10 to 15 percent of Americans died from heart disease and strokes (and much of that was from rheumatic heart disease). Today it's 45 percent. Back then, less than 6 percent died of cancer, while today the figure is exceeding 25 percent.

This isn't nature's way. We weren't meant to die in such numbers from heart attacks, strokes, diabetes, and from cancer of the lungs, breast, prostate, and colon. Significant cardiovascular disease began to emerge in America after World War I. It became rampant only after World War II, when people could afford diets rich in animal products and when the food industry began producing highly processed foods crammed with calories and emptied of nutrition.

PURE CORN

Last year Americans grew almost 8 billion bushels of corn—but less than 1 percent of this crop was sweet corn, the kind we eat as a vegetable. The rest was used for animal feed, soft drinks (as corn syrup), gasoline additives, and paper.

"This is what the kingdom of God is like. A man scatters seed on the ground. Night and day, whether he sleeps or gets up, the seed sprouts and grows, though he does not know how. All by itself the soil produces grain—first the stalk, then the head, then the full kernel in the head. As soon as the grain is ripe, he puts the sickle to it, because the harvest has come." Mark 4:26-29

Could this be coincidental?

Hardly. This problem is unique to Westernized people. Rural populations in China and Southeast Asia who have little access to rich foods experience few heart attacks. Similarly, most people in rural Africa and South and Central America have little fear of diabetes and cardiovascular disease. Yet in North America, Australia, New Zealand, and the increasingly affluent countries in Europe and Asia, where diets are rich in fat and cholesterol, heart disease and diabetes are epidemic.

The villains, low fiber, high fat, and cholesterol, take their toll by damaging the body's vital oxygen-carrying arteries and by upsetting important metabolic functions. Because of thickened, narrowed arteries, 4,000 Americans have heart attacks every day, every third adult has high blood pres-

In 1900 people got 70 percent of their protein from plant foods. Today we get 70 percent of our protein from animal products—high in fat and cholesterol.

sure, and thousands are crippled from strokes. Because of disordered metabolisms from unbalanced lifestyles, obesity is epidemic, and a new diabetic is diagnosed every 50 seconds.

How did these dietary changes come about?

Before 1900 the North

American diet consisted mostly of foods grown in local gardens and nearby farms, supplemented with a few staples from the general store. Their meat came from barnyard animals and range-fed cattle. Our grandparents didn't have thousands of beautifully packaged and highly promoted food products waiting at the supermarket. Fast-food restaurants didn't beckon from nearly every street corner.

The backbone of their diet was kernels—kernels of wheat and other grains growing in reassuring profusion. Families ate freshly cooked food and thick slices of home-baked bread around their own tables. They enjoyed hot cereals, cornbread, and biscuits. They ate rice, pasta, and corn, along with beans, potatoes, vegetables, and fruit. These nutritious high-fiber foods made up 53 percent of their daily calorie intake.

But times and tastes have changed dramatically. Cereals like oatmeal have been replaced by cold, presweetened flakes. Lunch

15

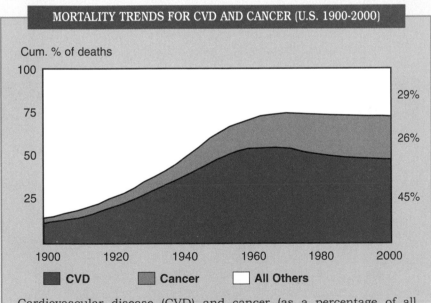

LIFESTYLE MEDICINE INSTITUTE

MORTALITY TRENDS FOR CVD AND CANCER (U.S. 1900-2000)

Cum. % of deaths

100

75 — 29%

50 — 26%

25 — 45%

1900   1920   1940   1960   1980   2000

■ CVD   ■ Cancer   □ All Others

Cardiovascular disease (CVD) and cancer (as a percentage of all causes of death) have increased over the years. While CVD at the turn of the century accounted for 10 to 15 percent of deaths, it now accounts for almost every second death. Similar increases are shown for cancer, which is continuing to rise despite heroic after-the-fact medical interventions. (US 1900-2000)

LIFESTYLE MEDICINE INSTITUTE

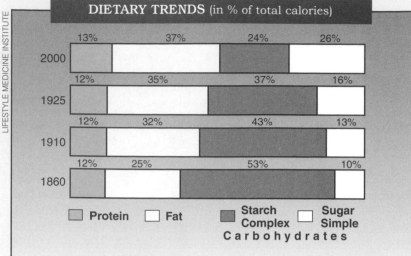

DIETARY TRENDS (in % of total calories)

Year	Protein	Fat	Starch Complex Carbohydrates	Sugar Simple Carbohydrates
2000	13%	37%	24%	26%
1925	12%	35%	37%	16%
1910	12%	32%	43%	13%
1860	12%	25%	53%	10%

☐ Protein ☐ Fat ■ Starch Complex ☐ Sugar Simple
C a r b o h y d r a t e s

The standard American diet (SAD) has been shifting, resulting in a dramatic change in its composition. Today more calories come from sugar (simple carbohydrates) than from starch (complex carbohydrates) and more than one third of the calories come from fat. (U.S. 1860-2000)

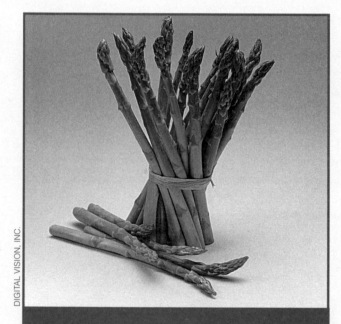

DIGITAL VISION, INC.

FOOD "as grown" is nutritionally balanced. Refinement, however, strips food of most of its fiber and nutrients. Processing adds calories, subtracts nutrition, and contributes myriads of chemical additives.

typically consists of a salad soaked in oily dressing, a hamburger, and a soda. And dinner often comes frozen in a cardboard box or from the Colonel. Between meals there are sodas, chips, Ding Dongs, and dough-nuts. Nutritious, high-fiber foods now represent only 24 percent of our daily calories, while fat and sugar intake have increased up to 250 percent.

That's frightening! What can be done?

Education is the key. As people learn that refinement robs food of most of its fiber and nutrients, and processing adds calories, subtracts nutrition, and contributes scores of chemical additives, many are willing to make changes.

People are also realizing that meat and dairy products should be used sparingly. While they carry nutrients, most are too high in fat, cholesterol, protein, and calories, are loaded with hormones and pesticides, and contain virtually no fiber.

Today's people are increasingly giving up their preoccupation with rich animal products and processed foods. Instead, they are eating more complex carbohydrates—whole plant foods, usually rich in fiber. Since 1970 the consumption of meat, whole milk, and eggs has decreased, and so has the number of heart attacks and strokes.

People know it, and science confirms it. The road to better health and longer life detours around fast-food outlets, feedlot animals, and shops full of contrived and depleted foods. Instead, the road leads us back to the gardens and farmlands of our country—to the fresh fruits and crisp vegetables, and to the kernels of golden grain.

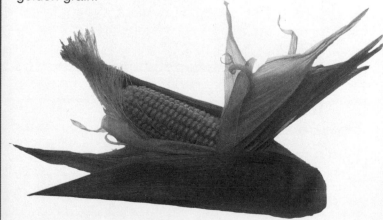

The Choice Is Yours

One hundred years ago very few Americans suffered from coronary heart disease, stroke, and cancer. Today these lifestyle-related illnesses account for the majority of deaths in North America. The good news is that you don't have to become a statistic. By adopting a better diet and wiser lifestyle habits, you can live longer and enjoy a healthier, more productive life.

You Can Do It

Simply by changing your habits of diet and exercise, you can have the same freedom from coronary heart disease, stroke, diabetes, and cancer that our ancestors enjoyed. It's possible. You need only three essentials.

The Three Essentials

Desire: To modify a habit, you must want to change. Old patterns are comfortable. To break their grip, you need a strong desire to energize yourself.

Knowledge: Desire alone can't change entrenched lifestyle patterns. You must also know what to change and understand why you should change it.

For instance, although most people want to avoid clogged arteries, achieving this is impossible without a knowledge of the harmful effects of excess cholesterol and fat in the diet.

YOUR FRESH FRUIT LIST:

Write them down in this space:

_____

_____

_____

_____

_____

Skill: Just knowing what to do isn't enough. You need to know how to do it. And then you need to practice it until the new behavior becomes automatic.

Skills that promote health include learning how to cook cholesterol-free, low-fat meals, developing a program of regular exercise, reading food labels to avoid highly salted products, and becoming skilled at choosing healthful food at restaurants.

Try this simple experiment. Eat one or two servings of fresh fruit every morning for the next three weeks. Eat as many different kinds as you can find.

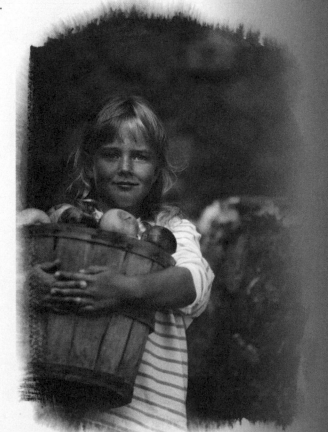

MODERN NUTRITION

Seven Wrong Roads

Many of us are digging our own graves with knife and fork.

A s Americans, we pride ourselves on being the best-fed nation on earth. But we are paying a high price for the privilege—in needless disease, disability, and premature death.

What are we doing wrong?

Americans are eating too much of nearly everything—too much sugar, too much fat, too much cholesterol, and too much salt. We eat too many calories. And we eat too often.

Such abundance has helped lay the foundation for coronary artery disease, stroke, high blood pressure, arthritis, adult-onset diabetes, obesity, and several kinds of cancer. These diseases are responsible for three out of four deaths. They are related to our lifestyle, especially to how we eat.

Disease from food? You must mean pesticides and preservatives!

Surprisingly, pesticides and preservatives aren't the worst offenders. Here are some of the more serious culprits:

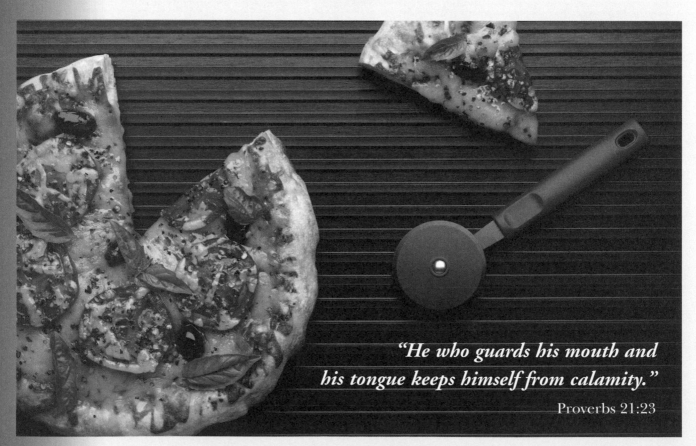

"He who guards his mouth and his tongue keeps himself from calamity."

Proverbs 21:23

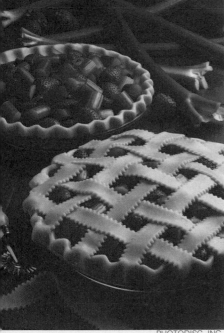

PHOTODISC, INC.

hemorrhoids, diverticulitis, and constipation.

3 *SALT.* Most Westerners consume 10 to 20 grams (two to four teaspoons) of salt a day. This is many times more than is actually needed and contributes prominently to high blood pressure, heart failure, and kidney disease.

4 *FAT.* Most people don't realize that they are consuming an average of 37 percent of their daily calories as fat. This is much more than the body can properly handle. As a result, blood vessels plug up, impotence sets in, and

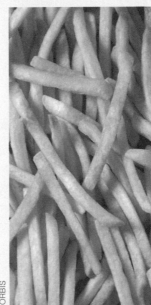

CORBIS

hearts and brains suffer. A high-fat diet also contributes to overweight, adult diabetes, and certain cancers.

5 *PROTEIN.* A diet heavy in meat and animal products provides more protein, fat, and cholesterol than the body can use. Westerners eat two to three times more protein than is recommended. Scientists now recognize that a diet containing less protein and much less fat and cholesterol is essential for improved health and longevity.

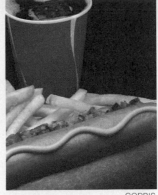

CORBIS

6 *BEVERAGES.* North Americans seldom drink water. Instead, they average several servings of soda pop, beer, coffee, tea, and sweet drinks every day. Because most of these drinks are loaded with calories from sugar and alcohol, they can play havoc with blood sugar levels and sabotage weight-control efforts. Caffeine, phosphates, and other chemicals found in beverages pose additional health risks.

7 *SNACKS.* Engineered taste sensations are taking the place of real food. Schools, day-care centers, even hospitals require snacks to be available. The coffee break remains standard at work, and snacks reign supreme after school and at home. Well-planned family meals are now the exception. Snack attacks disrupt digestion,

1 *SUGAR.* The National Research Council reports that refined sugars and sweeteners account for up to 20 percent of many people's daily calories. Devoid of fiber and nutrients, refined sugars are empty, or naked, calories. But because of their caloric density, they are well suited to promote obesity.

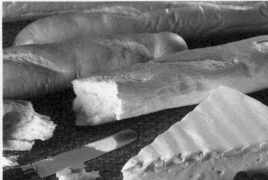

CORBIS

2 *REFINED FOODS.* People used to think refinement was good because it got rid of useless roughage. Now we're learning how necessary fiber is in protecting us from certain cancers, stabilizing blood sugar, controlling weight, and preventing gastrointestinal problems such as gallstones,

CORBIS

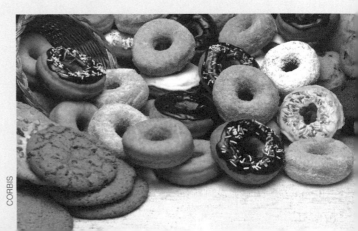

What you don't know about eating could hurt you.

overburden the stomach, and are a frequent cause of bloating and indigestion.

Is there anything *safe* to eat?

Think fruit—hundreds of varieties, spectacular colors, and every imaginable texture and flavor. Go for vegetables, potatoes, and yams. Include legumes—all kinds of beans, lentils, chick-peas —in scores of shapes, colors, and flavors. And don't forget the grains—the mainstay of a good diet and a gold mine of delectable and healthful foods.

Eating a variety of whole-plant foods will furnish all the fat, pro-tein, fiber, and nutrients the body needs. It's also ecologically sensitive and will cut the food budget in half.

The best news is that this kind of dietary lifestyle helps delay and often prevents the onset of most Western killer diseases. Eating full-fiber plant foods not only allows people to eat larger quantities of food without having to worry about weight gain, but also can promote optimum health and energy for a lifetime.

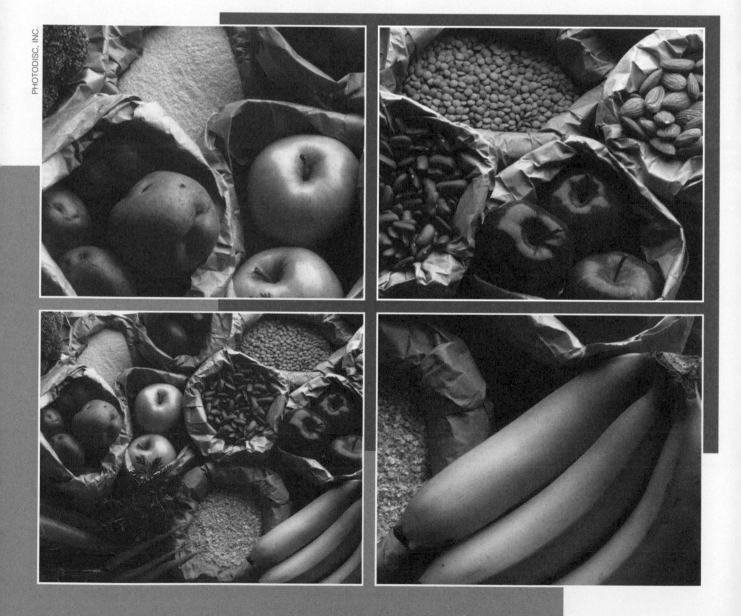

Too much! Too much sugar, refined foods, salt, fat, protein, beverages, and snacks in our diet is a deadly mix. Only by eating less of these substances and eating more whole plant foods can we enjoy optimum health and energy.

Is There Too Much on Our Plate?

A "Fat Tooth"?

Americans eat too much fat, and they pay for it with heart attacks, strokes, obesity, and other diseases.

Slim Your Salad Down

Four tablespoons of regular blue cheese or ranch dressing adds more than 500 calories to a salad.

That is 500 calories you don't need. This week try your salads with lemon, or mix up some super salad dressing using this recipe:

Super Salad Dressing

1/4 c. water

1/4 tsp. Italian seasoning

1/4 tsp. garlic powder

1/4 c. lemon juice

1/4 tsp. onion powder

1/4 tsp. salt *(optional)*

Combine all ingredients and shake well. Let it sit; it'll get even better with age.

Write the letter of the correct description in each blank.

___ Sugar   ___ Snacks   ___ Fat

___ Salt   ___ Protein   ___ Beverages   ___ Refined Foods

A. Americans consume these instead of water. Most are loaded with calories and chemicals.

B. Fiber, which protects us from certain cancers, stabilizes blood sugar, and helps control our weight, is removed from these foods.

C. North Americans eat up to 20 times more than they really need. It contributes to high blood pressure, heart failure, and kidney disease.

D. Many people get close to 40 percent of their daily calories from this. It plugs arteries and contributes to overweight and adult (Type II) diabetes.

E. It makes up more than 20 percent of America's daily calories, yet provides no fiber or nutrients.

F. Americans eat two to three times more of this than is recommended. Scientists now recognize that too much can be harmful.

G. These often take the place of real food. They are low in nutrition, high in price, and can disrupt digestion.

CHILDREN AT RISK

Growing Healthy Kids

The news is not good. "Heart disease begins in childhood," reports the National Institutes of Health. A recent examination of 360 randomly selected youngsters ages 7 to 12 revealed that 98 percent of the children already had three or more risk factors.

But we keep hearing that people are getting healthier!

It's mainly the grown-ups who are exercising, losing weight, quitting tobacco, and becoming more health-conscious.

But it's a different story for kids. "Since the early 1960s the general health of adolescents has declined," says the American Academy of Pediatrics. "Today's kids are flabby. They don't have the proper cardiovascular tone. They are not physically fit."

Remember the simple pleasures of just being a kid?

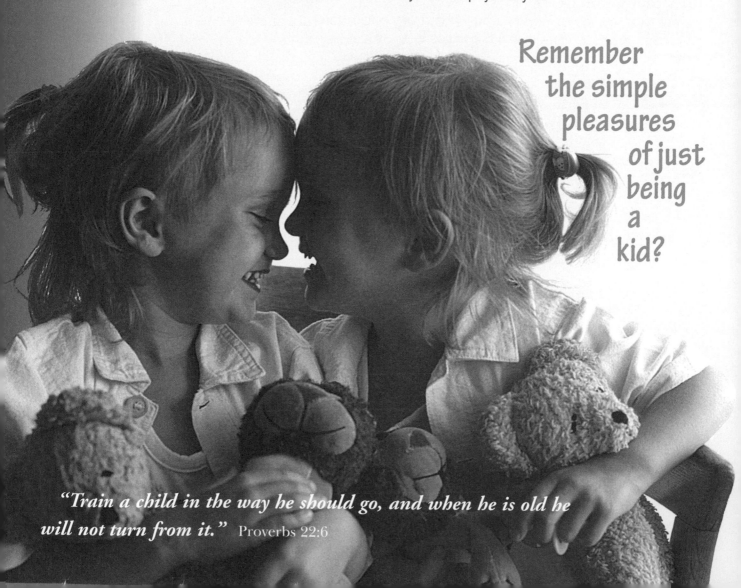

"Train a child in the way he should go, and when he is old he will not turn from it." Proverbs 22:6

Too much television?

Television certainly has had an impact. Time spent in front of the TV set is time taken away from body-building, calorie-burning physical activities such as bicycling, skating, basketball, or climbing trees. That sets the stage for excessive weight gain, which in itself is a risk factor for high blood cholesterol and heart disease.

Exercise physiologist Kate O'Shea warns that "the junior couch potato of today is the fat farm candidate of tomorrow."

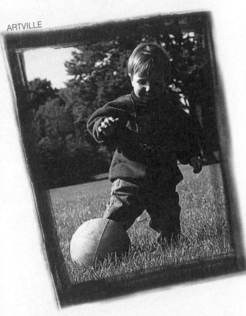

ARTVILLE

Don't school PE programs help?

Only a few require students to take physical education in all grades. In an era of tight budgets and teacher shortages, health and physical education programs are often among the first to go.

What about children's eating habits?

With nine out of 10 Saturday-morning food advertisements on the networks hawking processed foods, high in sugar, fat, and salt, television significantly influences the food preferences of children from their earliest years.

Home-cooked, sitting-down-around-the-table meals are now the exception in most American homes, being largely replaced by fast foods and engineered foods. More than half of today's high school kids head off to fast-food chains and snack machines instead of school lunch rooms.

Any good news?

The good news is that children can be taught—and the younger they get started, the better.

Here are some tips for building good health habits early in life:

- Daily exercise—preferably outdoors—for at least an hour.
- Three meals a day, at regular times, with lots of whole grains, fruits, and vegetables. Discourage snacks, and the child will have a better appetite for nutritious food at mealtimes. If a snack is needed, offer a piece of fresh fruit.
- Plenty of water. Save sodas for special occasions.
- Control TV. The hours a child watches TV relate directly to weight gain and elevated blood cholesterol levels.
- Adequate rest. Most children are chronically tired—not surprising when you remember that teenagers do best on nine hours of sleep a night, and younger ones need more. Put the kids to bed early enough so they awaken naturally in time for a healthy

ARTVILLE

breakfast.

- Cultivate a wide range of interests—schedule library visits, music lessons, arts and crafts, hobbies, and family outings. Children who spend time with their parents and develop deep spiritual roots experience less stress and improved mental health.
- Set a good example. The life choices you are modeling day by day are the strongest determinants of your children's future behavior.

Is it worth the effort?

"Fitness can be fun," says Arnold Schwarzeneggar, who was President Bush's spokesman for the Council on Physical Fitness and Sports. "Stay away from junk food, get off the couch, unplug the Nintendo, turn off the TV, and go out and get some exercise. A body is a terrible thing to waste."

2
3

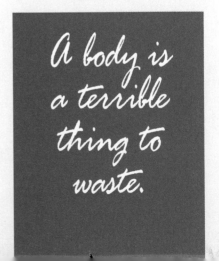

A body is a terrible thing to waste.

How to raise GOOD kids

- Be good parents; set the example.
- Maintain consistent united discipline.
- Clearly explain boundaries and expectations.
- Teach responsibility early.
- Let children work for money.
- Have a good attitude toward your kids.
- Think positive with them.
- Teach spiritual values.

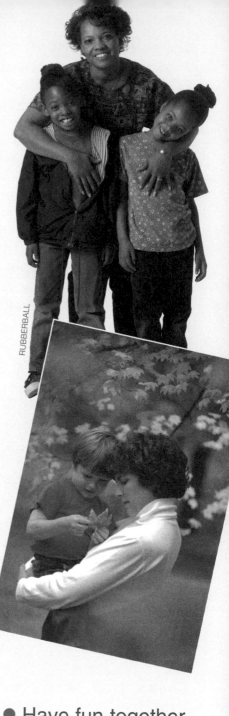

RUBBERBALL

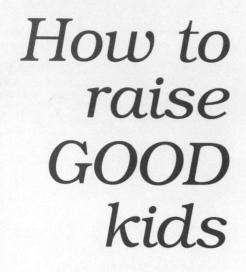

CORBIS

CORBIS

- Have fun together.
- Learn to listen— *really* listen.
- Give them unconditional love.

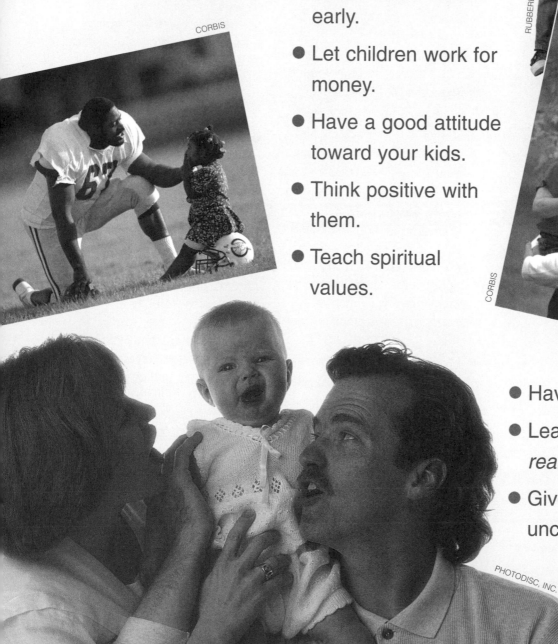

PHOTODISC, INC.

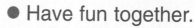

Application

Time spent with children encourages greater trust and better communication. Teaching and modeling spiritual values deepens spiritual roots. Children need these basics to cope with the stresses of growing up into balanced, mentally healthy adults.

HOW MANY THINGS can you think of that will help relationships with the children in your life?

Write them down in this space:

1) _____

2) _____

3) _____

4) _____

5) _____

6) _____

7) _____

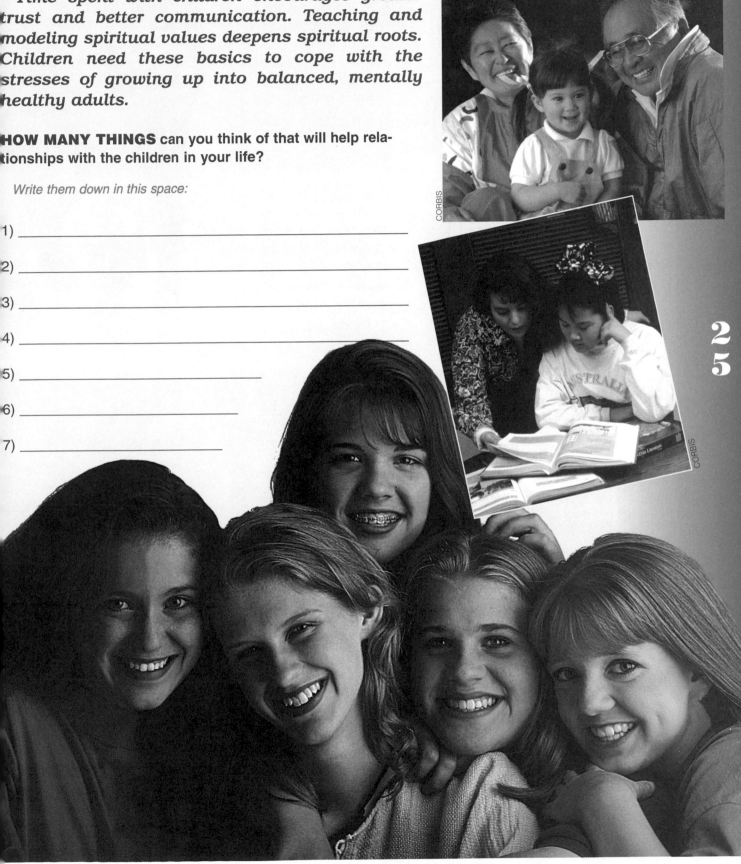

CORBIS

CORBIS

2 5

AGING

Older Can Be Better

"Grandchildren are the crown of the elderly."

Proverbs 17:6, Clear Word

Everyone hates getting old. People want to stay young or at least middle-aged. But time keeps marching. With the 65-and-older segment getting larger in North America, what are the prospects for the golden-agers in today's world?

An increasing trend is to date people by their intellectual and social capabilities rather than by chronological age. Health, rather than years, usually determines one's status.

Old age sets in when disease and disability limit

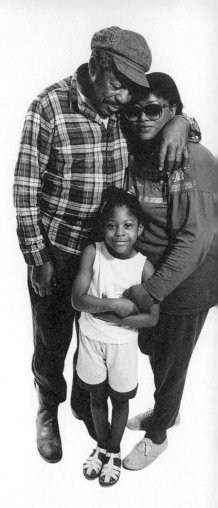

CORBIS

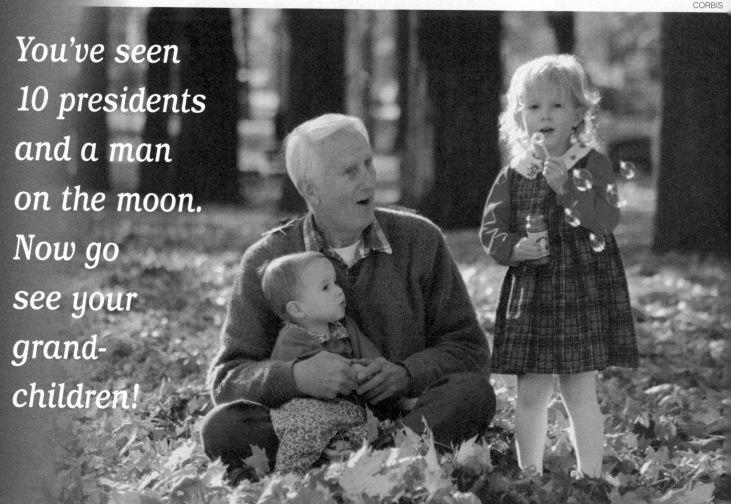

You've seen 10 presidents and a man on the moon. Now go see your grand-children!

Research shows that a healthy lifestyle can hold back the aging process as much as 30 years.

everyday tasks. Some people are old while still relatively young in years. These are usually people who are chronically ill, injured, or victims of a major tragedy, many of whom withdraw and give up on life. Others remain youthful, vital, interesting, and productive into advanced age.

ALL PHOTOS PHOTODISC, INC.

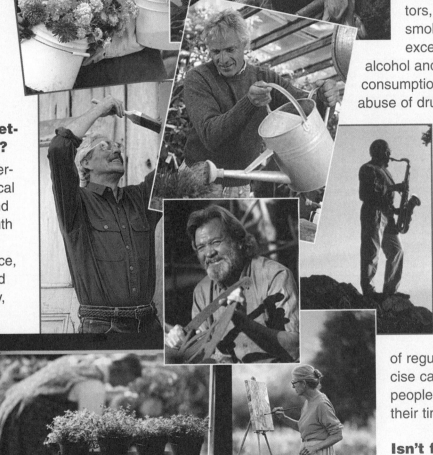

Some people claim older is better. Can that be?

It's a matter of perspective. For physical strength, energy and fewer ailments, youth is better. But for increased confidence, better judgment and insight, less anxiety, and more freedom, older can be better. And experience helps too. Most philosophers, composers, painters, and writers, for instance, improve with time.

Don't most people over 65 suffer from chronic illnesses?

In affluent Western society, about 80 percent of the 65-and-over group have some

kind of health problem, such as high blood pressure, arthritis, diabetes, depression, or heart disease. But most of these illnesses are not incapacitating. About 95 percent of older people live in

their communities, and most have their own households.

Premature aging and disability are largely the result of lifestyle factors, such as smoking, excessive alcohol and caffeine consumption, and the abuse of drugs. Being overweight speeds up physical and sexual decline. A diet of rich, refined foods and lack of regular exercise can make people old before their time.

Isn't forgetfulness a bad sign?

Forgetfulness in older people is exaggerated. Stress, anxiety, fast-moving events, memory overload, and lack of interest can cause forgetfulness at any age. Depression, which affects many older people, is often

27

It's true — many things get better with age.

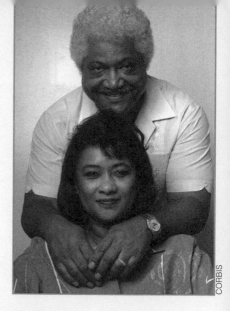

misdiagnosed as senility. Only a few people develop Alzheimer's disease or other genuinely senile dementias. Most people retain remarkable memory function for a long time, especially when they stay active and fit.

Don't many older people end up in nursing homes?

Actually, in North America only 2 percent of people 64 to 75 years of age live in nursing homes. Only after age 85 does the figure reach 20 percent.

Today is a good time to be alive! Productive social activities are pushing back the aging process. So are exercise, a better understanding of the role of diet, earlier attention to health problems, and advances in modern technology. People today are often staying physically and mentally fit into their 80s and 90s. Many remain sexually active as well.

There is more. Scientists are discovering that an optimistic, positive attitude actually boosts the body's immune mechanism. This sophisticated defense system is proving to be one of the major keys to good health.

The Good Book said it long ago: "A merry heart does good, like medicine" (Proverbs 17:22, NKJV).

Beautiful young people are accidents of nature. Beautiful old people are works of art.

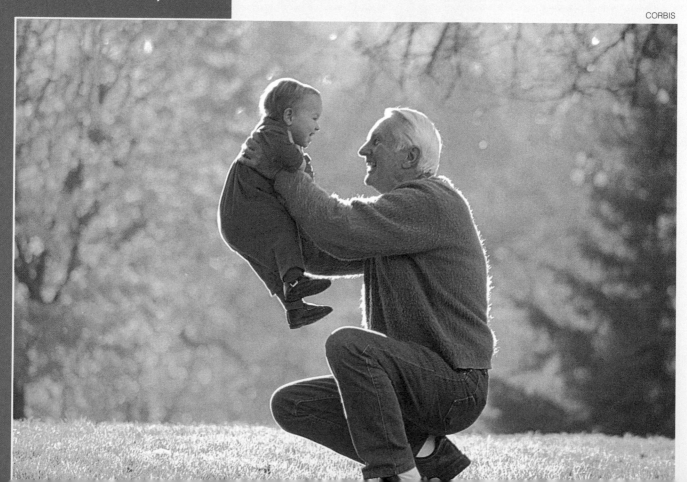

Application

A diet of rich, refined foods and a lack of exercise can make you old before your time. But with a healthy lifestyle, worthwhile goals, and a positive mental attitude, it is possible to enjoy life well into your golden years.

Super Seniors!

At age 66, **HULDA CROOKS** decided to take on a new challenge— mountain climbing. Over the next 25 years she scaled some of North America's tallest peaks, plus Mount Fuji, the tallest mountain in Japan.

MARTIN KNOPPER

What's in Your Future?

Take a moment to imagine yourself on your ninetieth birthday. Are you standing atop a mountain? painting a picture? celebrating life with family and friends? Or are you ill and isolated?

A positive attitude is important for physical health and happiness. Without purpose, goals, and productive social activities, we age quickly. Do you have interests and goals that will carry you through your lifetime?

List three interests or goals you would like to pursue. Is there something you've always wanted to try? Someplace you wanted to visit? Something you hoped to contribute?

1. _____
2. _____
3. _____

Choose one of the goals you've listed. If you were going to pursue it, what would be the first steps you would take?

1. _____
2. _____
3. _____

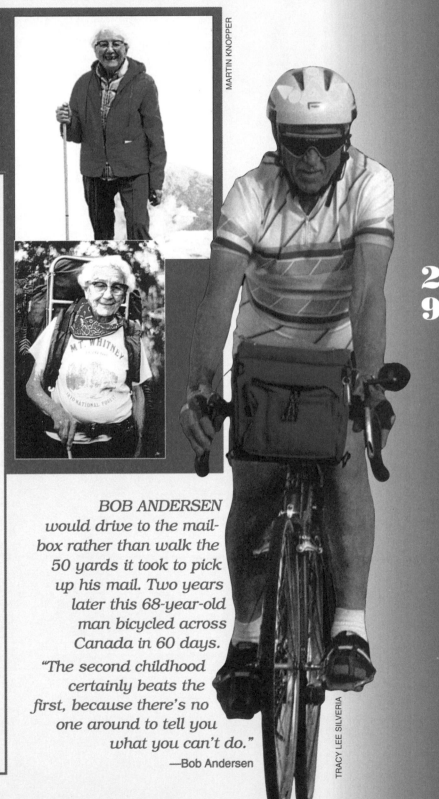

BOB ANDERSEN would drive to the mailbox rather than walk the 50 yards it took to pick up his mail. Two years later this 68-year-old man bicycled across Canada in 60 days.

"The second childhood certainly beats the first, because there's no one around to tell you what you can't do."
—Bob Andersen

TRACY LEE SILVERIA

Want to enjoy the "good life" with good health?

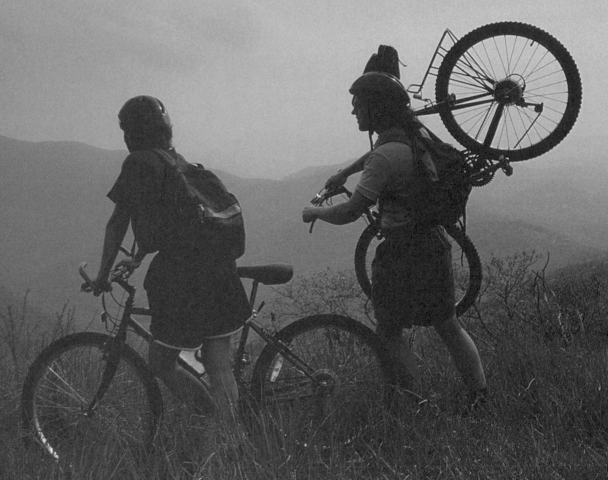

MODERN MEDICINE has made great strides. But some of the greatest strides have been found to relate back to rather simple things: what you eat, what you drink, what you think, and what you do.

DISEASES OF LIFESTYLE

- **Coronary Heart Disease**
- **Reversing Heart Disease**
- **Hypertension**
- **Stroke**
- **Cancer**
- **Diabetes**
- **Osteoporosis**
- **Arthritis**
- **Obesity**
- **Alcohol**
- **Tobacco and Disease**
- **Caffeine Addiction**
- **Legalized Drug Abuse**

**3
1**

"Don't you know that you yourselves are God's temple and that God's Spirit lives in you?" 1 Corinthians 3:16

CORONARY HEART DISEASE

Killer for Dinner

Hundreds of thousands of people die every year from heart attacks without a murmur of protest from the public, the press, or government agencies. Yet the nation's number one killer can be found right on the American dinner table!

Do you mean that what we eat causes heart attacks?

Not everything. The main culprits are excessive amounts of fat and cholesterol. The underlying problem is narrowing, hardening, and, eventually, plugging up of vital arteries that supply the heart with oxygen. The process is known as atherosclerosis.

People are born with clean, flexible arteries. They should stay that way throughout life. The arteries of many North Americans, however, are clogging up with cholesterol, fat, and calcium—a concoction that gradually hardens and eventually chokes off needed oxygen supplies.

During and after World War II most Europeans were forced to change their eating habits from their customary diet of meat, eggs, and dairy products to a more austere diet of potatoes, grains, beans, roots, and vegetables. The result? A dramatic decrease in atherosclerosis-related diseases, such as heart attacks, strokes, diabetes, gallstones, as well as certain cancers and arthritis. The marked drop in these diseases was felt for as long as 20 years after World War II.

Since then, massive amounts of data have accumulated from research on animals and humans around the world. The results are essentially the same: diets high in fat and cholesterol produce elevated levels of blood cholesterol and heart disease. Diets low in fat and cholesterol reduce blood cholesterol levels and heart disease and even facilitate plaque reversal.

How can I tell if I have atherosclerosis?

There simply aren't any hints of the problem until your arteries are seriously narrowed, or they plug up with a sudden plaque

"Heart disease before age 80 is our fault, not God's fault, or nature's will."

—Paul Dudley White, M.D.

"Above all else, guard your heart, for it is the wellspring of life."

Proverbs 4:23

break-off. Some people begin to experience angina (heart pain) on exertion. For many people a heart attack is the first sign of trouble. About one third of heart attacks result in sudden death.

Who is at risk for heart attack?

The risk factor concept is a good way to determine the likelihood of coronary heart disease:

- The most serious risk factor by far is an elevated blood cholesterol. Men, 50 years and older, with cholesterol levels over 295 mg% (or 7.6 mmol/L) are 10 times more likely to develop atherosclerosis than men the same age with levels under 200 mg% (or 5.1 mmol/L). A 20 percent decrease in blood cholesterol levels lowers the risk of a coronary by 50 percent.

- By age 60, smokers are 10 times more likely than non-

smokers to die from heart disease. More than 160,000 coronary deaths a year are directly related to smoking, about 30 percent of the total.

- In North America every third adult has high blood pressure. This triples the likelihood of coronary death when compared to a person with normal blood pressure.

- Obese men are five times more likely to die of heart disease by age 60 than men of normal weight.

- Other risk factors are diabetes, elevated triglycerides, sedentary lifestyle, stress and possibly an elevated homocysteine blood level. Fortunately, all of these risk factors can be controlled by

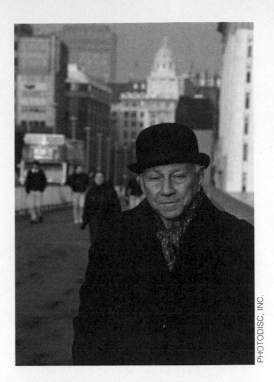

changes in diet and lifestyle. Heredity, age, and gender are risk factors a person cannot control, but they are usually the least important ones.

What about medications and surgery?

For those with dangerous cholesterol levels that do not respond adequately to diet, medications may be needed. Medications, however, are expensive. Furthermore, most have serious side effects. They require frequent laboratory tests and physician checkups.

More glamorous are the surgical procedures: bypass operations, roto-rooter cleanouts, and balloon stretching. Some results have been spectacular. But as time goes on and statistics accumulate, it is becoming apparent that most of these operations do not prolong life or even necessarily improve it. Medical treatment is temporary at best. The only long-term solution is a serious lifestyle change.

Four thousand times a day someone in the U.S. has a heart attack.

33

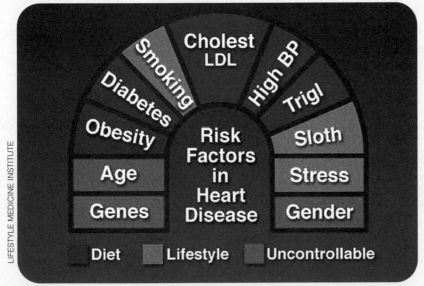

The higher on the arch, the higher the contribution of the risk factor to heart disease. Five of the eight controllable risk factors are largely under the control of diet.

Progression of Coronary Artery Disease

AGE　10　　　　20　　　　40　　　　60　　　　70

LIFESTYLE MEDICINE INSTITUTE

"People in Framingham with cholesterol levels below 150 mg% had no heart attacks."

—William Castelli, M.D.
Reporting on the famous
Framingham Heart Study

So what is the best approach?

It is always better to prevent than to repair. But if heart disease has developed, as suggested by the presence of coronary risk factors and documented by diagnostic tests, it still isn't too late to make lifestyle changes. You can actually clean out your arteries, lower your risk of dying of athero-sclerosis, and extend your active, produc-tive years. You can markedly change your risk factors no matter how old you are, often in just a few weeks.

Start with healthful, home-cooked meals that are very low in fat and cholesterol, yet high in unrefined complex carbohydrates and fiber. Such a diet can lower cholesterol levels by 20 to 30 percent and reverse many cases of diabetes in less than four weeks (see page 52). When combined with salt restriction, this diet will also help normalize blood pressure and control obesity (see pages 40 and 64).

Begin an active daily exercise program.

If Americans would lower their cholesterol to below 180 and their blood pressures to under 125 mmHg and quit smoking, it has been estimated that 82 percent of all heart attacks before age 65 could be prevented. These simple changes in lifestyle would do more to improve the health of our nation than all the hospitals, surgeries, and drugs put together.

Seeing is Believing . . .

This *HeartScreen* test will help you identify and understand your own risk factors, and guide you in dealing with them. It will approximate your relative risk and will help you identify areas that you may want to work on. In this test, eight risk factors are listed, and scores from 1 to 8 are assigned to each factor.

HeartScreen: Interpreting Your Score

0-6　**IDEAL** — Development of heart disease or stroke is extremely unlikely, especially if your cholesterol level is below 160.

7-14　**ELEVATED** — The development of heart disease or stroke is about one third of the U.S. average, yet three times higher than for the ideal group.

15-22　**HIGH RISK** — This is the average. You cannot afford to be average, because your risk is 10 times higher than the ideal group.

23-30　**VERY HIGH RISK** — The development of heart disease and stroke is about three times the U.S. average, or 30 times higher than the ideal group. Action is imperative! You may be able to drop four points on this test within four to eight weeks by lowering cholesterol and blood pressure through dietary change.

31-38　**DANGEROUS** — The likelihood of having a heart attack or stroke is about four to six times the U.S. average and about 50 times higher than the ideal group. Set goals and take action without delay!

Application

HeartScreen
Self Scoring Test of Heart Attack and Stroke Risk

Risk Level and Score

Risk Factor	0	1	2	3	4	5	6	7	8
1. Cholesterol* (mg%)	under 160	160-179	180-199	200-219	220-239	240-259	260-279	280-299	300 plus
2. Blood Pressure* (mmHg)	under 110	110-119	120-129	130-139	140-159	160 plus			
3. Smoking (cig./day)	none	up to 5	5-9	10-19	20-29	30+			
4. Overweight† (in %)	0-4%	5-9%	10-14%	15-19%	20-29%	30%+			
5. Triglycerides* (mg%)	under 100	100-149	150-249	250-349	350+				
6. Diabetes (duration)	None	under 5 years	5-10 years	10+ years					
7. Resting Pulse (beats/min.)	under 56	56-62	63-69	70-80	80+				
8. Stress	Rarely tense	Tense 3x/wk	Tense 2-3/day	Tense and rushed	on tranquilizers				

Risk Factor	Score
1. Cholesterol	___
2. Blood Pressure	___
3. Smoking	___
4. Overweight	___
5. Triglycerides	___
6. Diabetes	___
7. Pulse	___
8. Stress	___
Total Score:	___

* To determine your cholesterol, triglycerides, and blood pressure, just see your physician. The blood test is very simple and inexpensive, and takes about five minutes. What you learn may save your life! If you take blood pressure pills, score four points regardless of your blood pressure level.

† To determine your percentage of overweight, look up your ideal weight, take its midpoint, and subtract it from your actual weight. Divide the difference in pounds by your ideal weight and multiply by 100.

35

REVERSING HEART DISEASE

Eat Your Way Out

The sports world rejoiced when former Yale president, Bart Giamotti, became commissioner of baseball. A few months later a shocked nation wept when this respected man died suddenly at age 51, attacked by his heart.

Scenarios like this one are repeated thousands of times each day across North America. Heart disease now strikes a deadly blow to four out of every 10 Americans.

Is there no way out? Does it have to be like this?

Yes . . . and no.

As long as Americans continue to eat their rich, fatty diet, the statistics will remain the same. We've known for years that a diet high in fat and cholesterol is the primary and essential cause of coronary heart disease.

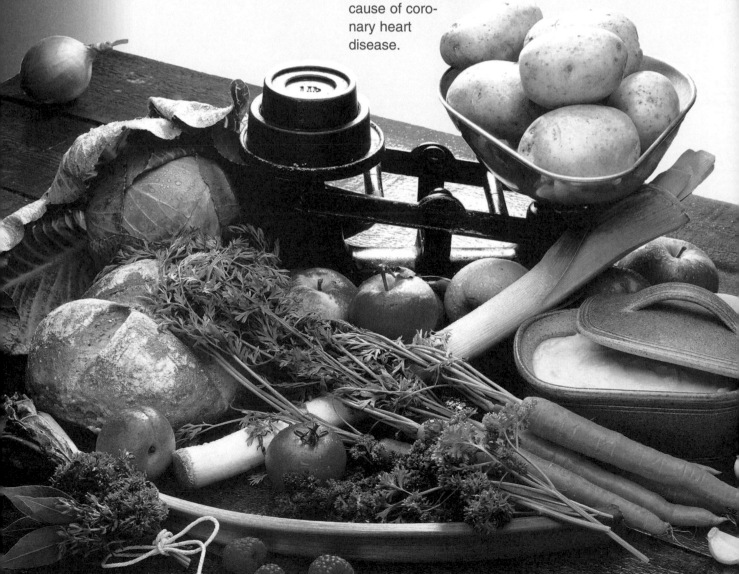

But there is a way out: it requires that we *lean out* our high-fat diet. To the extent that we commit to do this, we can help prevent and even *reverse* heart disease.

Are you saying that heart disease may be curable?

It looks more and more that way.

The idea took on a life of its own when a young cardiologist, Dr. Dean Ornish, published a report in the *Lancet* medical journal, in 1990, that shook up the medical community. Dr. Ornish spent one year studying 50 men with advanced heart disease, many of whom were candidates for coronary bypass surgery.

He randomly assigned the men to two groups. Both groups were asked to quit smoking and to walk daily. In addition, the first group practiced stress management and followed a strict vegetarian diet with less than 10 percent of calories as fat and with virtually no cholesterol.

The second group was given the standard American Heart Association's "Prudent Diet" for heart disease. This diet allowed 30 percent of calories as fat and up to 300 milligrams of cholesterol a day. At the end of the year, when the results were presented at the Scientific Session of the American Heart Association in Washington, D.C., they became front-page news all over America.

Dr. Ornish reported that those on the very-low-fat vegetarian diet not

EAT AT YOUR OWN RISK

Despite subhuman diets and torture, survivors of the Holocaust were surprisingly free of atherosclerosis. It was the first indication— later confirmed by angiographic examinations of American POWs in Vietnam—that the process of atherosclerosis is reversible. Those held longest in captivity had the cleanest arteries.

Keys to Reversing Heart Disease

It may be the nation's leading cause of death, but it needn't be yours. And you can actually reverse it!

1. Reduce blood cholesterol to less than 160 mg% with a very low-fat, high fiber vegetarian diet and with cholesterol-lowering medication if necessary.

2. Lose weight by eating more foods-as-grown and less refined foods and animal products.

3. Drop your high blood pressure by cutting the salt to less than 5 grams (or 5000 milligrams) a day, and by getting into a daily exercise program.

4. Stop smoking and reduce alcohol intake. Alcohol is toxic to a struggling heart.

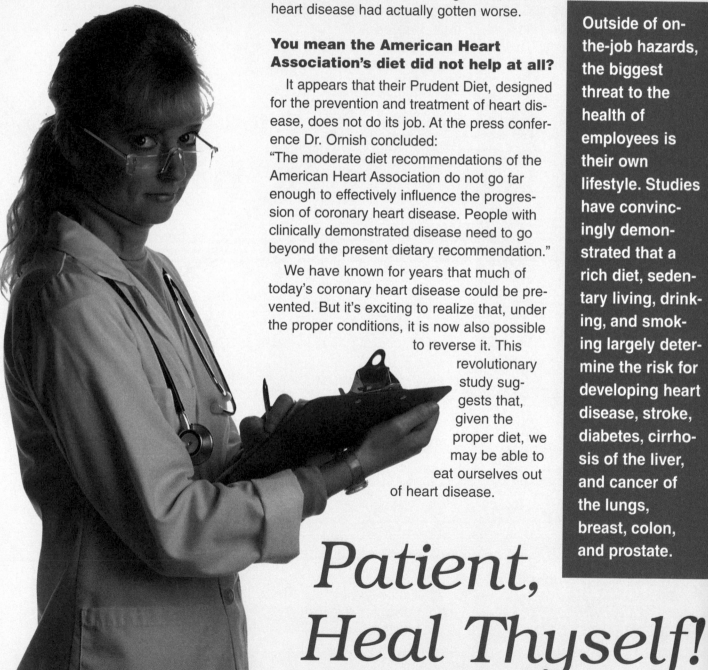

A Healthy Lifestyle Lowers Coronary Risk by Lowering Homocysteine

A study done at the Lifestyle Center of America showed that by changing diet and exercise, homocysteine levels in the blood could be lowered by as much as 20 percent in only 14 days.

only dropped their dangerous LDL-cholesterol levels by 37 percent, but 82 percent of their narrowed, plaque-filled arteries had actually widened, allowing more blood and oxygen to the heart muscle. The heart disease had, in fact, begun to reverse itself. And the older men with the most advanced disease actually had the best results.

The group on the so-called Prudent Diet, however, had virtually no cholesterol drop, and most of their coronary arteries showed increased narrowing. In general, their heart disease had actually gotten worse.

You mean the American Heart Association's diet did not help at all?

It appears that their Prudent Diet, designed for the prevention and treatment of heart disease, does not do its job. At the press conference Dr. Ornish concluded: "The moderate diet recommendations of the American Heart Association do not go far enough to effectively influence the progression of coronary heart disease. People with clinically demonstrated disease need to go beyond the present dietary recommendation."

We have known for years that much of today's coronary heart disease could be prevented. But it's exciting to realize that, under the proper conditions, it is now also possible to reverse it. This revolutionary study suggests that, given the proper diet, we may be able to eat ourselves out of heart disease.

Outside of on-the-job hazards, the biggest threat to the health of employees is their own lifestyle. Studies have convincingly demonstrated that a rich diet, sedentary living, drinking, and smoking largely determine the risk for developing heart disease, stroke, diabetes, cirrhosis of the liver, and cancer of the lungs, breast, colon, and prostate.

Patient, Heal Thyself!

Application

We are born with clean, flexible arteries, but excessive fat and cholesterol in the diet can clog them. Eventually this chokes off the oxygen supply to vital organs. Dr. Ornish's study found that plaque-filled arteries in patients on very-low-fat vegetarian diets actually began to open up, allowing more blood and oxygen to the heart and other vital organs.

A Killer on the Loose

Heart attacks are the leading cause of death in the United States—and too much fat is the leading cause of heart attacks. It's been said that excess fat is the most harmful element in the Western diet. Isn't it time you reduced the amount you are eating?

Getting the Fat Out

Here are four general strategies you can use to reduce the fat in your diet.

Substitute: Drink skim milk instead of whole milk. Or, better yet, use a nondairy substitute. Try a bowl of chilled fruit instead of ice cream for dessert. Look for healthful substitutes for the high-fat items in your diet, such as cheeses, meats, dressings, and oils.

Reduce: Instead of ordering an eight-ounce steak, try a smaller portion with pasta or a vegetarian lasagna. Instead of a whole piece of pie, take just a sliver. Eating smaller portions of your favorite high-fat foods allows you to savor a few decadent bites while still cutting fat from your diet.

Eliminate: Eliminate as many temptations as possible. If you don't buy it and bring it into the house, you won't eat it.

Eliminating high-fat foods can work wonders. In Dr. Ornish's headline-making study, the subjects that reversed the narrowing in their arteries were those who had eliminated meat and high-fat dairy products entirely.

Construct: Processed foods are stuffed with added fat. If you want to regain control over what goes into your body, cook for yourself. Get a good low-fat cookbook and learn how to prepare delicious new dishes. It's the surest way to protect yourself from the deadly effects of too much fat.

Get Started!

List some specific ways you can apply the principles of substitution, reduction, elimination, and construction to your diet:

Substitution:

_____

_____

_____

Reduction:

_____

_____

_____

Elimination:

_____

_____

_____

Construction:

_____

_____

_____

HYPERTENSION

The Silent Killer

CORBIS

Every third adult in North America has high blood pressure. These hypertensives are three times more likely to have a heart attack, five times more likely to develop heart failure, and eight times more likely to suffer a stroke than people with normal blood pressure.

How can I know if I have hypertension?

Hypertension is defined as a systolic blood pressure reading (the top number) consistently over 130, and/or a diastolic (lower number) reading of 85 or above. The optimal level is now below 120/80. Even though high blood pressure has no symptoms (that's why it is called the *silent disease*), it can cause progressive changes in the blood vessels until the first sign hits, usually a stroke or a heart attack.

What causes the blood pressure to go up?

Certain kinds of tumors will do it; also diseases within the kidney itself. But in 90% of everyday hypertension, no specific organic causes can be determined. For this reason this kind of hypertension is called *essential* hypertension.

The following factors contribute to essential hypertension:

- **High Salt Intake.** Surprisingly, hypertension is uncommon in 80 percent of the world's population where salt intake is also very low. In places where salt intake is high, as in Japan, the disease is epidemic, affecting approximately one half of adults. Americans consume an average of 10 to 15 grams of salt per day. That's two to three teaspoonsful, or about 10 to 15 times more than the body actually needs!

- **Low Potassium.** The potassium/sodium ration is of critical importance. Eating more

What's Your Risk?

High Blood Pressure (greater risk of disease)   130 and above or 85

High Normal BP (some increased risk of disease)   120 to 129 or 80 to 84 (high normal)

Optimal Blood Pressure   below 120 and below 80

SYSTOLIC   DIASTOLIC

130   85

120   80

NEIL NEDLEY, *PROOF POSITIVE*

Numbers apply to adults who are not taking drugs to lower their blood pressure.

If your systolic and diastolic pressure fall into different categories your risk depends on the higher category.

While sodium is essential for body metabolism, too much can cause trouble. Excess sodium can stay in body tissues and hold extra water. This causes swelling, which raises the blood pressure, which in turn increases stress on the heart.

pressure in order to deliver necessary oxygen and food to body cells.

- *Lack of exercise.*
- *Smoking.*
- *Alcohol.* Scientific studies have demonstrated that even moderate use of alcohol may account for 5 to 15 percent of all hypertension.

AMERICANS eat 10 to 15 times more salt than they need. And they pay for it with high blood pressure, heart failure, and other problems related to fluid retention.

vegetables whilte reducing salt would greatly increase this ratio and lower elevated blood pressures.
- *Obesity.* Nearly everyone who is significantly overweight will eventually experience high blood pressure. It's just a matter of time.
- *Arterial Plaque.* Narrowed and plugged arteries force the body to boost the blood

Why do Americans eat so much salt?

In today's life it's hard to get away from salt. About 75 percent of our salt intake comes from fast and processed foods. A taste for salt is easy to develop, and salty snacks and foods abound to accommodate us.

What about medications for hypertension?

The past few years have produced an avalanche of new drugs that are effective in lowering blood pressure. Some are lifesaving. Most produce prompt results—the quick fix that Americans love.

But a closer look at hypertension medications reveals some disquieting facts: the drugs do not cure hypertension; they only control it. In some cases the medications need to be taken for life. Unpleasant

side effects may include fatigue, depression, and lack of sexual desire and impotence. While the drugs help protect against strokes, they do not protect against coronary atherosclerosis (the plugging of heart arteries). They may actually *promote* atherosclerosis, diabetes, and gouty arthritis.

What are the alternatives?

A number of major scientific studies have shown that simple dietary and lifestyle changes can reverse most essential hypertension in a matter of weeks without drugs.

- A large percentage of people are sensitive to salt and would benefit from its reduction in their diets.
- When the weight goes down, blood pressure levels usually fall.

4 1

OUR BEST GUESS is that roughly 30 million North Americans with mild essential hypertension could normalize their blood pressure by cutting their salt intake to one teaspoon a day.

PEOPLE NEED less than a half gram of salt a day—about one fifth of a teaspoon. Sodium occurs naturally in foods—more than enough to meet daily needs.

Reducing excess weight is often the only treatment needed to correct a rising blood pressure.

- A diet very low in fat yet high in fiber lowers the blood pressure about 10 percent even without weight loss or salt restriction. Thinning of the blood, which results from eating less fat, probably produces these favorable changes.
- Deleting alcohol from the diet will lower blood pressure and do the body a favor in several other areas as well.
- Physical exercise lowers blood pressure by reducing peripheral arterial resistance. In addition, regular exercise promotes general health and well-being.

People taking blood pressure medications should not play doctor and change doses or stop medicines on their own. But those who are willing to make healthful lifestyle changes will usually find their physicians glad to help them eat and exercise their way out of hypertension.

Reducing Blood Pressure!

- *Eat lots of fresh, raw foods, both fruits and vegetables. They need no added salt. They also increase potassium stores, which helps lower blood pressure.*
- *Look for unsalted snacks (if you need them).*
- *Undercook vegetables and eat them a bit crispy. They will require less salt.*
- *Learn to flavor foods with lemon juice, parsley, tarragon, garlic, or onions, instead of salt.*
- *Take advantage of the excellent salt-free gourmet cookbooks available on the market today.*

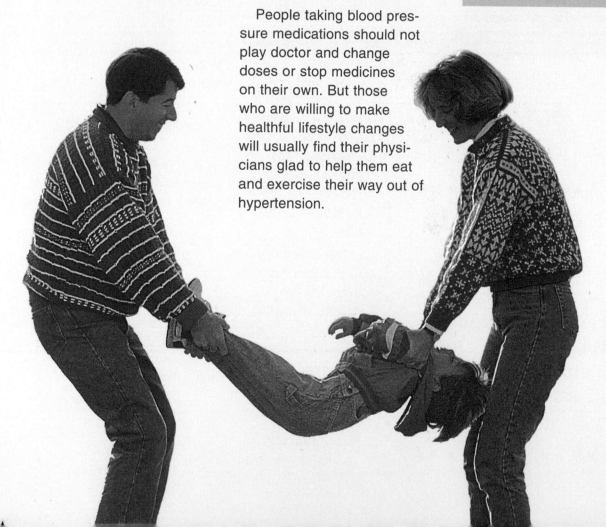

Application

Every third adult in North America has high blood pressure. This puts them at risk of heart failure, stroke, and other debilitating diseases. Obesity, narrowed arteries, smoking, lack of exercise, estrogen, alcohol, and high salt intake all contribute to the problem. Fortunately, most cases of hypertension can be reversed in weeks by simple dietary and lifestyle changes.

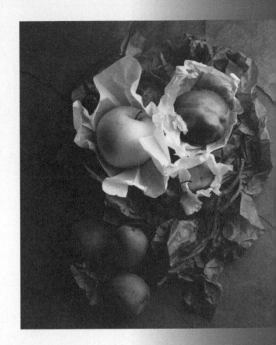

A Tremendous Step

Become a Label Reader

By carefully reading labels, you can select products low in sodium. Watch for words like "salt," "sodium," and "soda," and avoid products in which these terms are listed among the first five ingredients.

Be aware of the FDA's packaging terminology. Under these guidelines, words appearing on a package have very specific meanings.

How About You?

Are you surprised? Does it seem like just about everything contains enough salt to pickle your insides? Don't despair. By eating an abundance of fresh and unrefined foods, you automatically cut the sodium (and fat) in your diet, and you'll get plenty of protective potassium.

FDA's Proposed Packaging
GUIDELINES

	Per Serving
Sodium-free	under 5 mg
Very Low Sodium	under 35 mg
Low Sodium	under 140 mg
Reduced Sodium	a 75 percent decrease

Getting the Salt Out

Not salting your food is a good way to start protecting yourself from stroke. Unfortunately, only 25 percent of the salt we eat comes from the shaker. Much of the rest is hidden in processed foods and snacks. Here are a few examples.

SOME PROCESSED FOODS	SALT (mg)
Apple Pie (1 slice)	800
Canned Chili and Beans (1 cup)	4,100
Minute Rice (1 cup)	120
Wheaties (2 oz)	1,100
Potato Chips (Pringles) (7 oz)	3,000
Tomato Sauce (1 cup)	950
Canned Tomato Bisque (1 cup)	1,125
Corned Beef (3 oz)	1,685
Cheese, American (2 slices)	1,800
Kentucky Fried Chicken (3-piece meal)	5,600

STROKE

Stalking a Crippler

NOT ONLY CAN YOU SURVIVE THIS GRIM CONDITION— YOU CAN PREVENT IT.

Two million Americans lie crippled from paralyzing strokes. After AIDS and cancer, stroke is probably the most dreaded and disabling disease to afflict Westernized civilizations.

What are a person's chances of developing a stroke?

Some 730,000 Americans suffer strokes each year and 160,000 die from them. As with heart attacks, serious and even fatal strokes can occur without warning. Around one fourth of victims under age 70 die from the first attack; after that the figure doubles.

"You worry about heart attacks when you pass 50. Strokes, you begin to worry past 60."

— Don Smith, M.D.
Colorado Neurological Institute

Of those who survive, 40 percent need some degree of on-going special care, but only 10 percent require institutionalization.

The remaining 60 percent represent the good news. Some recover completely; nearly all improve enough to care for themselves; most are able to resume their normal activities.

What causes strokes?

A stroke, or Cerebral Vascular Accident (CVA), is most commonly related to atherosclerosis—a thickening, narrowing, and hardening of arteries supplying the brain with

"Let the morning bring me word of your unfailing love, for I have put my trust in you. Show me the way I should go, for to you I lift up my soul." Psalm 143:8

In the U.S., stroke is the leading cause of adult disability.

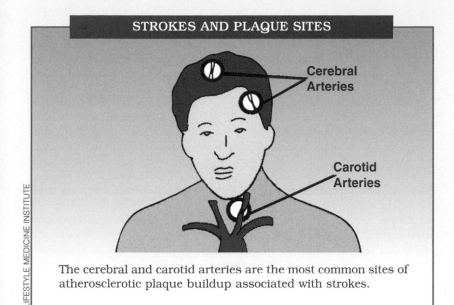

STROKES AND PLAQUE SITES

Cerebral Arteries

Carotid Arteries

The cerebral and carotid arteries are the most common sites of atherosclerotic plaque buildup associated with strokes.

LIFESTYLE MEDICINE INSTITUTE

Stroke Warning Signs

Call "911" immediately if any of the following warning signs appear. "Clotbusters" can neutralize many strokes if given in time:

- *Sudden dimness or loss of vision, particularly in one eye.*

- *Loss of speech, or trouble talking or understanding speech.*

- *Sudden weakness or numbness of the face, arm or leg on one side of the body.*

- *Unexplained dizziness, unsteadiness or sudden falls, especially with any of the above-mentioned symptoms.*

4 5

oxygenated blood. This atherosclerotic process can occur both in arteries within the brain and in arteries leading to the brain. The roughened, ragged inner surfaces of damaged arteries become seedbeds for clot formation and plaque buildup. When obstruction is complete, the artery is said to be *thrombosed.*

Sometimes pieces of plaque or a blood clot break off from other parts of the circulatory system and travel to smaller brain arteries, producing obstruction. These are called *emboli.* Some 80% of CVAs result from either thrombotic or embolic arterial blockage.

Hemorrhages, or blowouts, cause the rest of the strokes. Most of these are associated with uncontrolled high blood pressure which forces blood through cracks in stiffened artery walls. A few blowouts are caused by *aneurysms.* These are ballooned-out areas in certain arteries that

eventually rupture. Either way, the result is bleeding into the brain.

Strokes do their damage by preventing fresh blood from reaching an area of the brain, which soon dies from lack of oxygen. If a large portion of the brain is affected, the stroke will be severe or fatal. A smaller area of brain damage will cause lesser symptoms.

Who is at risk for strokes?

Most strokes are directly related to high blood pressure. People with hypertension are eight times more likely to suffer a stroke than are people with normal blood pressure. The presence of atrial fibrillation (irregular heart beat) increases stroke risk six times.

Blackout spells, called *Transient Ischemic Attacks* (TIAs), may be early warnings. These are small strokes that start suddenly and disappear

in less than 24 hours. Most last only a few seconds, and recovery is complete. Persistent TIAs, however, increase the chances for a complete stroke, much as angina attacks increase the chances of a heart attack.

Other risk factors include elevated blood cholesterol and triglycerides, smoking, diabetes, obesity, and sedentary lifestyle. All of these contribute to the atherosclerotic process. In fact, the risk factors for stroke are basically the same as those for coronary heart disease since both diseases are caused by underlying damage to vital, oxygen-carrying arteries.

Reducing the Risk

- *Know your blood pressure. If you're over age 40, have it checked at least twice a year. If it's high, make lifestyle changes, especially toward a very-low-sodium and -fat diet.*

- *Normalize weight.*

- *Find out if you have atrial fibrillation (irregular heart rate).*

- *If you smoke, stop.*

- *Find out if you have high cholesterol; then do something about it!*

- *Actively exercise daily.*

Can strokes be prevented?

Yes, most strokes can be prevented. In fact, strokes, like certain other lifestyle diseases, could become relatively uncommon within a generation if people would begin adopting, early in life, the healthful lifestyle practices already known today. These include the following:

❑ Don't smoke. One out of every six CVA deaths is directly related to tobacco use.

❑ Check blood pressure regularly. Hypertension has no symptoms, and it can sneak up on the unaware.

❑ Learn to use much less salt. In areas of the world where salt intake is low, hypertension is virtually unknown. In Japan, where salt intake is high, stroke is the leading cause of death.

❑ Normalize weight. Obesity promotes atherosclerosis, hypertension and most diabetes.

❑ Eat a diet very low in fat and cholesterol, yet high in fiber. Experiments have shown that keeping fat below 15 percent and cholesterol as low as possible protects the arterial linings from atherosclerosis.

❑ Exercise actively and regularly. Exercise improves circulation and helps control weight and hypertension.

What about people who have already had strokes? Is there help for them?

Definitely. The lifestyle that helps prevent strokes will also hasten recovery, as well as help prevent recurrent strokes.

Acute strokes require good nursing care and energetic rehabilitation. In selected cases, certain surgical procedures such as endarterectomy (cleaning out the arteries), may be of value.

Small doses of aspirin have been shown to help prevent some strokes in susceptible people, especially people with atrial fibrillation. Remember, however, that aspirin may also promote bleeding tendencies (hemorrhagic strokes) and aggravate stomach ulcers.

But the best news is that arterial blockages are reversible. Thickened, narrowed arteries slowly open again when a *very* low-fat, vegetarian diet is consistently followed, along with the other health practices. While these studies, so far, center on coronary arteries, similar results are expected in arteries affecting the brain, since the underlying problem is basically the same.

Everyone is born with soft, flexible, elastic artery walls. Many populations around the world retain their healthy arteries and low blood pressures throughout their lifetimes. We can, too, if we get serious about pursuing healthful lifestyle practices before the damage is done.

New guidelines put the moderately overweight in the danger zone.

Application

Stroke is one of the most dreaded and disabling diseases afflicting Westernized countries, but it is not a disease that attacks indiscriminately. In many populations around the world, stroke is virtually unknown. You can reduce your risk by adopting a lifestyle that promotes healthy arteries and low blood pressure.

Change Your Bad Habits to Good

Getting the Salt Out

We all need to reduce the amount of salt we eat. Don't worry about not getting enough. If you are like most Americans, you eat up to 20 times more than you need. Three culprits responsible for much of this harmful excess are:

The Saltshaker. Throw it away. You already get a dangerously high amount of salt from the food you eat. Don't add to the problem by pouring more on top. Your food will seem bland for a few weeks, but your taste buds will soon adjust, and you will begin to enjoy the subtle flavors of foods. The day will come when foods you now think of as delicious will taste salty.

Salty Snacks. Things like potato chips, pretzels, and salted nuts are so dangerous they should have a surgeon general's warning on the box: "Warning: salty snacks are linked to hypertension, stroke, and heart disease. Eat at your own risk." If you must snack, use substitutes like carrot sticks and sliced apples.

Fast Foods. If we would cut salt intake to five grams a day (one teaspoonful), hypertension would virtually disappear. We will never reach that goal, however, until we break the fast-food habit. A McDonald's cheeseburger alone contains two grams of salt. And a three-piece chicken dinner from Kentucky Fried Chicken has a whopping 5.6 grams of salt—more than you should eat for an entire day.

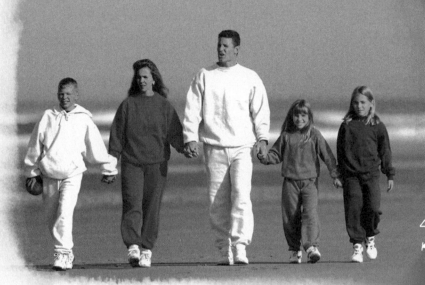

Substitute

Get yourself started in a new direction. Use salt-free spice blends, such as Mrs. Dash, to liven up your food.

How About You?

List several things you can do to reduce your risk of stroke:

_____

_____

_____

_____

_____

_____

_____

_____

PHOTODISC, INC.

CANCER

Many cancers are turning out to be do-it-yourself diseases. We promote them by chronic exposure to certain environmental factors. What we eat and drink, where we live and work, and what we breathe may well determine whether we become a cancer statistic.

Are you saying that we bring cancer on ourselves?

Medical science continues to make strides toward earlier detection and improved treatments for many cancers. But these efforts are largely after the fact. The sad truth is that the overall death rates for many cancers continue to rise. One in four American lives are now being claimed by cancer.

This trend, however, could be reversed. If we would simply take the precautions that we already know about, 70 to 80 percent of the cancers that afflict Americans could be prevented.

Won't people do just about anything to avoid such a terrifying disease?

Almost anything, it seems, except change their lifestyles.

Take lung cancer (the cancer that kills more men and women in the United States than any other) for example. Ever since the surgeon general's report in 1964 we've known that lung cancer is directly related to cigarette smoking. It's true that millions have quit smoking, yet every fourth adult in North America still smokes! Close to 90 percent of the cancers of the lung, lip, mouth, tongue, throat, and esophagus could be prevented if people simply stopped using tobacco. It would also prevent half the bladder cancers.

Do-It-Yourself-Cancers

DEATHS FROM SMOKING/YR	
Lung cancer	115,000
All other cancers	33,000
Cardiovascular disease	181,000
Respiratory diseases	88,300
Smoking-related fires	1,500
Babies because of smoking mothers	2,000
Passive smoking	4,200
TOTAL FROM SMOKING	**425,000**

"Test everything. Hold on to the good. Avoid every kind of evil."

1 Thessalonians 5:21-22

BREAST CANCER TRENDS

1960 = 1 in 20   1980 = 1 in 11   2000 = 1 in 7

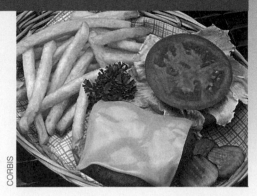

CORBIS

Cancer Mortality Risk Differential of Japanese Immigrants

Cancer Type	Japanese in Japan	Japanese in Hawaii	Caucasians in Hawaii
Breast	1x	4x	6x
Colon	1x	5x	5x
Prostate	1x	11x	3x
Rectum	1x	3x	2x
Lung	1x	2x	4x

Are some cancers related to diet?

In men, the second and third most frequently occurring cancers are those of the prostrate and colon. For women it's cancers of the breast and colon. Extensive evidence links nearly 50 percent of these cancers to overnutrition—too much fat and too much weight.

That sounds like a long shot. Wouldn't a more likely culprit be the many chemicals that find their way into our food supply?

Carcinogens (cancer-producing chemicals) are a concern—especially with the array of additives, preservatives, flavor enhancers, pesticides, and other chemicals that we use in producing and marketing food. However, only 2 percent of all cancers can be reliably linked to these substances.

In contrast, evidence of the connection between cancer and such dietary factors as fiber and fat grows stronger every day. Compared with diets around 1900, the average American now eats one-third *more* fat, and one-third *less* fiber. In areas of the world in which fat intake is low and fiber consumption is high, the incidence of colon, breast, and prostate cancers are negligible. In countries such as the United States, Canada, and New Zealand, where diets are low in fiber and high in fat, the rates for these kinds of cancers are much higher.

Could ethnic variations, rather than diet, account for these differences?

Researchers asked the same question. They found, for example, that Japanese living in Japan had very few of these cancers. In Japan, fiber consumption was high and fat intake low (15 percent). But when these Japanese migrated to Hawaii and adopted Western eating habits and lifestyles, their rates for these cancers increased dramatically and soon equaled those for other Americans.

How can such things as fiber and fat influence cancer?

Not all the answers are in yet, but cancer is associated with carcinogens—chemical irritants that can produce cancerous lesions over time.

Bile acids are an example. The amount of fat in the diet affects the amount of bile the body produces. In the intestinal tract some of these bile acids can form irritating carcinogenic compounds. The longer these compounds stay in contact with the lining of the colon, the more irritation results.

This is where fiber comes in. With a low-fiber diet, material moves slowly through the intestines, often taking from 72 hours to five days to complete the journey from entry to exit. Most fibers absorb water like a sponge. This helps fill the intestines and stimulates them to increased activity. With a high-fiber diet, food travels through the intestines in 24 to 36 hours.

4
9

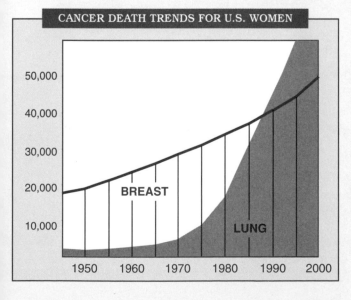

CANCER DEATH TRENDS FOR U.S. WOMEN

BREAST

LUNG

50,000
40,000
30,000
20,000
10,000

1950   1960   1970   1980   1990   2000

Most Cancer Is Preventable

This helps the colon in two ways. It shortens the exposure to irritating substances, and it dilutes the concentration of the irritants thanks to fiber's water-holding ability and insulating effect.

How does diet relate to breast and prostate cancers?

A high fat intake depresses the activity of important cells in the body's immune system. This effect has been studied extensively in connection with breast cancer and may affect other types of cancer as well.

Are other lifestyle areas connected to cancer?

Excessive alcohol consumption increases the risk for cancer of the esophagus and pancreas, and does so dramatically for those who smoke as well. Excess weight raises the risk of cancer of the breast, colon and prostate. Then there are such things as exposure to asbestos, side-stream smoke and toxic chemicals.

Just four lifestyle factors—no smoking, no alcohol, a vegetarian diet very low in fat and high in fiber, and normal weight—could prevent close to 80 percent of cancers found in Western society today. Instead of one American in four dying of cancer, the risk could be reduced to one in 20.

It's not an impossible dream.

THE RISKS OF CANCER

TOBACCO
Smoking causes one of every three cancer deaths in North America.

RED MEAT
Regular meat eaters have a three times higher risk of developing colon cancer when compared with occasional meat eaters.

JUNK FOOD
Those who fill up on doughnuts, sodas, and potato chips lose out on the cancer-fighting substances found in fruits and vegetables.

INACTIVITY
Those who log at least four hours of exercise a week cut their risk of breast and colon cancer by more than a third.

OVEREATING
Among women, being heavy adds markedly to the danger from breast, colon, and endometrial cancer. And men are pushing their luck with prostate and colon cancers.

ALCOHOL
Heavy drinking has been clearly linked to cancers of the liver, throat, and esophagus. In women, even a daily drink or two raises breast cancer risk.

Percent of fatal cancers related to alcohol

Esophagus .75%
Mouth 50%
Larynx 50%
Liver 30%

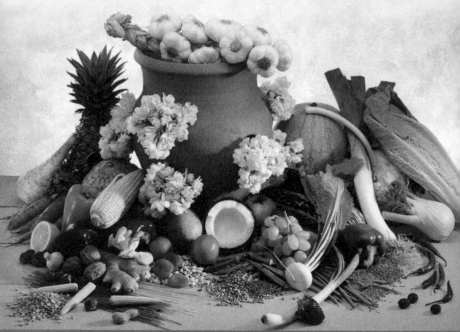

The Newest Cancer Fighter

Application

Lifestyle factors, such as smoking, obesity, consumption of alcohol, and a diet that is high in animal products and fat, account for up to 80 percent of all cancers.

Miracle Cure?

Imagine the announcement of a pill that would make people immune to cancer. It would be the news story of the decade. People would flock to their doctors for a prescription, and the inventors would be wealthy beyond belief.

No such pill exists. But there are a number of things we can do for ourselves to prevent the majority of adult cancers.

A good place to start is with our food. We can begin eating a diet considerably lower in fat and cholesterol. Many studies have shown that such a diet reduces the risk of heart disease, diabetes, stroke, and many types of cancer.

But making lifestyle changes is not as simple as swallowing a pill. It involves learning new habits and skills. For example, cutting the fat and cholesterol in our diet means preparing more meatless dishes.

One sensible way to develop these skills is by designating a day or two each week for vegetarian-style meals. This gives you a chance to experiment with healthful ways of cooking while gradually building up a new repertoire of favorite new recipes.

Good Eating Begins With Good Recipes

A good cookbook is an investment that will repay you many times over. There's no better tool when it comes to changing your eating habits. (See Educational Resources, page 253-256.)

LIFE-SAVING TESTS

Beat cancer by detecting it early. The odds of surviving colon cancer are nine in ten when it's discovered before it spreads, but only one in 14 afterward.

What's more, a full 97% of women diagnosed with localized breast cancer are alive five years later, compared to only 20% of those found to have metastasized breast cancer.

BREAST

Self-examination monthly from age 20. Any new or suspicious lumps should be checked by a doctor.
Breast exam every three years from age 20 to 39, then annually.
Mammogram every year or two from age 40.

CERVIX

Pelvic exam with Pap smear annually from age 18 and for younger women who are sexually active. After three consecutive normal results, some doctors recommend testing less frequently.

SKIN

Self-examination once a month. Look for unusual pearly bumps or red scaly patches. Also check for moles that have changed size or color, or have begun to ooze or bleed easily.

COLON

Fecal occult blood test annually after age 50.
Digital rectal exam, performed as part of a standard physical exam, annually after age 40.
Sigmoidoscopy, a rectal exam using a flexible lighted tube, every three to five years after age 50.

PROSTATE

Prostate-Specific Antigen (PSA) test annually after age 50.
Digital rectal exam, as part of a standard physical exam, annually after age 40.

Moving Toward the Optimal Diet

- *Use whole-grain breads and cereals.* They have the vitamins, minerals, and fiber that products made with refined flour lack.

- *Enjoy a variety of fresh fruit each day*.

- *Eat a wide variety of vegetables*. Dark-green leafy vegetables are essential for the total vegetarian. (One cup of greens contains more calcium than milk.) Yellow vegetables are high in vitamin A.

- *Use nuts sparingly*. They are high in minerals and vitamins but also contain lots of fat.

- *Use a wide variety of beans and peas*. They provide protein and fiber and are low in fat.

DIABETES

Disarming Diabetes

Since World War II diabetes has been advancing relentlessly in developed countries where it is now one of the leading causes of death. If present trends continue, babies born today will have a one in five chance of becoming diabetic in their lifetimes. Until recent times, there has been no known cure.

No more! Today many people are beating diabetes. They are normalizing their blood sugars and getting off insulin by making healthful lifestyle changes.

In America a new diabetic is discovered every 50 seconds.

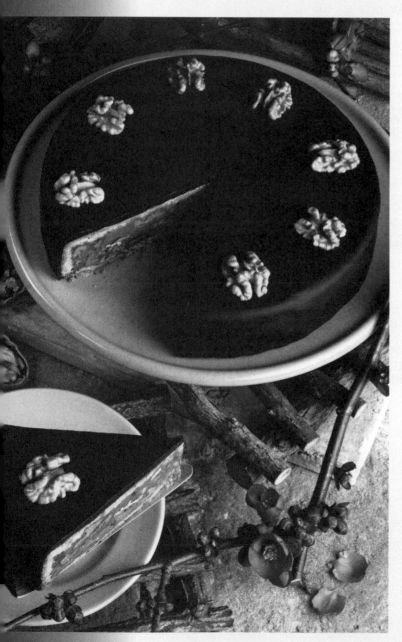

What exactly is Diabetes?

Diabetes occurs when the body becomes unable to handle glucose (sugar), which builds up to dangerous levels in the blood. A diagnosis of diabetes is usually made when a blood sugar test is consistently above 125 mg% (7.0 mmol/L) after an eight-hour fast. Fasting blood sugar (FBS) levels of 100-125 (5.6-6.9 mmol/L) are known as pre-diabetes.

There are two kinds of diabetes. Type I afflicts about 5 percent of diabetics. They are usually thin and rarely overweight. This type of diabetes usually begins in childhood and is commonly known as *juvenile diabetes.* Since these diabetics cannot survive without insulin, it is now officially called *insulin-dependent diabetes mellitus* (IDDM).

Type II diabetes is different. Called *adult-onset diabetes* or *noninsulin-dependent diabetes mellitus* (NIDDM), it is the most common kind, affecting more than 90 percent of diabetics. While this type generally hits around age 50 as people get older and fatter, some people with the recent epidemic of obesity are developing this disease now in their teens. In contrast to the juvenile diabetics, most Type II diabetics have plenty of insulin in their bodies when diagnosed, but something blocks the insulin so it cannot do its job properly.

The Bible says, "Your body is a temple" (1 Corinthians 6:19). *Treat it that way!*

What are the warning signs of diabetes?

The classical symptoms are polydipsia (excessive thirst), polyphagia (excessive appetite), and polyuria (excessive passage of urine). Early in the disease, however, few symptoms show up—perhaps some increase in urinary frequency and thirst. Of the 16 million diabetics in America it is estimated that 7 million don't know that they have it. As the disease progresses, its effects are devastating, affecting all organs of the body and gradually destroying them. Consider the risks of unrecognized or poorly controlled diabetes:

- Eight out of ten diabetics develop eye problems. Diabetes is the leading cause of new blindness in developed countries.

- Diabetics are 18 times more likely to experience serious kidney damage than are nondiabetics. Some 25 percent of kidney dialysis patients are diabetics.

- Diabetes is a potent promoter of atherosclerosis (plugging of the arteries). The result is that diabetes more than doubles the risk of heart attacks and strokes. It can also lead to sexual impotence, hearing impairment, intermittent claudication (disabling leg cramps) and gangrene (half of all foot and leg amputations in adults are from this cause).

What causes adult-onset diabetes?

Studies demonstrate a strong relationship to fat—both fat in the diet and fat on the body. The disease is rare in areas of the world where fat intake is low and obesity uncommon.

Normally insulin, a pancreatic hormone, enables body cells to use glucose and controls blood sugar levels. But most of the time the problem in adult-onset diabetes is not a defective pancreas unable to produce sufficient insulin, but a lack of sensitivity to insulin. This resistance of the cells to insulin appears to relate directly to obesity and to excess fat in the diet and possibly in the liver.

But isn't sugar the culprit?

James Anderson, M.D., professor of medicine and clinical nutrition at the University of Kentucky College of Medicine and a widely respected authority on diabetes, evaluated the effect of diet on blood sugar levels. Just as others had done before him, Dr. Anderson was able to turn lean healthy young men into mild diabetics in less than two weeks by feeding them a rich 65 percent fat diet. A similar group, fed a lean 10 percent fat diet plus one pound of sugar a day, did not produce

even one diabetic after 11 weeks when the experiment was terminated.

So what's the best way to treat this disease?

Several treatment centers have convincingly demonstrated that most Type II diabetics can normalize their blood sugar levels, often within weeks, by following a simple diet, very low in fat and high in fiber, coupled with daily exercise.

Lowering the amount of fat, oil and grease in the diet plays the crucial role. When less fat is eaten, less fat reaches the bloodstream and the liver. This begins a complicated process that gradually restores the sensitivity to insulin, which can then faciliatate the entry of sugar

53

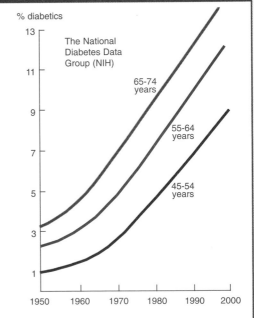

The percentage of diabetics for selected age groups has steadily increased; i.e., the diabetes rate for those 45 to 54 years has gone from 1% in 1950 to 9% in 2000, an increase of 900%. (U.S. 1950-2000)

from the bloodstream into the body cells. The effect is often dramatic. A Type II diabetic who lowers daily fat intake to about 10 percent of total calories can often bring blood sugar levels to normal ranges in less than eight weeks. Many are eventually able to get off diabetic medication entirely—both pills and injections.

Eating more natural, fiber-rich foods plays an important role by helping stabilize blood sugar levels. When foods are eaten without their normal complement of fiber, blood sugar levels can quickly shoot up. Normally a surge of insulin counteracts this. People who consume refined foods, drinks, and snacks high in calories but low in fiber may experience hikes and dips in blood sugar levels all day long. High-fiber foods, on the other hand, smooth out these blood sugar fluctuations and stabilize energy levels.

Active physical exercise has an insulin-like reaction in that it *burns up the excess fuel* (blood sugar and fatty acids) more rapidly.

The foremost recommended lifestyle modification for diabetes, however, is losing excess weight. Obesity is far and away the most common non-genetic component contributing to the development of diabetes.

Normalizing body weight is often all that is necessary to bring the blood sugar back to normal. The low-fat, high-fiber diet will greatly aid this effort, as will regular, active exercise.

> A STUDY CONFIRMS that even small amounts of weight gain can increase your risk of developing Type II diabetes, according to the American Journal of Epidemiology. A five-pound gain increases your risk for diabetes by 10 percent.

> The earlier that diabetes is detected, the more likely lifestyle modifications are going to be effective.

What about Type I diabetes?

Insulin-dependent, or juvenile, diabetics will need to take insulin for life until pancreatic transplants become feasible and affordable. However, the high-fiber, very low-fat diet will help reduce the amount of insulin required to maintain stable blood sugar levels and reduce the ever present threat of vascular complications.

A protein has been identified in cow's milk that can increase the risk of diabetes in small children. The American Academy of Pediatrics recommends that cow's milk NOT be given to children until at least one year of age. Breast-fed infants have a measure of protection against this kind of diabetes.

The Outlook

The earlier the detection of diabetes, the more likely lifestyle modifications will be effective. Earlier detection thus takes much of the emphasis off drugs and insulin injections, both of which come with undesirable side effects.

Remember that the same lifestyle measures that are disarming and normalizing many cases of Type II diabetes are preventive as well. Even losing as little as 10 extra pounds and taking a brisk walk a few times a week can help stave off the disease.

Start now. Beat diabetes before it happens.

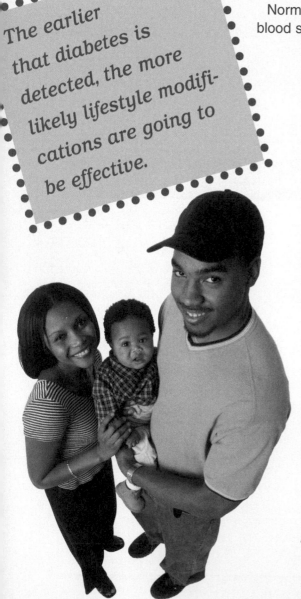

It's your future.
Be There!

Application

One in five people in North America develop diabetes at some point in their life, yet this disease can be prevented and sometimes even cured. Low fat, both in the diet and on the body, is the secret.

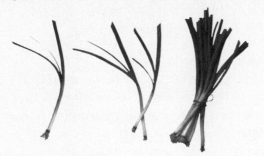

Low-fat Checklist

The main villain in adult-onset diabetes is the enormous amount of fat in our diet. One way we can reduce this overabundance is by using less fat, oil, and grease during cooking. How many of the following do you do?

____ Use nonstick (Teflon) cookware to minimize the amount of oil needed to keep food from sticking.

____ Cook onions, green peppers, and other vegetables in broth instead of browning in fat.

____ Use less oil, butter, or fat than a recipe calls for.

____ Eliminate the dabs of butter from casserole toppings and vegetables.

____ Use a nonstick spray or a film of lecithin instead of greasing a casserole dish.

____ Avoid frying.

____ Only cook very lean meat (or better yet, eat no meat at all).

____ Steam or microwave vegetables instead of sautéeing them in butter or oil.

What can you do?

What steps can you take to reduce the fat in your diet?

_____

_____

_____

How to Beat Diabetes (Type II)

Diabetes is a leading cause of new blindness, foot and leg amputations, and hearing impairment. The worst part is that many people suffer needlessly. Here is the formula that can help beat this disease.

1. Eat more natural fiber-rich foods, simply prepared, low in fat, grease, and sugar. Freely use whole-grain products, tubers and legumes, salads and vegetables. Eat a substantial breakfast daily—a hot multigrain cereal will curb your appetite for hours and stabilize your blood sugar.

2. Use fresh whole fruits, but not more than three servings a day (if you have diabetes).

3. Avoid refined and processed foods. They are usually high in fat and sugar, and low in fiber.

4. Markedly reduce fats, oils, and grease. If you use animal products, use them lean and very sparingly, more like a condiment. And avoid oily and creamy dressings and sauces.

5. Walk briskly each day. Two 30-minute walks every day are ideal to help burn up the extra sugar in your blood.

6. Work with a physician experienced in the effects of dietary therapy to monitor and adjust your insulin need.

OSTEOPOROSIS

Building Better Bones

Has ordinary, everyday calcium turned out to be the gallant gladiator that can deliver fair maidens from brittle bones, fractured hips, and deformed spines? That is what the calcium manufacturers and the dairy industry would like us to believe. In reality, osteoporosis is far more complicated than that.

What is osteoporosis?

Osteoporosis (literally, *porous bone*) silently and painlessly weakens the bones of 25 million Americans. Previously sturdy bones gradually become thin and fragile, their interiors soft and spongy. As a result, bones break, giving rise to the term *brittle bones.*

Osteoporosis may cause as many as 1.3 million fractures a year. Hip fractures can be both disabling and deadly. Spinal fractures, on the other hand, are often painless, but can rob a person of two to eight inches of height. The resultant spinal curvature is the source of dowager's hump.

How does osteoporosis develop?

Normal bones continue to increase in strength and thickness until around age 35. Then the process gradually reverses itself, and small amounts of bone are being lost each year. This loss accelerates in women after menopause and can continue for 7 to 15 years. When risk factors are present, bone loss occurs even faster, and osteoporosis may develop. Although usually considered a disease of older women, 20 percent of victims are men.

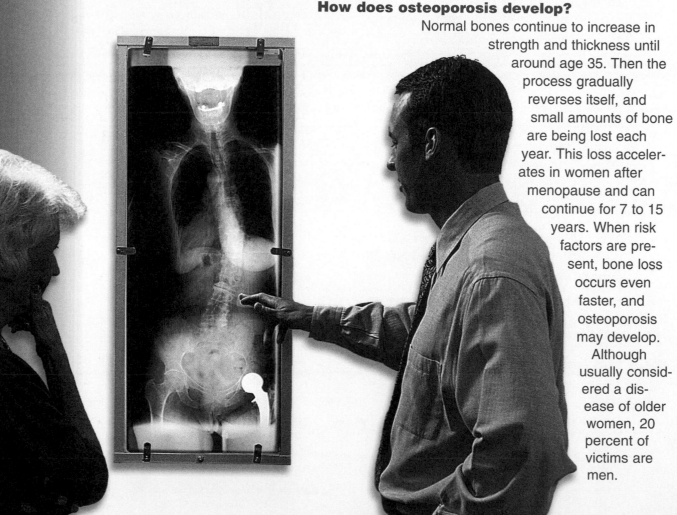

How can I tell if I have it?

Without professional help, you can't—not until you fracture a bone or start shrinking in height, and that's quite late in the disease. Earlier diagnosis is best done by physicians at reliable medical centers.

Protein is an essential component of a healthy diet. But we eat too much of it, especially animal protein. And that can be harmful.

USE IT OR LOSE IT

In its efficiency the body deposits minerals when there is extra demand placed upon the bones. Exercise stresses bone structure, producing small electrical charges that cause calcium and other minerals to be drawn in and held. "Use it or lose it" is an adage that certainly applies to keeping bones strong.

If you are middle-aged or older and you have two or more of the following risk factors, you should be tested:

● *sedentary lifestyle*
● *early menopause*
● *chronic use of corticosteroids*
● *cigarettes, caffeine, or alcohol use*
● *standard American diet high in animal protein, salt, and phosphoric acid*

Lean Caucasians and Westernized Asians are more susceptible than other races, probably because they have smaller bones.

What can be done to treat this disease?

Several treatments are being used:

✔ *Estrogen therapy.* When used, it slows down bone loss, but increases the risk for uterine and breast cancer, thrombophlebitis (blood clots) and gallbladder disease. It may also aggravate diabetes and hypertension, and women sometimes face periodic uterine biopsies. Over the years, adding progesterone was designed to blunt some of these disturbing side effects. The results of the recent Women's Health Initiative, however, have raised so much concern about the use of these hormones that many physicians prescribe them now only for special clinical conditions, such as severe hot flashes, and even then, only for a short time.

✔ *Vitamin D.* The body uses vitamin D to absorb calcium, but most Americans get more than they need if they have sufficient sun exposure; additional supplements, in general, have not proven very beneficial.

✔ *Calcium.* Various U.S. governmental agencies have recommended 800 to 1,500 milligrams a day. The World Health Organization, however, recommends only 500 milligrams since calcium deficiency has never been documented anywhere in the world, even with calcium intakes of as little as 300 milligrams a day.

✔ *Exercise.* Bones will not thicken and strengthen without regular, weight-bearing exercise, such as walking. To retain their minerals, bones *need* to be pressed, pushed, pulled, and twisted against gravity.

5 7

HOW EASY IT IS TO EAT TOO MUCH PROTEIN!

Breakfast	Protein (gm)	
3-egg ham and cheese omelette	46	
Hash brown potatoes	3	
Toast (2) with butter and jelly	5	
Coffee with cream	1	
Orange juice	1	
Lunch		
Big Mac	26	
French fries	3	
Milkshake	11	
Dinner		
Fried chicken	55	TOTAL
Peas	5	**178 gms**
Mixed salad with dressing	4	
Baked potato with sour cream	9	*Recommended*
Milk (2%), 1 glass	9	50 gms

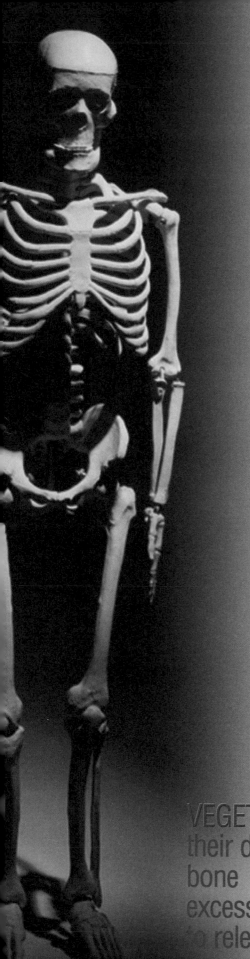

The gravity factor was well demonstrated by the early astronauts. Even though they exercised faithfully while in space, their bones showed startling osteoporotic changes on their return. While nearly all types of aerobic exercise are beneficial to the body, what the bones need most is a good daily shake-up.

- **If you smoke, stop!**

  It will do your bones a big favor.

- **Reduce the amount of animal protein, salt and caffeine in the diet.**

  Osteoporosis appears to be a disease of affluence and excess, rather than one of deficiency. Osteoporosis is a rather complex disease largely related to our dietary lifestyle. The Standard American Diet, high in animal protein, salt, phosphorus (meat, certain soft drinks), and caffeine, causes calcium to be leached from the bones and excreted in the urine. These lifestyle-induced calcium losses seem to override any amount of calcium consumed or swallowed.

What's the evidence for this connection?

Eskimos consume diets extremely high in both protein (250 to 400 grams/day) and calcium (1,500 to 2,500 milligrams/day). In spite of their high calcium intake and the very active lives they lead, they have one of the highest rates of osteoporosis in the world.

The Bantu tribes in Africa, on the other hand, consume an average of 47 grams of protein and less than 400 milligrams of calcium a day, predominantly from plant foods. Yet, even though Bantu women bear an average of 10 children, making special demands on calcium reserves, they are essentially free of osteoporosis. In contrast, relatives of the Bantu who have migrated to the United States and adopted the American dietary lifestyle eventually experience a rate of osteoporosis comparable to that of the rest of the American population.

How about prevention?

Most populations around the world average 400 milligrams of calcium a day without any evidence of osteoporosis. It's strangely paradoxical that osteoporosis has become epidemic in the United States, where the consumption of calcium-rich dairy products and calcium supplements is the highest in the world.

North Americans eat two to three times more protein than they need. Reducing protein intake to the Recommended Daily Allowance (RDA) of 50 to 60 grams a day, along with daily active exercise and a healthful diet low in salt, phosphorus, and caffeine, holds promise of turning the tide in the battle against brittle bones.

VEGETARIANS HAVE AN ADVANTAGE in that their diet is more alkaline, a condition that favors bone density. Part of the body's response to excess acid-forming foods like animal protein is to release calcium from the bones.

Application

Osteoporosis is epidemic in North America, even though the consumption of calcium-rich dairy products and supplements is the highest in the world. By reducing the intake of animal protein, salt, and caffeine and adopting a program of daily exercise, the tide can be turned in the battle against this crippling disease.

The Case of the Unsuccessful Savers

Janice and Steve have trouble saving money. Once the bills are paid, nothing ever seems to be left. After some serious discussion, Janice decided to take a part-time job, and Steve asked his boss for more overtime hours.

What a difference! The next month their paychecks were larger than ever before. But once again, no money was left once the bills had been paid. Janice and Steve had increased their spending to match their new income.

Spending Calcium

Something similar happens to people eating a diet high in protein and salt. The body "spends" calcium as it processes animal protein, salt, and caffeine. When there is not enough calcium available in the diet, it "borrows" from another source—the bones.

The Western diet provides two to three times the Recommended Daily Allowance of protein. At the same time, it provides 10 to 20 times more salt than the body requires. At this level it is almost impossible to get enough calcium to balance the losses. Slowly over the years the bones become brittle and weak.

The solution is not to take more calcium, but to eat less protein, salt, and caffeine. This allows the body to conserve the calcium already stored in the bones.

High-Calcium, High-Protein Foods

Chart 1 lists some typical sources of calcium. Notice how high they are in protein. With some of these foods you get a lot of calcium, but you may lose even more as the body has to deal with the excess animal protein.

High-Calcium, Low-Protein Foods

Chart 2 also lists good sources of calcium. But this time, note the moderate amounts of protein provided by these foods. Another bonus is that they are all low in fat and are cholesterol-free.

1 — Calcium in Concentrated Protein Foods

	Serving size	Calcium (in mg)	Protein (in gm)
Beef, Chicken	5 oz.	15	34-45
Cheddar cheese	4 sl.	900	35
Whole milk	3 glasses	875	27

Save More Than You Spend

Everyone knows that you can't save money when you spend more than you make. The same principle applies to calcium: You can't keep bones strong if you're flushing the calcium out of them with a diet high in animal protein, salt, and phosphorus.

2 — Calcium in Unconcentrated Protein Foods

	Serving size	Calcium (in mg)	Protein (in gm)
Collard greens	1 cup	360	5
Spinach, Broccoli	1 cup	175	5
Bread	2 sl.	50-90	5

How Tough Are Your Bones?

Try to cut down on calcium-robbing, high-protein meats and dairy products. Instead, look to lower protein sources of calcium found in whole grains, dark-green leafy vegetables, and beans.

ARTHRITIS

Disease With a Thousand "Cures"

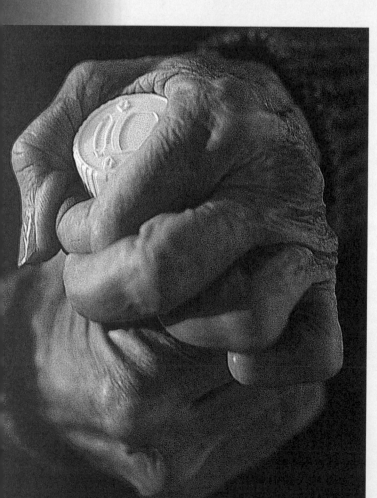

Because arthritis is a chronic disease that never quite seems to go away, even with good medical treatment, hundreds of folk remedies have grown up around it. And there are hundreds more unproven, expensive, and often outright quack treatments being offered today to vulnerable arthritis sufferers by unscrupulous promoters.

How would you define arthritis?

Arthritis is a general term for diseases or other abnormal processes occurring in the joints. An estimated 40 million Americans suffer from some form of arthritis.

Our joints and ligaments, like our muscles, wear with use and need to be constantly repaired—a process that normally occurs during sleep. Repair of any body part requires free access to oxygen and other nutrients. When circulation of the blood becomes inadequate, ligaments weaken, joint fluids decrease, and cartilage wears away.

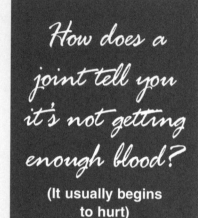

How does a joint tell you it's not getting enough blood?

(It usually begins to hurt)

What is the most common form of arthritis?

Osteoarthritis is the most common type, and in some degree is almost universally present in our older populations. It can also occur at any time after an injury or excessive wear and tear to a joint, as often happens in football. Arthritis resulting from injuries is also known as *traumatic arthritis.*

Osteoarthritis usually occurs when a joint's blood supply becomes inadequate for its needed function. Just as a heart will weaken and ultimately fail when the coronary arteries clog up with plaque, so joints begin to break down when the arteries supplying them become narrowed or obstructed. For this reason most osteoarthritis responds to measures that improve circulation, such as lowering the amount of fat in the bloodstream, regular exercise, and hydrotherapy (water treatments).

Osteoarthritis of weight-bearing joints, such as the spine, knees, and hips, is commonly aggravated by caloric overload (obesity). Just as a bridge has a load limit, so do the joints.

The most common symptoms of osteoarthritis are pain and stiffness, which tend to decrease as the joint is warmed up with activity.

Are backaches caused by arthritis?

Backaches afflict more than 5 million Americans every year—four out of five people will suffer from them at some-time in their lives. Back problems are important because they are a leading cause of disability, missed workdays, and many lawsuits.

Surprisingly, up to 80 percent of low back sufferers are victims of overworked or underexercised muscles. A strained muscle may suddenly go into a sustained contraction or spasm and become a hard knotty mass, signaling body distress by sharp pain.

Another 10 percent of back problems may be caused by osteoarthritis or a disc problem. Only a very few who suffer from back pain have a specific serious injury.

When a backache occurs, it's important to rule out an identifiable injury before anything else is done. Without an evident serious problem, the important thing is *not* to do what you feel like—retiring to a soft sofa. One day of rest after

The surprising answer to arthritis pain: *Exercise!*

Since cartilage (the pad between the bones) doesn't have a blood supply, it has to get its nutrients from the joint lining, which occurs only when the joint is used.

injury or onset of pain—two at the most. Ice bags are helpful at this stage, along with doctor-prescribed muscle relaxants and nonsteroidal anti-inflammatory medications.

Then it's time to get up on your feet and start walking. Walk through the pain. Back specialists say that prolonged bed rest will do more harm than good, because rest causes your back muscles to weaken rapidly. Instead of becoming *reconditioned,* you become *deconditioned.* After a while even light activity may sprain or strain muscles barely able to carry their own weight.

Fortunately most back problems resolve themselves in four to 12 weeks. Here are a few tips to prevent recurrence, or to prevent backaches entirely.

- Keep your weight down— the biggest favor you can do for your back.

- Avoid high heels (over one inch). They tilt the pelvis and throw the back out of alignment.

- Strengthen your back and abdominal muscles with special exercises. Walk, swim, or jog at least 20 minutes five times a week.

- Eat a diet very low in fat and high in fiber to improve your circulation, better allowing the blood to carry extra oxygen and nutrients to the compromised areas.

These measures are important for all kinds of arthritis as well as for back pain.

What about the painful, swollen big toe?

You mean gout, or *gouty arthritis.* From antiquity this disease has been associated with the lifestyle of the rich: too much rich food and too little activity. You can still see pictures in old history books of such kings, with a foot propped up on a footstool, protecting that painful big toe.

Sometimes the afflicted royal person was sent to live and work with the peasants. This was effective because a simplified diet and a more active life eventually reversed the disease.

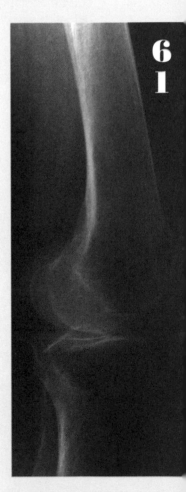

6 1

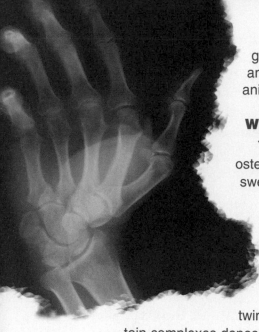

We now know that some metabolic weakness may be involved in gout. But we also know that it can be controlled by simplifying the diet and by eliminating the offending purines (largely from the breakdown of animal protein) and normalizing weight.

What about red swollen joints?

You are probably thinking of *rheumatoid arthritis*. This is different from osteoarthritis in that it results from inflammation of the joints with redness, swelling, pain, and fever, rather than from injury or wear and tear.

Rheumatoid arthritis is an autoimmune disease, related to asthma, hay fever, eczema, and other diseases that have an allergic component. Acute attacks tend to recur over the years, producing nodules and gradually stiffening and disfiguring the joints, most notably the wrist and finger joints.

Rheumatoid arthritis has long been known to be closely intertwined with the body's immune (defense) system. Certain immune protein complexes deposited in the joints play a key role in the marked destruction of cartilage that takes place. We now know that these protein antigens (perpetuators of allergies) can be absorbed intact from the small intestine without being digested, thus causing the problems.

Dietary habits are believed important because studies of rural populations in undeveloped countries show a fraction of the incidence of rheumatoid arthritis that is found among their urban counterparts. Other studies have demonstrated that when eating foods associated with few allergic symptoms, patients experience less stiffness and pain, and improvement in muscle strength. In addition, any lifestyle measures designed to improve circulation are important as well.

The best long-term results are seen in patients willing to adopt a very strict vegan diet (without any animal products). This is not surprising, since milk is the most common cause of food allergies, with eggs close behind. Studies have shown, for example, that more than 100 antigens (perpetrators of allergies) may be released *during the digestion of cow's milk alone.*

Fight for your health. Stay active. The people who get better are the ones who take an active role in bringing about positive, permanent changes in their lifestyles.

"*At age 89 it's a wonderful thing to get up in the morning and not hurt anywhere.*"
— Mavis Lindgren,
marathon runner

Healing Moves for Aching Joints

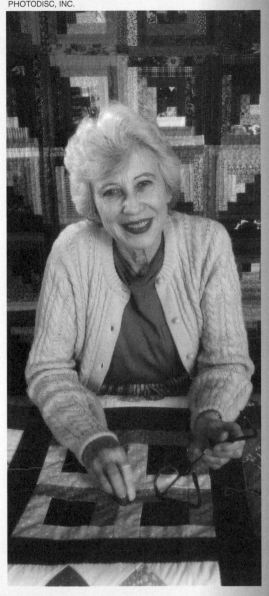

6 3

Can you summarize some practical guidelines for preventing or reversing the effects of chronic arthritis?

Despite the many different forms of arthritis, here are some general principles that are effective in most cases:

1. Normalizing weight is perhaps the most important. Every extra pound increases the wear and tear of the main weight-bearing joints—the hips, knees, and spine.

2. A simplified diet, low in fat and high in fiber, has been shown to improve circulation to the joints. In time, this kind of diet may help open up some of the narrowed arteries. Eliminate all dairy products for three weeks and evaluate your response.

3. Regular, active exercise at least five days a week, to keep muscles strong. Weakened muscles do not adequately protect the joints. When joints are painful, swimming and water aerobics are ideal.

4. Use affected joints only within the limits of their blood supply. Resting during acute episodes, then quickly returning to activity, is very important in preventing chronic disability.

5. Medications such as analgesics, muscle relaxants, and nonsteroidal anti-inflammatory drugs may help, especially in the acute phase. Steroid therapy can produce dramatic improvement; but in the long run it usually does more harm than good.

6. If joint destruction is advanced, the joint may need to be fused or replaced with an artificial joint. Also there are surgical procedures available to correct deformities and to repair injuries.

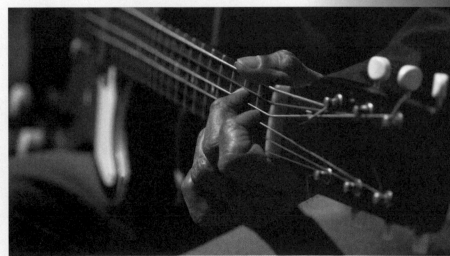

OBESITY*

Creeping Fat

AMERICANS are the fattest people on earth

"When you sit down to dine with a ruler, note well what is before you. . . . Do not crave his delicacies, for that food is deceptive."

Proverbs 23:1-3

Americans are the fattest people on earth. Obesity is one of our leading public health problems. So serious is this disease that 36 million people are at significant medical risk.

That's frightening. No wonder weight-loss diets are so popular!

Yes, and far too many people fall prey to fads and eating plans that offer quick results. Like a conditioned reflex, extra pounds spell d-i-e-t to most people. A recent survey found that 40 to 50 percent of Americans between the ages of 35 and 59 were on some kind of diet at any given time.

The sad truth is that unless people make lasting changes in their lifestyles and consistently choose healthful foods on a regular basis, their efforts are largely wasted. Up to 90 percent of dieters regain their lost weight within a year, usually with a bonus. Constantly losing and regaining weight is frustrating and demoralizing, and does more damage than good.

Would it be better to just stay fat?

For many people, remaining overweight would be less harmful than endlessly playing the rhythm game of girth control. Before running up the white flag of surrender, however, take a careful look at the health risks of being overweight.*

When compared with people of normal weight, obese people are:

- three times more likely to suffer from heart disease;
- four times more likely to suffer from high blood pressure;
- five times more likely

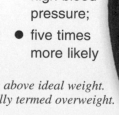

* Obesity, by definition, is being 20 percent or more above ideal weight. Being 10 to 19 percent above ideal weight is usually termed overweight.

Excess weight lays the foundation for nearly every degenerative disease except osteoporosis.

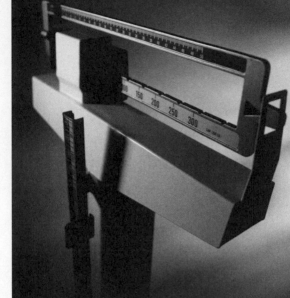

to develop diabetes, and elevated blood cholesterols;

- and they are also at higher risk of developing cancer of the colon, rectum, prostate, breast, cervix, uterus, and ovaries, and to suffer osteoarthritis and low back pain.

Overweight people are like ticking bombs waiting for one or more of these diseases to explode in their lives. In addition, extra weight affects self-image. In today's appearance-oriented society it can be a great psychological burden.

What causes obesity?

The key to the problem is calories—too many of them. Overweight happens when you eat more calories than your body can use. Whether calories come from fat, protein, sugar or starch, the leftovers are turned into fat. Some of this fat floats around in the blood, plastering and gradually plugging vital oxygen-carrying arteries.

The rest of the leftover fat ends up in the body's central fat bank, located around the midsection. Embarrassing branch offices often pop up in other parts of the body. For every 3,500 excess calories received by the body, one pound of fat is placed on deposit.

Would losing just a few pounds do any good?

The answer is yes. Excess fat relates so directly to health that a little bit goes a long way. A 10 percent weight reduction in men 35 to 55 years of age will result in a 20 percent decrease in coronary heart disease. On the other hand, a 10 percent increase in weight produces a 30 percent increase in coronary disease. This is just one example of many such relationships. Every pound counts, one way or the other.

> ## Extra Weight Shortens Life!
>
> *Every extra pound shaves about one month from your life span. Sixty extra pounds, in other words, can cost you five years!*

What are some positive ways to deal with obesity?

The strategy for successful weight control is threefold:

- Eat more food "as grown," simply prepared, without all the sugar, grease, and salt.

---

10 Basic Habits to Form for Permanent Weight Control

1. Eat lots of foods "as grown." These are the complex carbohydrate foods, high in fiber and nutrients, yet low in calories and price, and devoid of cholesterol.
2. Never skip breakfast. A hot cereal with fruit is great!
3. Eat three meals a day at regular times.
4. Eat slowly. Take time to enjoy your food.
5. End your main meal with a piece of fruit. Save deserts for special treats.
6. Skip snacks and night munchies (or eat a piece of fruit or some raw veggies).
7. Drink water instead of juice or sodas.
8. Daily active exercise (30-60 minutes).
9. Allow no harmful substances into your body (alcohol, tobacco, caffeine, drugs, etc.).
10. Develop hobbies — music, books, sports, etc.

THINK LONG-TERM

Improving your health and energy is a more successful motivator over time than wanting to get thin for a wedding or a college reunion. Personalize the risk of being overweight. Pay attention to your blood pressure, your blood cholesterol and triglycerides, and your family history of disease. Losing just 10 percent of your body weight can significantly improve your health.

- Increase the rate at which calories are burned by increasing physical activity and muscle size.
- Make the above two lifestyle practices a permanent part of life.

Begin by eating generous amounts of high-fiber foods like whole grains, vegetables, fruits, potatoes, yams and beans. Omit as much fat and sugar from the diet as possible. Cut back on refined and processed foods and snacks. These engineered taste sensations are stuffed with calories and depleted of nutrients.

Use animal products such as meat, eggs, ice cream and cheese very sparingly. They have no fiber and are loaded with fat. You really don't need them at all!

This kind of eating plan, plus a brisk daily walk, will help you lose one to two pounds a week.

You can fight creeping fat, push up your energy level, improve your digestion and feel good every day. Beginning right now!

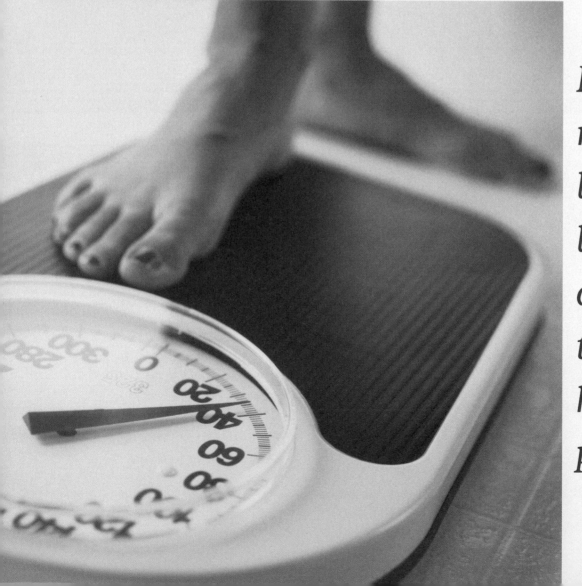

Fat, regardless of location, causes the same health problems.

Application

Being overweight hurts your self-image and lays the foundation for many diseases. The secret of lasting weight loss begins with eating generous amounts of high-fiber foods while limiting animal products and refined foods. Combine this with a brisk, daily walk, and you will easily drop those extra pounds at a healthy rate of one to two pounds a week.

Different Problem, Same Cure

Over and over you've heard the same advice: Change your lifestyle to prevent heart disease, stroke, hypertension, diabetes, and a host of other life-shortening diseases.

Why do all these problems have the same solution? Because a diet of whole-foods, very low in fat, sugar, salt and cholesterol, is not a gimmick or fad—it's the diet your body was designed for.

It should come as no surprise, then, that the same diet that keeps your arteries clean and reduces the risk of cancer also helps you lose weight—and keep it off for good.

Fats Make Fat

Ounce per ounce the American diet packs a lot of calories. That's because it's high in fat. Look at the comparison: a gram of fat contains more than twice the calories of an equal amount of protein or carbohydrate.

CALORIES PER GRAM

Fat	9
Alcohol	7
Carbohydrate	4
Protein	4

Count Those Calories

Which of the following contains the most calories: Salties, Vegi-o's, or Yummies? Compute and figure out the total calories per food:

	Salties	Vegi-o's	Yummies
Carbohydrate	8 g	4 g	2 g
Protein	4 g	5 g	5 g
Fat	2 g	5 g	7 g
	14 g	14 g	14 g
Calories:	_____	_____	_____

Eat More, Weigh Less

If you picked Yummies, you were correct. Although the weight was the same for all three, Yummies carry a higher proportion of that weight as fat. As a result, a serving of Yummies contains 91 calories as fat while Vegi-o's carry 81 and Salties only 66 calories.

Keep this in mind when you choose your food. You don't have to eat less to cut calories. In fact, if you choose foods that are high in unrefined complex carbohydrates and low in fat, you can actually eat more than ever and still lose weight. That's good news if you're one of the many who think going hungry is the only way to get thin.

Your Challenge:

When you shop, check the labels to see how much fat, carbohydrate, and protein the foods you buy contain. Choose those that are high in carbohydrates and low in calorie-dense fats. Remember, if you eat products that carry most of their weight as fat, soon you will be doing the same.

Esau's Pottage (Genesis 25:34)

1/3 c. brown rice (raw)

4 c. water

1 c. sautéed onions

1 c. lentils

herbs to taste: marjoram, thyme, Mrs. Dash

Add ingredients to Crockpot and cook until tender. Add herbs shortly before serving. Garnish with parsley and slices of red bell pepper.

ALCOHOL

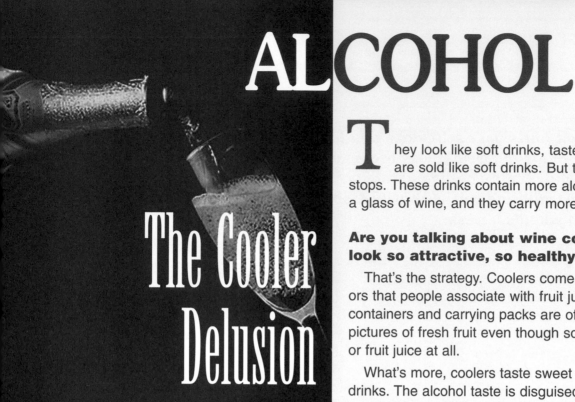

The Cooler Delusion

They look like soft drinks, taste like soft drinks and are sold like soft drinks. But there the similarity stops. These drinks contain more alcohol than a beer or a glass of wine, and they carry more calories.

Are you talking about wine coolers? They look so attractive, so healthy!

That's the strategy. Coolers come in a rainbow of colors that people associate with fruit juices. In fact, the containers and carrying packs are often plastered with pictures of fresh fruit even though some contain no fruit or fruit juice at all.

What's more, coolers taste sweet and fizzy, like soft drinks. The alcohol taste is disguised, making them attractive to people who do not ordinarily drink alcohol. Then, too, coolers are not packaged like other types of alcoholic beverages, but like soft drinks.

Do coolers carry less risk than other alcoholic beverages?

The worst part of the cooler caper is the illusion that coolers are low in alcohol. They're not. Coolers average 6 percent alcohol by volume, whereas beers average 4 percent.

And because coolers usually come in 12-ounce bottles, the amount of alcohol in a serving can exceed that of a gin and tonic (with one ounce of liquor) or a glass of wine served at dinner.

How are coolers affecting today's young people?

Teens, especially teenage girls, are attracted to coolers. They like the name; it suggests a light, refreshing drink. And they like the taste. "Coolers are a hazard for kids because they're so easy to drink," says

> ALCOHOL IS CLOSELY LINKED WITH VIRTUALLY EVERY NEGATIVE ASPECT OF SOCIETY: SUICIDE, VIOLENT CRIME, BIRTH DEFECTS, INDUSTRIAL ACCIDENTS, DOMESTIC AND SEXUAL ABUSE, DISEASE, HOMELESSNESS, AND DEATH. IT IS THE NUMBER ONE DRUG PROBLEM FOR PEOPLE FROM ALL WALKS OF LIFE. IT KNOWS NO RACIAL, ETHNIC, SOCIAL, OR ECONOMIC BARRIERS.
>
> — National Council on Alcohol and Drug Dependency

ALCOHOL FACTS:

- Two of every three adults drink.
- Alcohol is a factor in nearly half of America's murders, suicides, and accidental deaths.
- The economic costs to society of alcoholism and alcohol abuse are estimated at nearly $117 billion a year—including $18 billion from premature deaths, $66 billion in reduced work effort, $13 billion for treatments.

Most coolers have more alcohol than a beer or a glass of wine, more calories than a soda, and in some cases, not a drop of real fruit juice!

Two of every three high school seniors have drunk alcohol within the past month, and 5 percent drink daily; 40 percent of sixth graders have tasted wine coolers.

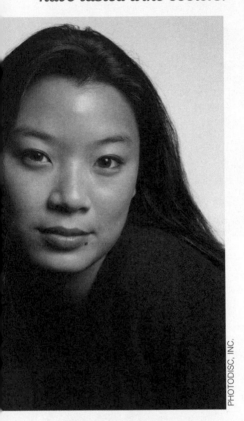

PHOTODISC, INC.

Diane Purcell of Chicago's Parkside Medical Services. "You can go from lemonade to a lemon cooler in one easy step. You don't have to acquire a taste for alcohol."

How serious is alcohol use among teens?

A recent survey revealed that at least 40 percent of sixth graders, and up to 80 percent of junior and senior high school students, have tried wine coolers. Of all 12- through 17-year-olds, 37 per-

cent currently use alcohol. And 5 million American teens already have serious problems stemming from alcohol use.

Are these kids in danger of becoming adult alcoholics?

Many kids are already alcoholics by the time they reach adulthood. Others are well on their way.

When it comes to alcohol, people carry their habits into adult life. And there are already 10.5 million adult alcoholics and 7.6 million more who have drinking-related problems. Half of all fatal auto accidents involve alcohol as do a growing number of air fatalities. Unless we can help our teenagers, things aren't going to get better.

Alcohol exacts a heavy price from personal health. Alcohol promotes high blood pressure and is directly toxic to heart muscle. Alcohol increases the risk of stroke, sudden death from heart arrhythmias and diseased heart muscle, congestive heart failure, cirrhosis and cancer. Alcohol also increases morbidity and hospitalization and reduces the drinker's years of useful life. And it ravages the lives of family and friends.

Perhaps the saddest statistics to emerge in recent years are those of damaged babies permanently mentally deficient as a result of their parents' alcohol use.

How can we best protect our young people?

The challenge to stay drug-and-alcohol-free is greater now than ever for America's teenagers. It is during their early teen years that most will face the critical decision of how they will personally respond to these issues. Each day billboards, magazines, and television, as well as many movies, tell our kids that drinking alcohol is synonymous with being accepted and having a good time. And peer pressure is enormous.

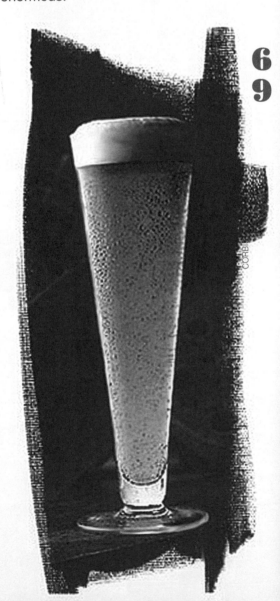

CORBIS

How Alcohol Affects Your Body

YOUR BRAIN—Alcohol, even in small amounts, causes irreparable damage to brain cells; some die and others are altered.

YOUR HEART—Alcohol increases the risk of hypertension, stroke, and damage to the heart muscle.

YOUR LUNGS—Alcohol depresses respiratory functions.

YOUR REPRODUCTIVE SYSTEM—In men, alcohol can damage cells in the testes, causing impotence, sterility, and possibly enlarged breasts. In women, alcohol can cause irregular menstrual cycles and malfunctioning of the ovaries. Alcohol has also been linked to birth defects in infants and to fetal alcohol syndrome.

YOUR LIVER—Because your liver must filter alcohol from the blood, alcohol affects it more than any other organ of your body:

- Excess calories in alcohol are stored as fat in the liver.
- Functioning liver cells die from alcoholic poisoning.
- Scar tissue replaces dead cells, causing cirrhosis.

YOUR IMMUNE SYSTEM—Alcohol weakens the body's defense against infection and breast cancer.

Yet today's youth can be very discerning. Most hold strong ideals about what is right and fair, yet they need guidance in making right choices.

- Their immediate need is for *education*—an honest, reliable, credible source of information. To be effective this education must start early, during the elementary years.

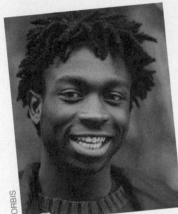

- Youth need support and encouragement—from grandparents, teachers, churches, mentors, and positive role models. This support must include the availability of positive activities to fill their free time, such as part-time jobs, sports, hobbies, crafts, library use, clubs such as Boy and Girl Scouts, and opportunities to work as community service volunteers.

- But most important of all is a *good parental example*. Nothing is more powerful than this! And the statistics show it. Young people who grow up in nonalcoholic homes are much less inclined to have problems when they reach adulthood.

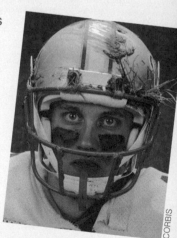

The Wise Man summed it up long ago:

"Wine is a mocker and beer a brawler: whoever is led astray by them is not wise" (Proverbs 20:1).

"Do not gaze at wine when it is red, when it sparkles in the cup, when it goes down smoothly! In the end it bites like a snake and poisons like a viper. Your eyes will see strange sights and your mind imagine confusing things." Proverbs 23:31-33

Application

Alcohol extracts a heavy price from personal health. This goes for teens as well as adults. Young people who grow up in nonalcoholic homes are less likely to have problems with alcohol when they reach adulthood. A parent's example can make a big difference.

The World's Most Abused Drug

Alcohol is not just a problem for young people; it's the greatest drug problem in the world for all ages. In the United States it's second only to tobacco on the list of "Most Deadly Drugs."

Despite the dangers, everyone in our society comes into contact with alcoholic beverages. If nothing else, we are exposed to commercials on television singing the praises of one brew after another.

Alcohol and Nutrition

Throughout this book we have urged you to avoid highly refined products that are high in calories but low in nutrition. Alcohol certainly falls into this category. Two cans of beer, for example, carry 300 calories; two jiggers of 100 proof whiskey, 250 calories; two glasses of dessert wine pack 280 calories—and they are all empty calories, providing none of the nutrients your body requires.

For men, alcohol accounts for 9 percent of the calories in the American diet. No wonder we are overfed and undernourished.

Your Challenge

Make this "ban the booze" week at your house. You should be able to get through it without any sort of urge or discomfort.

If you can't, you need to seriously consider who is the master: you or the alcohol. If you can get through the week with no problems, why not quit altogether? It will help keep your weight under control, improve your nutrition, and set a good example for the young people in your life.

Alcohol and Young People

Young people ages 14 to 24 account for more than 8,000 alcohol-related fatalities—about a third of the annual total.

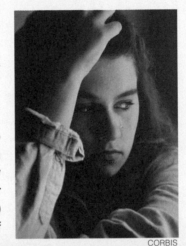

CORBIS

Those Lost Years

"When you're a teenager, it's hard to think of time ever being short; it's hard to realize what a precious commodity time is.

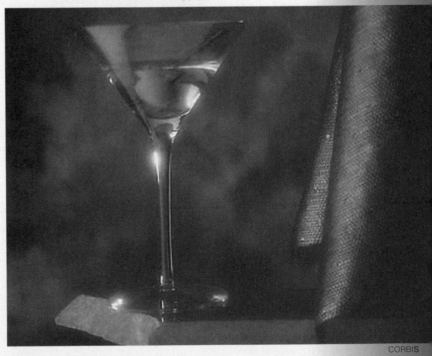

CORBIS

"Do not get drunk on wine, which leads to debauchery. Instead, be filled with the Spirit." Ephesians 5:18

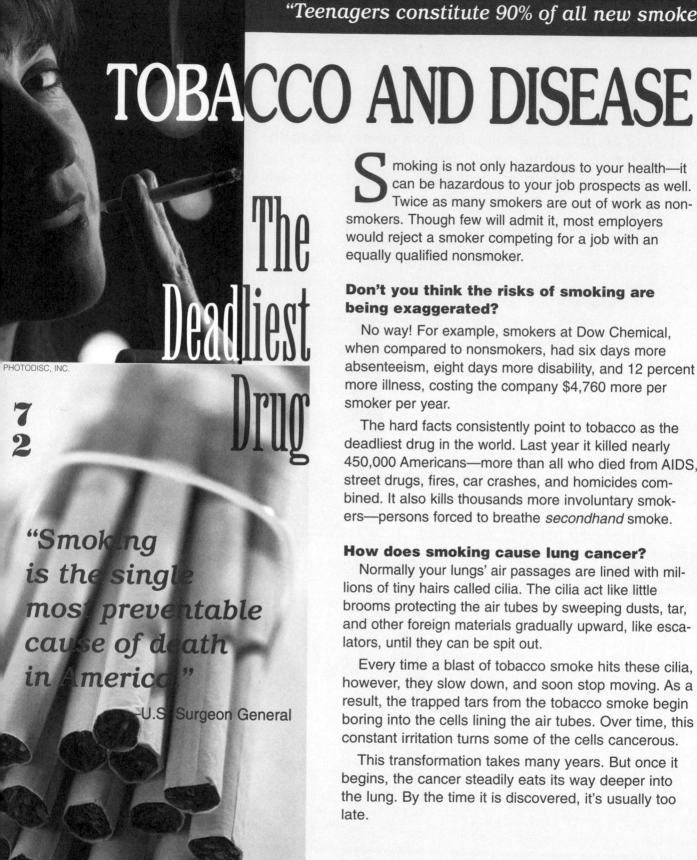

TOBACCO AND DISEASE

The Deadliest Drug

PHOTODISC, INC.

7
2

"Smoking is the single most preventable cause of death in America."

—U.S. Surgeon General

Smoking is not only hazardous to your health—it can be hazardous to your job prospects as well. Twice as many smokers are out of work as non-smokers. Though few will admit it, most employers would reject a smoker competing for a job with an equally qualified nonsmoker.

Don't you think the risks of smoking are being exaggerated?

No way! For example, smokers at Dow Chemical, when compared to nonsmokers, had six days more absenteeism, eight days more disability, and 12 percent more illness, costing the company $4,760 more per smoker per year.

The hard facts consistently point to tobacco as the deadliest drug in the world. Last year it killed nearly 450,000 Americans—more than all who died from AIDS, street drugs, fires, car crashes, and homicides combined. It also kills thousands more involuntary smokers—persons forced to breathe *secondhand* smoke.

How does smoking cause lung cancer?

Normally your lungs' air passages are lined with millions of tiny hairs called cilia. The cilia act like little brooms protecting the air tubes by sweeping dusts, tar, and other foreign materials gradually upward, like escalators, until they can be spit out.

Every time a blast of tobacco smoke hits these cilia, however, they slow down, and soon stop moving. As a result, the trapped tars from the tobacco smoke begin boring into the cells lining the air tubes. Over time, this constant irritation turns some of the cells cancerous.

This transformation takes many years. But once it begins, the cancer steadily eats its way deeper into the lung. By the time it is discovered, it's usually too late.

"Do you not know that your body is a temple? Therefore honor God with your body."

1 Corinthians 6:19, 20

Is lung cancer the leading cause of death in smokers?

No. Tobacco causes 128,000 lung cancer deaths per year in the United States. In contrast, smoking is responsible for 181,000 heart attacks and strokes.

The nicotine and carbon monoxide in tobacco smoke are the main culprits that promote vascular disease. Nicotine constricts small arteries depriving the heart, brain, lungs, and other important areas of vital oxygen. Nicotine also produces a sense of relaxation and well-being—smoking's main appeal. But nicotine is also addictive.

Carbon monoxide interferes directly with the ability of red blood cells to carry oxygen. This causes shortness of breath, lack of endurance, and acceleration of atherosclerosis (narrowing and hardening of the arteries).

That's a lot of bad news. Is there more?

Unfortunately there is a lot more.

● Smokers have much more cancer of the mouth, larynx, esophagus, pancreas, bladder, kidneys, and cervix than do nonsmokers.

● Emphysema gradually destroys lung tissue, producing death by suffocation. In the United States 71,000 of these grisly deaths occur each year as a result of smoking.

● Ulcers of the stomach and duodenum are 60 percent more common in smokers.

● Smoking pulls calcium out of the skeleton, accelerating the bone-thinning process known as osteoporosis.

● Smoking during pregnancy has an adverse effect on fetal development and increases the risk of death after birth up to 35 percent.

If a person has smoked heavily for a long time, does it pay to quit?

About 85 percent of lung cancers and 50 percent of bladder cancers could be prevented if people simply stopped smoking.

Smokers who quit begin to heal almost immediately. As the nicotine and carbon monoxide leave the body, the smoking-related risk for heart disease decreases dramatically. Although the risk for cancer decreases more slowly, the danger lessens as the weeks and months go by.

There are other payoffs to quitting: a sense of victory,

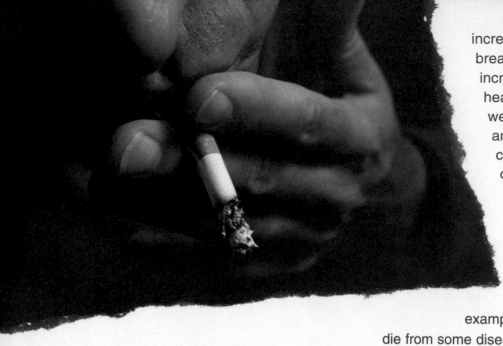

increased self-esteem, pleasant breath, better tasting food, increased endurance, improved health and energy, a feeling of well-being, and freedom from an inconvenient, unpopular, costly habit. Quitting may also open the way to more job opportunities.

Americans often overreact to the most trivial of risks while ignoring much more substantial threats to their health and safety. For example, every second smoker will die from some disease directly connected to the habit. Smokers will also lose an average of 8.3 years from their normal life expectancy, or 13 minutes for every cigarette smoked. Yet many people react more forcefully to evidence of a one-in-a-million risk of getting cancer from chemicals found in drinking water!

It's time to get life back into perspective. The biggest favor you can do for your body is to kick the habit and freely breathe clean air again.

Mess'n' With Death

Did You Know . . .

That smoking kills 1,200 Americans a day and costs $1 billion *a week* in extra health-care and insurance costs, while the U.S. government collects $12 billion *a year* in tobacco taxes.

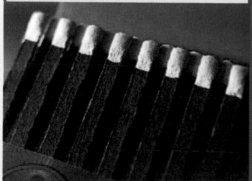

How Smoking Kills

Tobacco use kills and maims primarily by promoting vascular diseases and various cancers.

Vascular diseases

- Heart attacks—smoking is responsible for 30 percent of the annual 550,000 US coronary deaths.
- Stroke—responsible for 25 percent of the annual strokes.
- Peripheral vascular disease—about 90 percent of leg and thigh blockages occur in smokers.

Cancers

- Lung—85 percent because of smoking.
- Bladder and kidneys—3 times more frequent in smokers.
- Mouth, larynx, esophogus—2-25 times more prevalent in smokers.

Application

Tobacco is the deadliest drug in the world. In the United States alone it kills nearly 450,000 people a year. The biggest favor people can do for themselves is to break the smoking habit.

You Can Do It!

Kicking the Habit

The first step in breaking any habit is to decide that you are going to change. It's not enough just to want to change or to imagine that you will change someday. Breaking an addiction to tobacco requires positive commitment.

Reasons to Quit Smoking

Here are a few reasons that have convinced thousands to quit last year:

1. Quitting is the single most important thing you can do for your health and longevity.

2. Reduced risk of heart disease, stroke, and cancer of the lungs, mouth, throat, pancreas, bladder, kidneys, and cervix.

3. Reduced risk of emphysema and osteoporosis.

4. Elimination of the risk posed to the smoker's family from second-hand smoke.

5. Less chance of a smoker's children and grandchildren smoking.

6. Better breath, whiter teeth, and fewer wrinkles.

7. Less time spent sick: more physical endurance.

8. Lower medical and insurance costs.

The list goes on, and it grows every year as we learn more about the harmful effects of tobacco.

You have everything to gain by kicking the habit—longer life, better health, more vitality, fewer medical expenses . . .

. . . and the air is fresher, food tastes better, wallets are fatter, age is longer, life is sweeter!

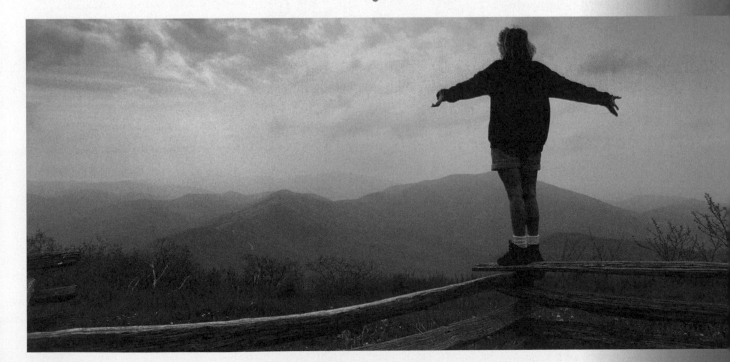

CAFFEINE ADDICTION

Nine out of 10 North Americans take a psychotropic (mind-altering) drug daily. The culprit? Everyday, ordinary, over-the-counter caffeine.

Are You Wired?

Does Caffeine Have You Running on Overdrive?

How can that be? Explain.

Do you know many people who don't drink at least one cup of coffee a day? Or tea? Or take an *extra-strength* pain reliever? Or guzzle down a cola? Although caffeine-free sodas are available, they are favored mainly for children and for people with medical problems that are affected by caffeine.

But I need a lift now and then! And caffeine isn't addictive, is it?

An addictive substance produces observable and measurable physical and mental effects when it is withdrawn. In this sense, even small doses of caffeine, taken regularly over time, will usually produce some degree of addiction.

A good way to check yourself is to stop all caffeine intake for a few days. The most common physical withdrawal symptom is headache, varying from mild to severe. Sometimes a migraine is triggered. Other physical manifestations include feelings of exhaustion, lack of appetite, nausea and vomiting. Symptoms last one to five days.

Psychological withdrawal can be even harder. Depression may occur. People become accustomed to reaching for the pick-me-up throughout the day. The urge can be compared to the desire for

EVERYONE WANTS to hear that coffee is good for us, but let's get real. We love the rich aroma and taste of coffee, and we do like something hot in the morning. But we're not fooling anyone— what we want is the buzz— the caffeine.

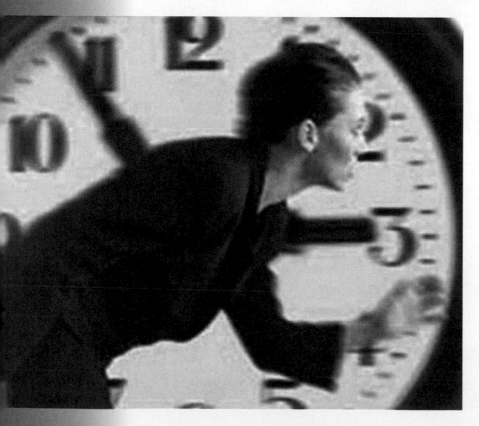

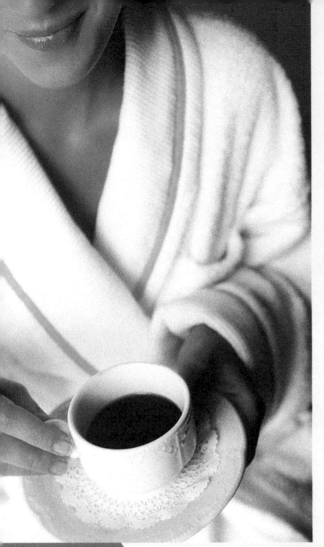

A person can get hooked with a relatively small amount of caffeine if it's on a fairly regular basis.

a cigarette—it may be difficult to resist.

Does caffeine damage the body?

● Most obvious is an overstimulated nervous system with tremors, nervousness, anxiety and sleep problems. In time these symptoms give way to chronic fatigue, lack of energy, and persistent insomnia.

● Caffeinated beverages can cause stomach irritation. While additives are primarily responsible for this effect, caffeine itself has a constricting effect on blood vessels. It can thus interfere with digestion.

● Caffeinated drinks stimulate the stomach to excrete excessive acid. This may aggravate ulcers.

● Caffeine has been found to interfere with calcium and iron absorption associated with osteoporosis and anemia.

● Caffeine increases energy by raising blood sugar levels. These, in turn, draw out an insulin response which not only cancels the surge but produces a letdown. This letdown triggers the yo-yo syndrome—reaching for another caffeinated drink, and then another, and yet another.

● Caffeine also irritates the kidneys and acts as a diuretic (increased urine output).

Caffeine can produce . . .

- Elevated blood sugar
- Increased blood pressure
- Elevated blood fats (triglycerides)
- Heightened symptoms of PMS
- Tremors, irritability, and nervousness
- Aggravation of anxiety disorders and panic attacks
- Increased stomach acid secretions
- Urinary calcium and magnesium losses
- Insomnia
- Irregular heartbeat
- Increased stimulation of the central nervous system (it overrules the need for rest)

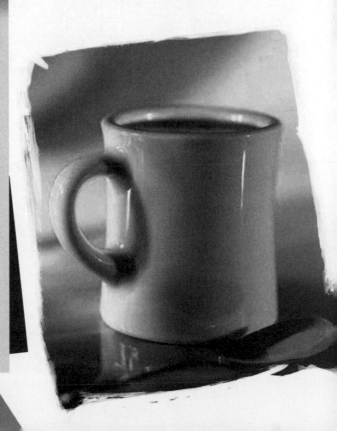

Where is the Caffeine?

COFFEE/TEA (average)

Cup drip coffee	145 mg
Cup brewed coffee	115 mg
Cup instant coffee	85 mg
Cup decaffeinated	3 mg
1.5-oz. shot espresso	100 mg
Cup hot tea	65 mg
Ice tea (12 oz.)	70 mg

Wake up and smell the caffeine, folks: America's drug of choice is not limited to your morning cup of coffee:

POPULAR HEADACHE MEDICATIONS (1 pill)

Vivarin	100-200 mg
NoDoz	100-200 mg
Excedrin	65 mg
Anacin	40 mg
Plain aspirin	0 mg
Tylenol	0 mg
Cold medications	0-30 mg

CHOCOLATE

1 oz. milk chocolate	6 mg
1 oz. unsweetened baking chocolate	25 mg
1/4 cup choc. chips	15 mg
8 oz. chocolate milk	10 mg

SODAS (12-oz. serving)

Java Water	100 mg
Jolt	100 mg
Sugar-free Mr. Pibb	60 mg
Mountain Dew	54 mg
TAB	45 mg
Coke & Diet Coke	45 mg
Pepsi Cola	40 mg

Are there some healthful alternatives to the caffeine high?

When you get up in the morning, follow your hot shower with a blast of cold water and towel off briskly.

At work, stand up, stretch, and take a few deep breaths every hour or so. Take a brisk walk at break time or during lunch hour. Drink a cup of cold (or hot) water several times a day. Rub a coworker's back and ask for a return favor. Walk to a window and relax your eyes on the distant landscape. Tidy up your work area. All these good things will make you feel better. Look for other creative ways to get a lift without the letdown.

In a crisis, would just a little caffeine really matter?

Occasional small doses of caffeine will hardly make a difference. The trouble is, most of us have a hard time knowing when to stop.

Java Water has grown steadily since it was introduced in 1996. A 17-ounce bottle of this flavorless spring water contains a hefty 140 milligrams of caffeine. On the way are caffeinated orange juice and lemonade.

CORBIS

PHOTODISC, INC.

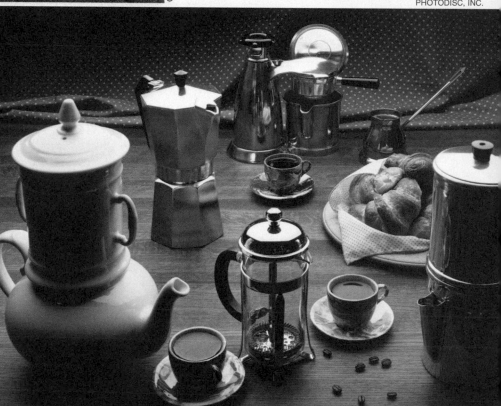

Application

Caffeine can be an addictive drug. Regular use over time often produces physical and mental effects when withdrawn. While an occasional small dose of caffeine may not make a difference, heavier use has been linked to health problems.

Coffee: Food or Drug?

Imagine going to buy coffee at the grocery store and finding the coffee section missing.

"What's going on?" you ask the clerk. "Where is the coffee?"

"Oh, haven't you heard? Coffee has been classified as a drug. The pharmacist sells it now."

Shaking your head in disbelief, you walk across the store to where the pharmacist dispenses medications, drugs, and—caffeinated beverages.

The pharmacist smiles at you knowingly. "You look like you're here for some coffee. I can tell from your expression."

You nod and tell him what brand you would like.

"That's fine," he says. "No prescription necessary—I just need to type up the warning label."

"Warning label?"

"That's right. Look at it. It says—

> *Warning:* **This drink contains caffeine. Possible side effects include addiction, tremors, nervousness, anxiety, insomnia, chronic fatigue, lack of energy, stomach irritation, vomiting, interference with calcium and iron absorption, and the aggravation of ulcers.**

He hands you the coffee, but you decline. "No thanks," you say. "I think I've changed my mind."

Are You an Addict?

You could be a caffeine addict without even knowing it.

One way to find out if you are addicted is to stop all caffeine intake for a week. If you're hooked, chances are good that you will notice physical symptoms like headache, lack of appetite, and nausea, which can last from one to five days. Psychologically, you may feel down and listless, and of course, there will be a strong urge for your favorite beverage.

Breaking the Habit

If you find you're a caffeine fiend, here are a few things you can do to ease through withdrawal.

1. Gradually reduce the amount of caffeine.
2. Replace it by drinking more water.
3. Slow down your daily activities.
4. Exercise in the fresh air.
5. Get the support of others around you.
6. Reward yourself for taking such a positive step.

Your Challenge:

Cut down on caffeinated drinks like tea, coffee, and colas, and eventually skip them altogether. See how you fare. At the end of a week, review this material and give serious consideration to making your body a caffeine-free zone.

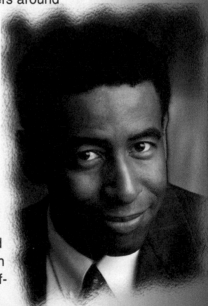

Are you living drug-free?

LEGALIZED DRUG ABUSE

Spiders and Sledge-hammers

*Many people believe medicines sold without prescription are safe and have no side effects. **NO DRUG IS COMPLETELY SAFE.** For example, acetaminophen (Tylenol) and ibuprofen (Advil, Motrin) used regularly for long periods of time have been shown to double the risk of kidney cancer and triple the risk of kidney damage.*

The way some people use drugs makes no more sense than using a sledgehammer to kill a spider. It's not just prescription drugs that pose problems, either. Common over-the-counter drugs can have unpleasant—even dangerous—side effects.

You must be exaggerating.

I wish I were! Take something as common as aspirin, for instance. Many people down it at the least sign of a headache, flu, or fever. As a matter of fact, every 24 hours Americans consume 45 tons of this drug!

Yet every year 10,000 people will be severely poisoned by aspirin or a related product. What's more, aspirin is known to promote stomach ulcers. It has also been associated with Reye's syndrome, an often fatal disease in children, and in older people it can trigger a hemorrhagic stroke.

Acetaminophen and ibuprofen, other common painkillers, can cause skin rashes and—in extreme cases—kidney and liver damage.

But prescription drugs are safe when you follow directions, right?

In the medical world new and more effective wonder drugs are being discovered and introduced almost daily, while older ones are improved and refined. Yet the perfect drug still eludes us—the one that will do its job with absolutely no deleterious side effects.

Consider blood pressure drugs. They are the most

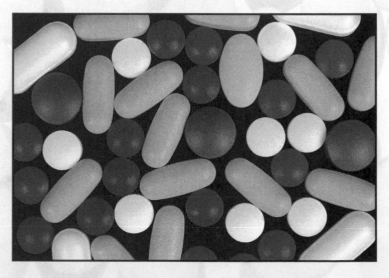

"Show me the way I should go, for to you I lift up my soul."
Psalm 143:8

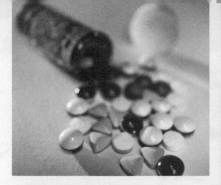

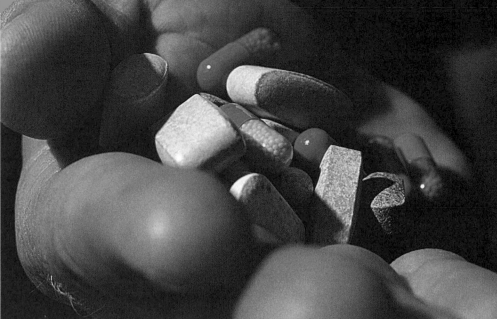

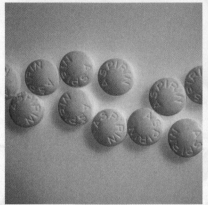

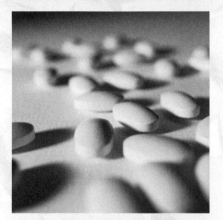

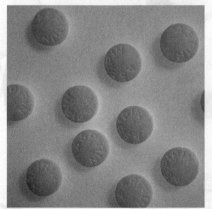

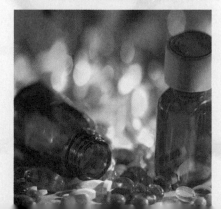

Many sedatives and tranquilizers are addictive when used over time.

widely used prescription medications on the market and among the most effective. Yet they carry a host of side effects. These can include weakness, fatigue, drowsiness, headache, mental depression, dizziness, bloating, sweating, indigestion, unstable emotional states, slurred speech, raised cholesterol levels, and impotence. People who need these drugs often must test several different kinds before they find one they can tolerate.

The point is, no drug is completely safe. Even lifesaving antibiotics carry potential problems such as nausea, vomiting, diarrhea, and allergic reactions.

Why then are people so anxious to take drugs?

While most of today's diseases respond to lifestyle measures (such as a better diet and regular exercise), physicians who advocate these principles often find themselves rowing upstream. Most people are impatient. They want quick fixes rather than real solutions. If one doctor doesn't produce the desired prescription, they often find another who will.

Simply put, people today too often want to believe there is a magic potion for their problem. With an almost childlike faith we swallow drugs to pep us up, calm us down, regulate our weight, and to ward off almost every conceivable ailment.

So why risk taking any drug?

When physicians prescribe drugs they must always balance risk against need. For

"I WOULD LOSE ONE THIRD TO ONE HALF OF MY PATIENTS IF I DIDN'T PRESCRIBE VALIUM OR SIMILAR DRUGS."
— *a frustrated physician*

8 1

instance, with a serious bacterial infection, the risk you run by taking an antibiotic is usually outweighed by the risk you run if you don't take it.

If you have a tension headache, on the other hand, you'd probably be better off taking a brisk walk or a nap.

What are some guidelines for using drugs intelligently?

A good rule of thumb is to reserve drugs for specific, identifiable needs that can't be met by lesser measures. Don't use a *big-gun* medicine like antibiotics, for instance, for a *flyswatter* problem like a head cold.

Likewise, a warm bath or a cup of herb tea is better than a sleeping pill if you can't get to sleep. And if you don't *want* to go to sleep, a cold shower or a brisk walk is better for you than a *wake-up* pill or cup of coffee.

When you *do* take a drug, be sure you know exactly what it's supposed to do. Understand its risks and side effects, how and when to take it, and the signs of overdosage. Don't mix medicines, and don't risk psychological dependence or physical addiction by taking any drug longer than needed. If you have more than one doctor, make sure your main doctor knows all the medications you are taking.

In short, give drugs the respect they deserve. Save them for the times they are truly needed. It's time to stop hitting spiders with sledgehammers.

Do you want health without drugs?

CORBIS

PHOTODISC, INC.

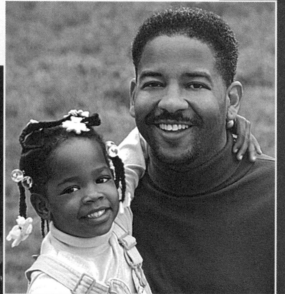

LEGALIZED DEATH

Cigarettes are among the world's most profitable drugs. They are also the only legal ones that, if used as intended, turn most of their users into addicts and kill every second smoker.

PRESCRIPTION DRUGS

You won't have the answers if you don't ask the questions. These are the questions you need to ask:

✔ What is the full name and strength of the medication?
✔ How will the medicine help me?
✔ What are the risks?
✔ What side effects can I expect?
✔ How, when, and for how long do I take it?
✔ What should I do if I miss a dose?
✔ Is there written information I can take with me?
✔ Is there a nondrug alternative for my problem?

This is the information you need to provide:

● About all other medicines you are taking, including self-medications with nonprescription drugs such as aspirin, vitamins, or cold/allergy pills.
● If cost is a concern to you.
● If you have any allergies or medical conditions, and how or if they are being treated.

Application

Many people have a childlike faith in drugs and medicines. They take them for every conceivable ailment. But using big-gun medicines for fly-swatter problems, or for problems that should be solved by lifestyle measures, can leave you tired, depleted and depressed. Use drugs sparingly and with care.

Pain is a Warning

Too many people run to the medicine cabinet whenever they feel the slightest ache or pain. They don't realize that pain often acts as a warning system telling us something is wrong.

We may be eating too much, drinking too much, smoking too much, or taking on obligations beyond our capacities. When pain is blocked by drugs, we ignore these causes rather than changing the behaviors that cause the pain in the first place. This kind of neglect sets the stage for more serious diseases.

Two Categories of Drugs

Some drugs attack the cause of a problem; others mainly relieve symptoms.

If you take any medications, list them in the spaces below. Write a "C" next to those that attack the cause of the problem. Put an "S" by those that simply help relieve symptoms.

_____

_____

_____

_____

UPPER DRUGS	DOWNER DRUGS
Caffeine	*Tranquilizers*
Tobacco	*Sedatives*
Some diet pills	*Alcohol*
Amphetamines	*Tobacco*
The Positives	*The Positives*
Sense of well-being	*Relaxes*
Decreased fatigue	*Relieves anxiety*
Sharpens mind	*False sense of*
	peacefulness
The Negatives	
Only temporary	*The Negatives*
Depletes resources	*Temporary effect*
Premature aging	*Solves no problems*
Depression	*Depression*

Your Challenge:

Don't go running to the medicine cabinet for every little ache and pain. The cure is often worse than the problem. When you must take a drug, be sure you get the answers to the questions on the drug checklist.

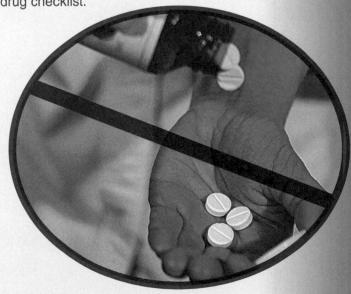

MODERN MEDICINE is a three-legged stool. Drugs and surgery are two legs—the third is what people can do for themselves:

- *Healthful lifestyle changes*
- *Regular active exercise*
- *Pursuit of spiritual goals*

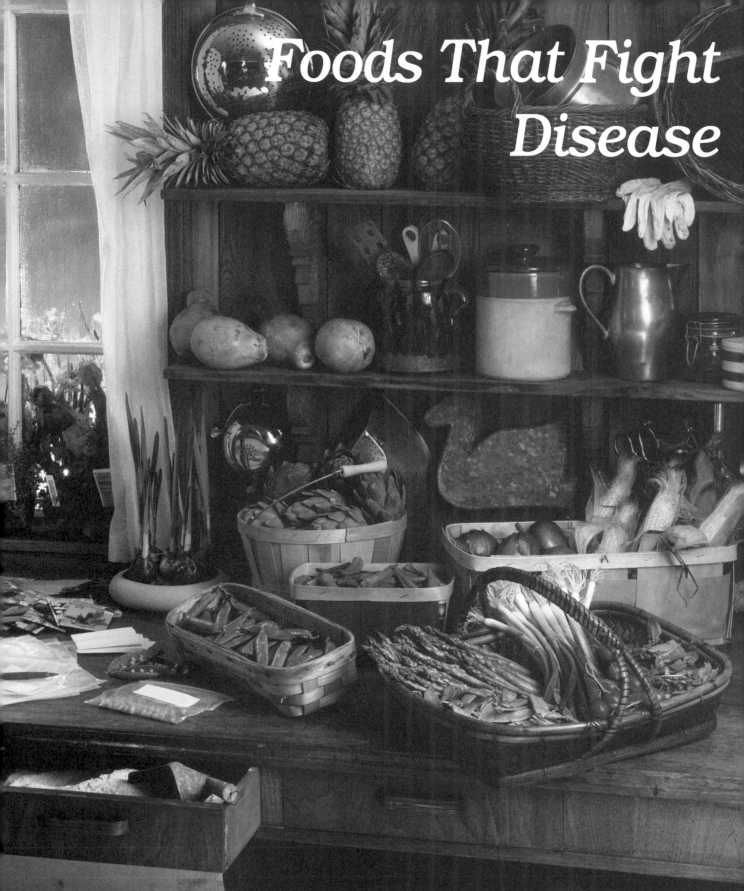

Foods That Fight Disease

GOD SAID: *"I give you every seed-bearing plant on the face of the whole earth and every tree that has fruit with seed in it. They will be yours for food."* Genesis 1:29

UNDERSTANDING FOOD

- Digestion
- Starch
- Sugar
- Bread
- Protein
- Milk
- Meat
- Fat
- Cholesterol
- Fiber
- Salt
- Vitamins, Minerals, Herbs
- Phytochemicals and Antioxidants

DIGESTION

What Follows the Swallows

Do you ever think about what happens to your food after you swallow it? Most of us take our digestive system very much for granted. We eat whatever we want, whenever we want. But how does our body handle the food it's given?

Proteins, fats and carbohydrates are the major constituents of food. They carry the food's energy to the body. The body digests each in an orderly fashion, yet at different rates. It digests simple carbohydrates (sugars) quickly, while fats take longer. Proteins and complex carbohydrates (starches) fall somewhere in between.

Is there some benefit in eating a starch food, for instance, at one meal and a protein food at a different time?

Nature doesn't support this idea. All plant foods and some animal foods are combinations of carbohydrate, protein and fat. Beans and peas, for example, have quite a bit of protein, and corn has a fair percentage of fat.

To get a pure carbohydrate meal you would need to eat white sugar or the starchy residue that's left after removing the gluten from white four. A pure protein meal could be egg whites or dry cottage cheese curds. For the fat meal, a few tablespoons of butter or cooking oil would do. Pure foods, in this sense, don't occur in nature, but they can be manufactured.

How does the stomach handle these different food constituents?

Digestion is the process by which the body breaks food down into its component parts, so that the sugars and starches of the carbohydrates become glucose, fats become fatty acids, and proteins become amino acids. The blood can pick up these smaller substances from the intestines.

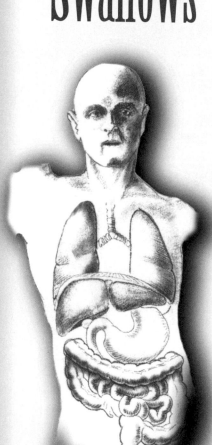

SWALLOWING IS SO EASY, but it is actually a very complicated physiological action. It requires the carefully coordinated efforts of more than 30 muscles or groups of muscles—and once it's begun, you can't stop it at will.

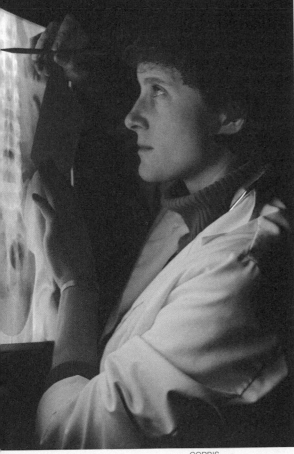

Only a part of digestion occurs in the stomach. The rest occurs in the mouth and intestines. In an amazingly orderly fashion, carbohydrate digestion begins in the mouth with the saliva and continues in the stomach. Protein digestion begins in the stomach and continues in the intestines. Fat is largely digested in the intestines.

Does the acidity or alkalinity of foods affect this process?

The stomach has three basic functions:

● It breaks food particles down to a more uniform size by muscular action.

● It brings the food mass to the needed consistency by adding or absorbing fluid.

● It brings the stomach contents to the necessary degree of acidity by secreting acidic digestive juices. This

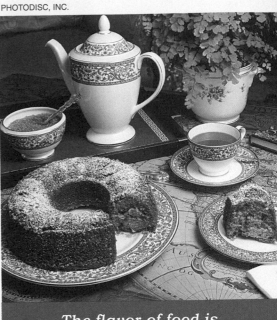

The flavor of food is appreciated through taste buds, nearly 9,000 of which are located on the human tongue. Each taste bud connects with about 50 nerve fibers.

phase accomplishes those parts of digestion that require an acid medium.

When the stomach contents go on to the intestines, they become alkalinized by juices that the pancreas secretes. The digestive process is completed in the intestines.

Don't some foods bog down this process?

Foods high in fats are the worst offenders. The body cannot digest fats until they are alkalinized and emulsified by the intestinal juices (much as the grease on your hands cannot be removed until it is emulsified with soap and hot water).

O ne of our worst habits relates to the TIME we eat. It's not just WHAT we eat, but WHEN we eat. The digestive machinery works best when given time to digest one meal before the next meal comes along.

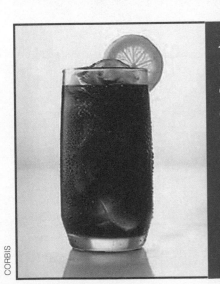

Drinking fluids with meals dilutes the digestive juices — and slows down digestion. It is best to drink water about two hours after a meal, and up to 15 minutes preceding it.

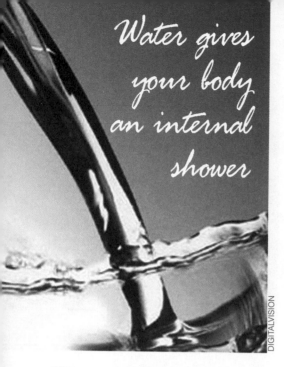

Water gives your body an internal shower

"Eat at a proper time — for strength and not for drunkenness."

Ecclesiastes 10:17

But the body has protective mechanisms that meter the fat from the stomach to the intestines so that the emulsification process isn't overwhelmed. If the amount of fat in a meal is not large, it will make little difference in digestion time. But a typical Western meal, however, because of its high fat content, may need 4 to 5 hours, or longer, to pass through the stomach.

Is there an ideal balance of foods?

The body can handle three or four kinds of whole plant foods with maximum efficiency and minimum stress. A more complex meal takes longer to digest and exacts a higher energy price from the body.

Eating snacks between meals disrupts the orderly digestive processes and stresses the stomach. Digestive problems will be slight if the stomach is presented with a simple meal, allowed to digest it, and then is given time to rest before adding more food. Ideally, meals should be four to five hours apart.

You mean we shouldn't eat anything between meals?

Take a drink of water. Water requires no digestion. It passes right through, giving everything a good rinse. If you just must have something more, choose a piece of fresh fruit or munch on some raw veggies.

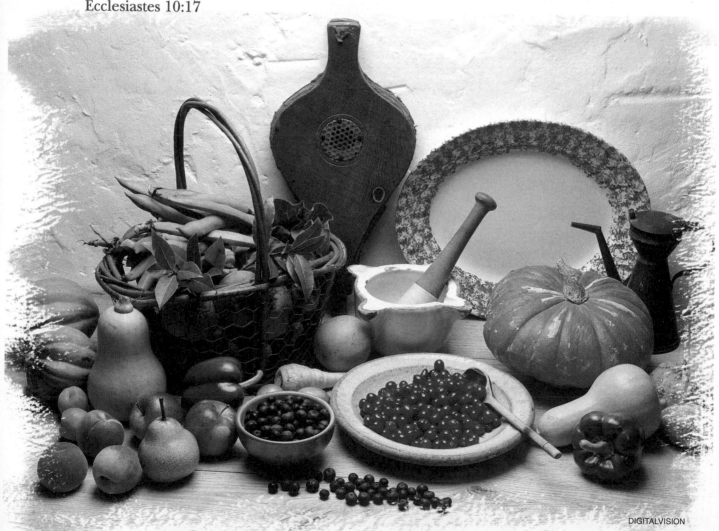

Application

How do you spell relief? If you are like most North Americans you spell it D-O-L-L-A-R-S. Each year we spend millions on pills and potions to quiet our angry stomachs. A better way would be: stop overloading your stomach and give it the rest it needs.

Sweetening a Sour Stomach

How often does your stomach protest?

__ Never
__ Several times a year
__ Several times a month
__ Weekly
__ Every day

If you frequently have indigestion or an upset stomach, and your doctor has ruled out more serious problems, it may be your eating habits that are causing you grief.

Answer the following questions with a YES or NO.

1. ___ *Do you have regular eating times?*

Your body thrives on a regular schedule, not only of eating, but of waking, sleeping, and exercise.

2. ___ *Do you often eat between meals?*

When new food shows up in a stomach that is already working, digestion must slow down until the system deals with the new arrival.

Imagine a washing machine working on a load of clothes. If you come by every 10 minutes, turn the dial back, and dump in more clothes, you would never finish a load. A washing machine, just like your stomach, needs time to finish its cycle.

3. ___ *Are your meals spaced four to five hours apart?*

Spacing meals several hours apart allows the stomach to work at its own pace. Food from one meal is completely digested before the next one arrives.

4. ___ *Do you drink coffee?*

Coffee, even decaf, contains substances that can irritate the lining of the stomach. Too much of this substance can send your stomach into rebellion.

5. ___ *Do you eat right before going to bed?*

The stomach, like the rest of your body, needs rest. A meal or snack late in the evening forces it to work overtime.

Dealing With Gas

Many people adjusting to a high-fiber diet experience problems with intestinal gas. This is especially true when legumes are on the menu. Here are some suggestions that can help:

● For occasional intestinal gas, try some pharmaceutical-grade charcoal. It adsorbs gas and provides a measure of relief. It is available as powder, tablets, syrup, or capsules and is sold over the counter.

● To reduce gas caused by cooked dried beans, try soaking them overnight, discarding the soak water, and replacing it with fresh water for cooking.

Your Challenge:

Give your stomach a break by spacing meals further apart. Not interrupting the digestive cycle with snacks will sweeten the disposition of a cranky stomach.

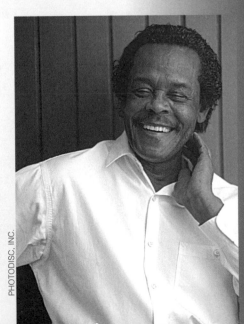

PHOTODISC, INC.

STARCH

The Body's Premium Fuel

Starchy foods, notwithstanding the low-carb promoters, are now the superstars of the food galaxy. The scientific community tells us that the road to better health is paved with potatoes, whole wheat pasta, brown rice, beans and good bread.

What about protein? Everybody needs protein!

Yes, but not so much. For a long time people assumed that because muscles are predominantly protein we needed to eat a lot of it to be strong.

But the body is like a car. Once the car is built, only a few additional parts are needed here and there for maintenance. Similarly, a human adult needs relatively little protein for daily maintenance—about 45 to 60 grams per day. That's about two ounces of pure protein.

What the car does need on a regular basis is good clean gasoline. And carbohydrates are the gasoline of the body, the high-octane fuel that keeps it running smoothly.

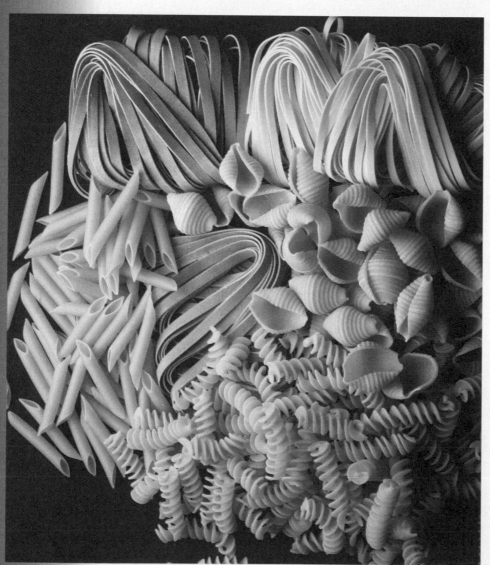

Isn't fat also a body fuel?

Fat, in general, is stored fuel, carried as baggage. It's the *reserve tank.* If the body runs out of carbohydrate fuel it can dig out the spare stuff. But fat doesn't burn as cleanly as carbohydrates and it's not as energy-efficient.

What are carbohydrates?

Carbohydrates are the sugars and starches in the foods we eat. A lot of people don't understand the relationship between sugars and starches, and the confusion is compounded when terms like *simple carbohydrates* and *complex carbohydrates* are used.

In general, simple carbohydrates are the sugars and complex carbohydrates are the starches. All carbohydrates, both sugars and starches, are broken down by the digestive tract

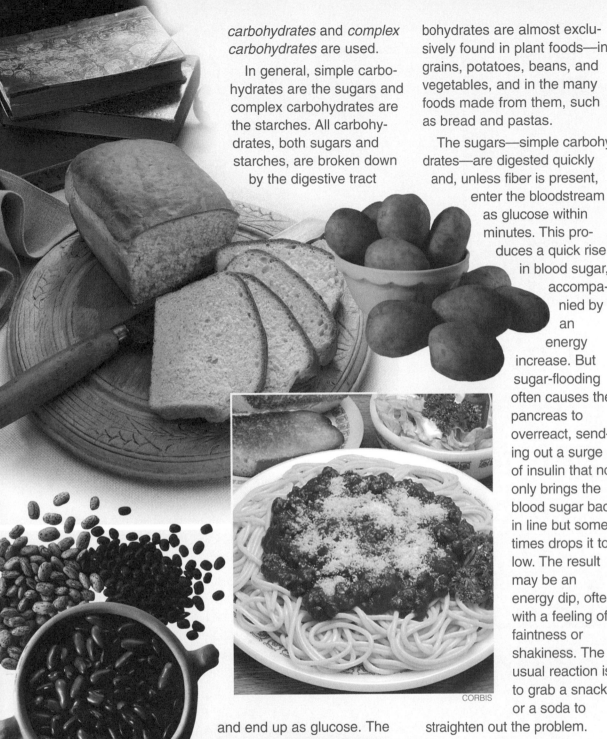

CORBIS

and end up as glucose. The blood absorbs this glucose from the intestines and uses it for energy (fuel). Complex car-

bohydrates are almost exclusively found in plant foods—in grains, potatoes, beans, and vegetables, and in the many foods made from them, such as bread and pastas.

The sugars—simple carbohydrates—are digested quickly and, unless fiber is present, enter the bloodstream as glucose within minutes. This produces a quick rise in blood sugar, accompanied by an energy increase. But sugar-flooding often causes the pancreas to overreact, sending out a surge of insulin that not only brings the blood sugar back in line but sometimes drops it too low. The result may be an energy dip, often with a feeling of faintness or shakiness. The usual reaction is to grab a snack or a soda to straighten out the problem.

It works, doesn't it?

A better solution would be to eat an apple. In their natural forms nearly all carbohydrate foods contain liberal amounts of different kinds of fiber. Some kinds are not digested by the body. Instead, they absorb water and form a

Carbohydrate Family Tree
CARBOHYDRATES

Simple Carbohydrates
(Sugars)

Complex Carbohydrates
(Starches)

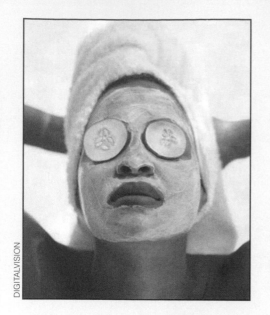
DIGITALVISION

soft mass in the intestines that acts to slow down the rate of sugar absorption.

Another solution would be to eat more unrefined complex carbohydrates, or starches. Starches are very complex molecules. Much larger than sugar molecules, they take considerably longer to digest. Thus they don't push up the blood sugar level as quickly. Moreover, fiber content of most unrefined foods is an additional help in leveling out the rates of digestion and the absorption of nutrients.

But aren't starches more fattening than other foods?

Fat is the most fattening food. One gram of fat carries nine calories, while a gram of carbohydrate carries only four calories. Much of the fat we eat goes right into the fat stores of the body.

It's the refining and processing of carbohydrates that causes problems: the volume of the food goes down, while its caloric concentration goes up. It's this caloric density that makes it so easy to eat too many calories! But when carbohydrates are eaten along with their fiber, then you can eat more food yet take in fewer calories.

So what can I eat?

Potatoes and whole wheat pasta, beans, barley, and brown rice, fill people's stomachs without overloading the system with calories. Add a variety of fruits and vegetables, and it's virtually impossible to eat enough to gain weight.

But top off these healthy foods with butter, gravies, sauces, salad dressings, sour cream or cheese, and a nutritious, low-calorie food becomes a caloric disaster.

Eating complex carbohydrates "as grown" with their full complement of fiber but without those fatty toppings, will not only allow you to eat a greater quantity of food and still lose weight, but it will provide you with more consistent energy levels and increased endurance. This kind of eating plan will keep your arteries clean and cut your food bill in half. Where can you find a better bargain than that?

Wouldn't it be great if you got hooked on foods that made you look and feel great

. . . and the more you ate them the healthier you became?

PHOTODISC, INC.

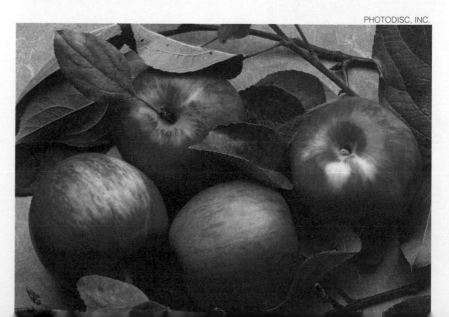

Application

Contrary to what many believe, we need less protein and more starch in our diets. Complex carbohydrates found in fruits, vegetables, and grains provide clean-burning energy and increased endurance. Building your diet around these foods helps keep your arteries clean, your food bill low, and your body healthy.

King Potato

The king of the starchy vegetables is the potato. It is filling, nutritious, and tasty. If you have a microwave, it takes only minutes to build a complete meal around this terrific tuber.

Are Potatoes Fattening?

A five-ounce spud contains only 80 calories. The potato's reputation as a fattening food comes from the way it is served—French-fried, baked, and slathered with butter or sour cream. It is the added fat, not the potato itself, that is fattening.

Topping Ideas

Lentils: Cook up a pot of lentils with onion and garlic. Ladle them onto a piping-hot baked potato. Served with a green salad and whole-wheat bread, this meal will satisfy even the heartiest appetite.

Salsa: Olé! It might sound a bit unusual, but salsa makes an excellent topping for a baked potato. It's available at many restaurants. Next time you eat out and the server asks "Butter or sour cream?" say, "Neither." Ask for salsa instead.

Mrs. Dash Seasoning (salt-free blend): Slice a cooked potato into wedges, sprinkle with Mrs. Dash (the one with the green cap!) seasonings, and bake until browned. It's the health-conscious chef's answer to French fries.

Leftover Soups and Stews: There are many wonderful recipes for meatless soups and stews that can do double duty as a topping. Get creative and see what you can come up with.

Your Challenge:

Add more complex carbohydrates to your diet. Enjoy whole-grain foods and potatoes. Complex carbohydrates will fill you up without weighing you down.

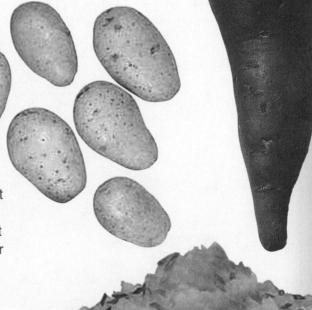

SUGAR

WE CAN'T GET ENOUGH OF THE WHITE STUFF, EVEN AS SCIENCE WARNS OF OBESITY AND OTHER HEALTH RISKS. ARE WE OFF TO THE SWEET HEREAFTER?

From Sugar Highs to Sugar Blues

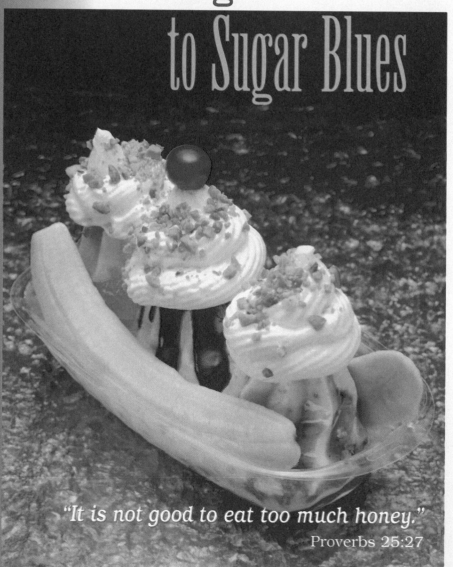

"It is not good to eat too much honey."
Proverbs 25:27

Americans consume an average of 150 pounds of sugars and sweeteners per year for each man, woman, and child. That's more than three fourths of a cup a day.

I don't buy that much sugar. Where does it all come from?

Most of the sugar we consume is hidden sugar. Here are some of the ways sugar slips into our diets:

● *Soft drinks.* Americans average 54 gallons of soft drinks per person per year. This works out to approximately two sodas per day. One 12-ounce soda may contain 12 teaspoons of sugar.

● *Desserts.* A piece of chocolate cake, for instance, contains 15 teaspoons of sugar; a cup of frozen yogurt has 12 teaspoons.

● *Ready-to-eat cereals.* Some, such as Shredded Wheat and Cheerios, are excellent. But look at cereals like Fruit Loops, and Sugar Smacks, with 48 and 64 percent of their calories coming from sugar. *This isn't cereal; it's candy!*

You'll also find hidden sugar in foods such as canned soups, potpies, TV dinners, and many brands of peanut butter.

Should I check labels for sugar?

Yes, but realize that sugar may also be hidden by giving it a different name. Sucrose, dextrose, lactose, fructose, and maltose, for instance, are all sugars. So are corn syrup, honey, and molasses. More than 100 substances that are called sugars exist.

Doesn't sugar produce quick energy?

Refined, concentrated sugars enter the bloodstream quickly. Up goes the blood

ARE YOU DRAGGING YOURSELF AROUND?

*Snapping at the kids? Feeling shaky and anxious?
It could be low blood sugar—the sugar blues.*

Blood sugar dips correspond to energy dips. The person
with sugar-rich, poor eating habits alternates between a
sense of well-being and an inevitable let-down.

sugar, resulting in a quick energy boost—a sugar high.

But the high is only temporary, because it triggers a surge of insulin. Insulin brings down blood sugar levels and, in the absence of the modulating effects of fiber, sometimes pulls it down too fast and too far.

A falling blood sugar often mimics symptoms of hypoglycemia, producing feelings of weakness, hunger, fatigue and let-

Soft drinks are the single biggest source of refined sugar in the U.S. diet.

down—the sugar blues. The usual reaction is to reach for another sugary snack, and then another, leading to a sort of grazing all day long.

Try eating an apple, a banana, or a bowl of brown rice. The fiber in these foods slows down the absorption of sugar into the bloodstream. The sugar levels won't jump around so much, your energy will stabilize, and you'll feel satisfied longer.

Is it true that the body can make sugar out of nearly everything we eat?

Everything but fat. For a long time people thought it didn't really matter what they ate because the body could turn it into whatever it needed. We now know that the way the body processes food, from the time it's eaten until it reaches the bloodstream, makes a great deal of difference.

The body's preferred fuel is glucose, which it makes largely from sugars and starches (carbohydrates). Although fresh fruits are high in natural sugars, they won't strain the body's blood sugar mechanism if they are eaten with their natural fiber.

SUGAR CONTENT

Food Portion	Size	Teaspoons of Sugar
Soft drinks	12 oz.	8-12
Jello, puddings	1 cup	9
Jelly, Jam	2 Tbsp.	10
Pies: apple, berry, cherry, coconut	1 slice	10
Chocolate mints	4	8
Marshmallow	10	15
Hard candy	4 oz.	20
Grape juice (commercial)	1 cup	7
Fruit cocktail (commercial)	1 cup	10
Donut (glazed)	1	6
Angel, pound cake	1 (6 oz.)	9
German chocolate cake	1 (8 oz.)	15
Ice cream, sherbet	1 cup	6-8
Ice cream cone, empty	1 triple	10

Scientists are taking a new look at our addiction to sweets and wondering exactly how giant sodas and oversized candy bars relate to our high rates of chronic disease.

Strip seven pounds of sugar beets of their bulk, fiber, and nutrients, and you will get one pound of "pure" white sugar.

Starchy foods have another built-in protective mechanism. Starches are broken down more slowly than sugars into the glucose the body needs. Eating starchy foods, especially unrefined starchy foods, along with sugar foods helps stabilize blood sugar levels for extended periods. The ups and downs of the blood sugar curve level off, and the insulin response is activated to a lesser degree, if at all.

What are some guidelines for eating sweet foods?

Education and moderation are the secrets.

If you have a sweet tooth, see your dentist . . . well, not really, but a sweet tooth can be reeducated. For instance, fruit is sweet, pleasant to the taste, and full of fruit sugars. Practice satisfying your sweet cravings by reaching for a bunch of chilled grapes instead of a doughnut. Sprinkle slices of strawberries and bananas on your cereal instead of sugar. In time your tastes will change, and you will actually prefer less concentrated sweets.

But this does not mean giving up favorite desserts altogether. Moderation is another guideline.

Begin by decreasing the frequency of eating sugared foods. Work from "several times daily" to "three times a week." When desserts are served less often, you and your family will begin looking forward to them and enjoy them more.

Another aspect of moderation is learning to be satisfied with smaller portions. Big servings and second helpings are just bad habits. You can learn to enjoy one piece of chocolate candy as much as eating the whole box. And you'll feel better! Half a normal slice of pie or cake, eaten slowly and with pleasure, can be more satisfying than a larger piece bolted down.

Reducing the amount of refined and concentrated sugars in the diet and eating more high-fiber foods, like whole grains, legumes, vegetables, and fruits, will produce the right kind of sugar highs. These highs will keep you energetic and feeling good all day long.

Food Processing Concentrates Calories

75 Calories

500 Calories

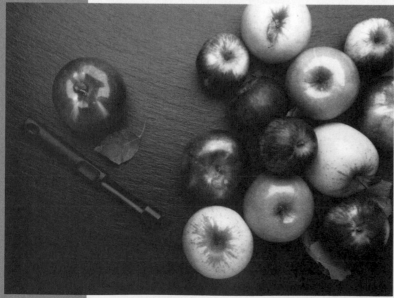

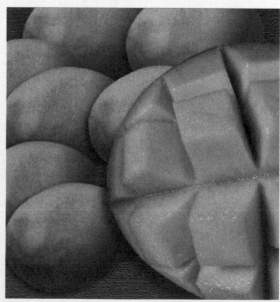

Application

Refined sugars make up around 21 percent of the calories most Americans eat—more than 30 teaspoonfuls per day. Much of this sugar is well hidden in food and beverages. To reduce the sugar in your diet, start by substituting naturally sweet foods for sugared snacks.

Reducing the Sugar in Your Diet

Sugar contains no nutrients or fiber. It's high in calories and can crowd more nutritious foods out of your diet.

If sugar has a grip on you, here are three simple tips to help you reduce your dependence without eliminating sweet treats altogether.

1. Indulge Less Frequently

How often do you eat desserts or sweet snacks?

__ 1-4 times/week   __ 1-2 times/day
__ 3-4 times/day   __ More than 4 times/day

If you answered more than once a day you would benefit from reserving treats for special times.

2. Eat Smaller Servings

When you do eat sweets and sugared foods, learn to savor small portions. Eat slowly, and make your portion last. You can train yourself to be satisfied with a smaller serving.

3. Make the Low-Sugar Choice

Choose low-sugar alternatives when shopping. It's not always easy to tell how much sugar a product contains, because sugar can be disguised as fructose, sucrose, corn syrup, and other ingredients. When possible, however, buy products you know are low in sugar.

Your Turn

Think of some ways you can reduce the amount of sugar you are eating. List them below:

_____

_____

_____

_____

_____

Your Challenge:

Try a fruit smoothie. Also, observe how many sweets and other sugary foods you are eating and then cut back to a healthier level.

Reeducate Your Sweet Tooth

A sweet tooth can be reeducated to enjoy less concentrated sweets. Fruit and desserts sweetened with fruit are good alternatives. Try this recipe for a special treat:

Fruit Smoothies

2 frozen, ripe bananas   1 c. pineapple juice
3 or 4 soft dates   2 c. frozen fruit*

Blend dates and pineapple juice until smooth. Add bananas and fruit. Blend until it is the consistency of soft ice cream. Delicious! It also makes a great topping for whole-grain waffles and pancakes.

*Try these flavors:

strawberries	blueberries
peaches	crushed pineapple
orange juice	fresh blackberries

moothies
Smoothies
Smoothies
Smoothies
Smoothies

BREAD

The Lowdown on "Wheat" Bread

"Imitation Bread—Stuff of Lies," is what a best-selling author calls today's white bread. "It's a bizarre combination of the least nutritious part of the wheat grain and a number of artificial chemicals, which can be harmful."

What's wrong with white bread?

Basically, what's wrong is what the milling process does to wheat. A grain of wheat is made up of an outer covering (bran), an embryo (wheat germ), and the endosperm.

The bran contains most of the fiber, generous amounts of vitamins and minerals, and a bit of protein.

The germ is a rich source of B and E vitamins, several minerals, and fiber.

On any given day, about 75 percent of the population eats white bread or rolls, while only 25 percent eat whole-wheat or rye.

The endosperm, which makes up roughly four fifths of the whole-wheat kernel, contains mostly starch. It is the only part used in making white flour. Ironically, the nutritious bran and wheat germ, which are removed during the milling process, are sold for animal feed.

The food industry further compounds the nutritional problems by using several artificial chemicals, such as:

- Propylene glycol (antifreeze) to keep bread white.

- Diacetyltartaric acid (an emulsifier) to save on shortening.

- Calcium sulfate (plaster of Paris) to make it easier to knead large batches of dough.

"Why spend money on what is not bread, and your labor on what does not satisfy? Listen, listen to me, and eat what is good." Isaiah 55:2

Should we avoid eating white bread?

No bread is all bad. Even the white, fluffy stuff is a high-starch and low-fat food. It's just that some breads are much better than others.

Take fiber, for instance. A slice of white bread contains about a half gram of fiber, while a slice of 100 percent whole-wheat bread contains two grams, and some whole-grain breads contain as much as four grams of fiber per slice. This means you'd need to eat eight slices of white bread to get the

Look past the hype. Because no bread is all bad, the makers of even the least nutritious loaves capitalize on this. The wrappers boldly proclaim "wholesome goodness," "natural," and "Fiber." Names like Roman Meal, 12-Grain, Stone-ground Wheat, Old-fashioned Oatmeal, Country, Rustic, Multi-grain — sound like they are overflowing with good stuff. Mostly, they are "overflow-ing" with white flour—with just a touch of some kinds of whole wheat or other whole grain.

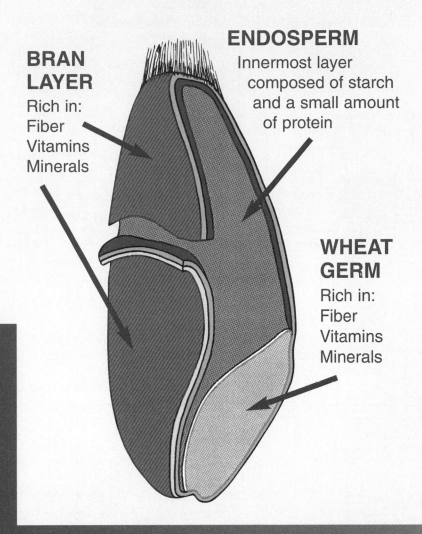

BRAN LAYER
Rich in:
Fiber
Vitamins
Minerals

ENDOSPERM
Innermost layer composed of starch and a small amount of protein

WHEAT GERM
Rich in:
Fiber
Vitamins
Minerals

A KERNEL OF WHEAT

fiber of one slice of whole-grain bread.

What about *enriched flour* and *enriched bread*?

During the milling of wheat at least 24 known minerals and vitamins are largely removed. When nutritional deficiency diseases emerged around the turn of the century as a result of commercial milling, the industry started an enrichment program. Four of the nutrients were restored—thiamin, riboflavin, niacin, and iron—and the bread was renamed "enriched." However, in most cases, not much was or has been done about the other nutrients lost or reduced in the milling process.

What kind of bread is the most healthful?

Truly healthful bread contains ground-up whole grains, with the bran, germ, and endosperm present. Such breads have double, triple, and in some cases quadruple

WHITE FLOUR, WHETHER IN A PRETZEL OR A BAGUETTE, IS DIGESTED RAPIDLY, SO IT CAN LEAVE YOU WITH ALMOST THE SAME ENERGY SHORTFALL YOU'D GET FROM A CANDY BAR. COARSE, SALT-OF-THE-EARTH BREADS PROVIDE HOURS MORE FUEL, MEANING HOURS MORE SUSTAINED ENERGY.

nutrient value when compared with their refined counterparts.

When combined with fresh fruit, cereals, vegetables, potatoes, and beans, bread makes interesting and satisfying meals and helps maintain good energy levels for long periods.

Look for the substantial-feeling loaves that aren't full of air. Look for 100 percent whole-wheat, stone-ground if possible. Sprouted-wheat breads are also excellent.

Find a reliable bakery. Better yet, make your own bread.

Whole-wheat flour seems to attract weevils!

Whole-grain flours have a healthy balance of starch, protein, natural fats, and fiber besides being loaded with vitamins and minerals. The bugs seem to know this. White flour, on the other hand, is such a nutritional minus that the bugs are too smart to touch it.

Store whole-grain flours in your refrigerator or freezer. Or buy the grains whole and grind them up into flour just before using.

Isn't bread, even whole-wheat bread, fattening?

It isn't the bread that's fattening, but what's done to it. A slice of whole-wheat bread has 70 calories—no more than an apple. If slathered with peanut butter and jam, the slice can pack close to 300 calories. It's not the raw materials but the overhead that can turn a low-calorie, nutritious, healthful slice of good bread into a caloric disaster.

Bread has traditionally been the backbone of human nutrition. Restoring good bread to its rightful place is a big step toward better health. Next time you shop for bread, go for the real staff of life.

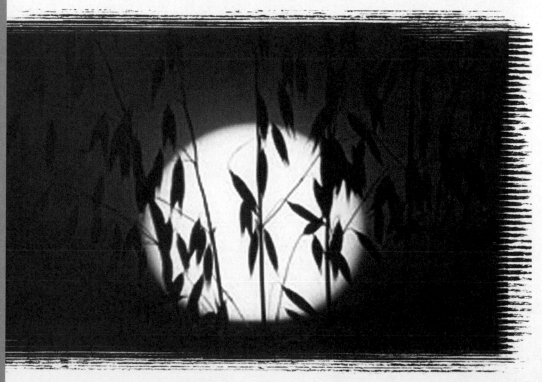

Application

During the milling process wheat loses much of its nutrients and fiber. That's why it is important to shop for 100 percent whole-wheatbread. It is better balanced and more nutritious than white bread.

Take a Closer Look

Below are the ingredient lists from three loaves of bread. Which one would you choose for optimum nutrition?

Loaf 1: Whole cracked wheat, unbleached enriched wheat flour (flour, malted barley flour, reduced iron, niacin, thiamin mononitrate, riboflavin), water, honey, raisin syrup, salt, butter, ground raisins, unprocessed millers bran, partially hydrogenated soybean oil, yeast, wheat gluten, wheat germ, vinegar, lecithin.

Loaf 2: Stone-ground whole-wheat flour, multigrain cereal (rolled oats, rye, corn meal, sunflower seeds, flax seeds, wheat germ, soyflour), honey, canola oil, yeast, sea salt, vinegar.

Loaf 3: Enriched bleached flour (barley malt, iron, niacin, thiamin mononitrate, riboflavin) water, corn syrup, soybean oil, yeast, salt, corn flour, whey, soy flour, corn starch, non-fat milk, fungal enzymes, ammonia chloride, calcium sulfate, potassium bromate, mono- and diglycerides.

WHICH LOAF DID YOU PICK?

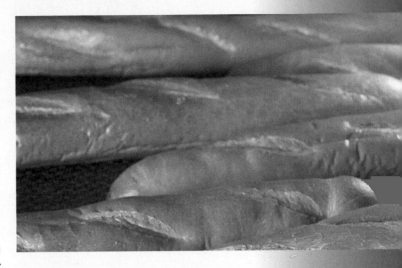

Did You Make the Best Choice?

Loaf 1: This loaf isn't bad. The first ingredient is whole cracked wheat. Its second ingredient, however, is enriched wheat flour—white flour. It lacks most of the vitamins and fiber of whole-grain flour.

Loaf 2: This is the best choice. Its first ingredient is whole-wheat flour. Its second ingredient is seven-grain cereal, which adds the nutrition of a variety of whole grains to the loaf. This loaf feels heavier and more dense than the others.

Loaf 3: This is a loaf of spongy white bread. It lacks vitamins and fiber. It's not the best choice for the health-conscious shopper.

Your Challenge:

Look for whole-grain breads when you shop. Read the labels carefully, and don't be misled by packaging that tries to pass off the "stuff of lies" as the "staff of life."

Delicious Fruit Spreads

Try these delicious toppings on whole-grain toast.

Strawberry Spread

1 c. strawberries   1 c. mashed, ripe banana

Blend ingredients in a blender until smooth. Pour in sauce pan, thicken with some corn starch. Bring to a rapid boil.

Apple Butter

2 c. chopped apples   1/2 c. pitted dates   1/2 c. water

Heat ingredients to a boil. Turn heat to low and simmer. Stir frequently until mixture reaches the desired thickness.

PROTEIN

Can We Eat Too Much?

Ask almost any 14-year-old boy whether he would rather grow bigger faster or live longer, and he would probably choose the former.

Is that a relevant question?

Yes, because in the 1930s studies on laboratory animals began to turn up evidence that high-protein diets accelerated growth rate and maturation, but shortened the life span.

In animals, maybe. But everyone knows that humans need plenty of protein!

Back in 1880 a German scientist, Dr. Justus von Liebig, determined that muscles were made of protein. His protegé, Dr. Karl Voit, watching coal miners, calculated that these strong, muscular men ate around 120 grams of protein a day. He concluded from this observation that this was the ideal amount to eat. Ever since, getting enough protein has been an obsession that persists to this day.

How much protein do we really need?

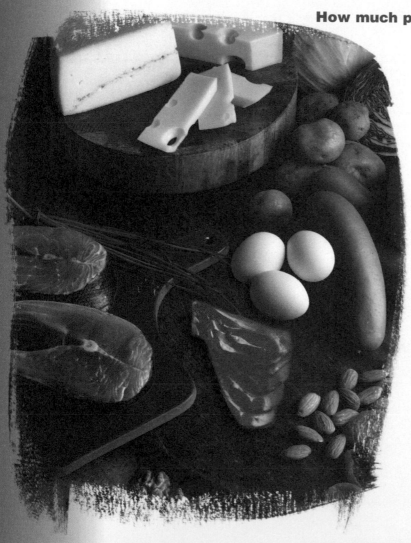

Modern scientific studies show that adults actually need only about 30 grams of protein a day. The human body very efficiently harvests and recycles its own protein. The only protein losses that need to be replaced are those that the body cannot retrieve, such as hair, fingernails and toenails, and skin.

So we need only 30 grams of protein a day?

The National Academy of Sciences sets the American Recommended Daily Allowances (RDA) for vitamins, minerals, and certain foods. The RDA for protein has been set at 0.35 grams per pound of body weight. This is more than the 30 grams/day minimum requirement, and works out to 60 grams for a 170-pound man and 45 grams for a 128-pound woman. Even so, the average Westerner continues to eat between 100 to 130 grams of protein a day.
(See page 104.)

Is that a problem?

● Most of the protein eaten by Westerners comes from animal sources and is loaded with cholesterol and fat. Because fat is well hidden, many people don't realize that meats and dairy products average from 50 to 85 percent of their calories as fat calories. Excess fat and cholesterol, and especially saturated fat, are known for their atherosclerosis-promoting effects, which lead to narrowing, hardening, and increase of plaque in vital oxygen-carrying arteries. This process accelerates aging and shortens life.

● A high-protein diet cuts endurance. Athletes now load up on complex carbohydrates rather than with protein.

● Excess protein places added burdens on the kidneys. Kidney disease is increasingly common in Western culture.

● High animal protein diets are associated with osteoporosis. The processing of excess protein by the kidneys requires calcium, much of which is leached from the bones.

● From 1850 to 1995 the average age of sexual maturity for teenage girls declined from 16.3 years to 11.9 years. The meat-centered diet is implicated.

● High intake of animal protein promotes the growth of several cancers.

Don't children need extra protein?

Yes, they do, especially during periods of rapid growth. The RDA of 0.35 grams per pound of body weight works out to 17 grams of protein a day for a 50-pound child—a little more than half an ounce. Since children in Western cultures eat the same high-protein diets that adults do, there is very little concern for not getting enough protein!

The problem may well be on the other side of the question. Accumulating evidence suggests that children eating high-fat and -protein diets tend to grow bigger and develop faster. Are they paying the price of a shortened life?

What about the amino acid arguments?

Proteins are made of some 20 amino acids. While the body can manufacture 12 of these building blocks, eight amino acids have been demonstrated to be essential for adults. They have to be provided by the diet. People used to believe that they had to eat meat and

> *UREA is produced in the processing of protein by the liver and in excess acts as a diuretic. A high protein intake may require up to seven times as much water to wash out the waste products from the kidneys.*

FOOD COMPOSITION
(in percent of calories)

	Protein	Fat	Carbo-hydrate
MEAT	**32%**	**68%**	**0%**
Steak, sirloin	25	75	0
Pork, medium	25	75	0
Chicken, roasted	45	55	0
DAIRY	**29%**	**41%**	**30%**
Milk, whole	21	48	31
Milk, skim	40	3	57
Cheese, cheddar	25	73	2
NUTS	**9%**	**87%**	**4%**
Almonds	12	82	6
Pecans	5	93	2
Walnuts	9	88	3
LEGUMES	**29%**	**12%**	**59%**
Soybeans	33	30	37
Pinto beans	26	3	71
Lentils	29	3	68
GRAINS	**13%**	**8%**	**79%**
Rice, brown	8	4	88
Oatmeal	14	16	70
Wheat, whole-grain	16	5	79
VEGETABLES	**14%**	**4%**	**82%**
Cabbage	22	7	71
Carrots	10	4	86
Potato	11	1	88
FRUITS	**6%**	**3%**	**91%**
Bananas	5	2	93
Peaches	6	2	92
Oranges	8	4	88

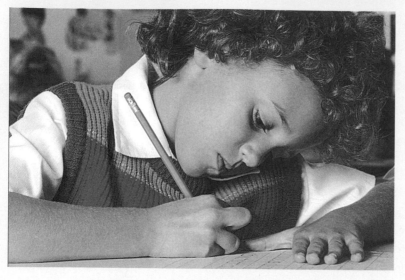

dairy products in order to supply these "essential" amino acids. The fact that these foods are high in fat and cholesterol, lack fiber, and have detrimental effects on health was, for many years, overlooked or considered irrelevant.

Now we know that these amino acids are easily available from a random selection of plant foods. This is shown in dietary patterns around the world. The staple food in Caribbean countries is black beans and rice. The amino acids low in rice are found in the beans, and vice versa. The same is true for the corn tortillas and pinto beans of the Mexicans, and the rice and soybeans relied upon by the Chinese.

The Western world is taking a fresh look at plant foods. They are low in fat, high in fiber, free of cholesterol, and have plenty of protein. The protein content of many vegetables exceeds 20 percent of total calories, while whole grains average about 12 percent and most legumes average 30 percent.

PROTEIN CONTENT IN FOOD PRODUCTS

U.S. Diet	Grams	Optimal Diet	Grams
3-Egg Ham and Cheese Omelet	46	Cooked Cereal	9
Hashbrowns	3	With Milk and 1/2 Banana	11
Toast (2) with Butter, Jelly	5	Toast (2) With 1/2 Banana	4
Orange Juice	1	Fruit (Orange)	1
Breakfast Total	**55**	**Breakfast Total**	**25**
		Pita Bread (3) Stuffed With	
Big Mac	26	Tomatoes, Sprouts, Cucumbers	8
French Fries	3	Three-Bean Salad	10
Milk Shake	11	Split-Pea Soup With Barley	12
Lunch Total	**40**	**Lunch Total**	**30**
Fried Chicken (basket)	48	Spaghetti With Tomato Sauce	10
Mixed Salad, Dressing	4	Tossed Salad	4
Baked Potato, Sour Cream	9	Broccoli Flowerets	5
Peas	5	Bread (2) With Garbanzo Spread	10
Milk	9	Baked Apple With Walnuts	1
Dinner Total	**75**	**Dinner Total**	**30**
Total Grams of Protein	**170**	**Total Grams of Protein**	**85**

Progressive nutritionists advise getting 10 percent of daily calories as protein. Even on a total vegetarian diet, getting this much protein is obviously no problem. In fact, when enough calories are available from a variety of unrefined plant foods, it's impossible to create a protein deficiency.

It's time to bury the myth and catch up with the times. With protein, as with much else in life, too much of a good thing is a bad thing.

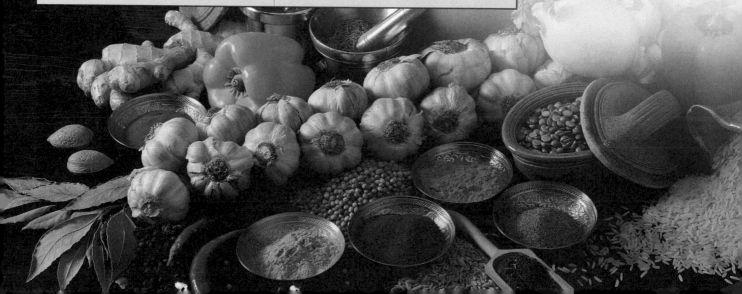

Application

Most North Americans eat two or three times more protein than recommended. This excess has been linked to kidney disease, gout, and osteoporosis. Large quantities of meat and dairy products are not needed—vegetable sources are ideal to provide your body with all the protein it needs.

The Protein Myth

What kind of foods come to mind when you hear the word *protein*? Beef? Eggs? Milk? Cheese? Advertisers spend millions each year making certain we feel these foods are indispensable for good health.

The fact is—animal products are not needed in the human diet. People may choose to eat them for reasons of flavor, habit, and convenience, but nobody should feel they must eat them to get enough protein or nutrients.

Plant Protein

All the protein you need is available from plant sources. Traditional "high-protein" foods are very high in fat. Plant foods, however, are naturally low in fat. If you eat a variety of grains, legumes, and vegetables, your diet will never lack the protein your body needs for optimal performance and well-being.

What Are You Eating?

Look at the two tables in this chapter. Which foods don't you usually eat? List them below.

_____

_____

_____

_____

Your Challenge:

Stretch the boundaries of your diet by sampling some of the foods you have listed. Experiment with the wide variety of tastes and textures available.

Easy Zucchini

6 small zucchinis
1/4 tsp. thyme

3 c. tomato juice
1/2 tsp. Mrs. Dash

Slice zucchini into 1/4-inch-thick slices. Place them into baking dish with other ingredients. Cover and bake at 375°F for 20 minutes.

MILK

Who Needs It?

EVERY-BODY KNOWS THAT MILK IS FOR BABIES..

Milk is the perfect food—for babies. But make no mistake: breast is best for each of the 4,300 species of mammals on earth, because each mammal's milk is precisely designed and balanced for its own young. That's why cow's milk is best for baby calves.

Are you saying that cow's milk shouldn't be given to human babies?

That's right! The American College of Pediatrics strongly urges that cow's milk should not be given to children until they are at least 1 year of age. There are many good reasons for this. A few examples:

● Allergies and asthma have reached epidemic proportions in the United States. Infants not exposed to cow's milk develop far fewer allergies; they also experience much less colic, eczema, and nasal and bronchial congestion.

● Babies need the antibodies (immunities) found in breast milk to protect them from infectious diseases. Scientists have discovered more than 90 elements in mother's milk, with concentrations changing to accommodate the needs of the developing child.

● Breast milk is sterile, unlike cow's milk, which is regularly contaminated.

● The protein in cow's milk is suspected of being able to trigger Type I (juvenile) diabetes.

● Despite antibiotics, infants fed formula or cow's milk are 70 percent more likely to develop diarrhea and ear infections when compared to babies exclusively breast-fed.

After the first year, then, isn't milk a healthful food?

Not really. For years we've been led to believe that milk is indispensable for sound health. The average Westerner, however, eats too much fat, too much cholesterol, too much protein, and not enough fiber. Whole milk, when calculated in percent of calories, is 50 percent fat (much of it saturated) and 20 percent protein. It contains cholesterol and has no dietary fiber. Drinking milk puts added burdens on an already overloaded metabolic system.

WHOLE MILK FAT CONTENT

Whole milk (2 glasses) = 3.7% fat *by weight*

Total Calories..300
Grams of fat...16.8
Calories of fat (16.8 gm fat x 9 cal/gm)...150

150 of the 300 calories in milk come from fat.

Whole milk = 50% fat *by calories*

The Federal Trade Commission (FTC) took the American Dairy Association to task for engaging in FALSE ADVERTISING by using the slogan "Everybody Needs Milk."

How about low-fat milk? Doesn't that solve most of the problems?

Low-fat milk is an improvement over whole milk, but not as great as it seems. The 2 percent fat in low-fat milk is calculated from the weight of the milk, not from its calories. By weight, this milk is 87 percent water and 2 percent fat. By calories, however, it is a 30 percent fat food.

Nonfat milk (skim milk) is the best choice for those who wish to drink milk. It has no fat, and is virtually cholesterol-free, yet retains its other nutrients.

products beyond all reason. For example:

● International studies have shown that a high calcium intake does not necessarily insure or protect against osteoporosis. Traditionally, Eskimos have eaten in excess of 2,000 milligrams of calcium per day, yet osteoporosis is rampant in that population.

● Generally speaking, cultures with the highest milk consumption have the highest rates of osteoporosis, a disease rarely found in non-milk-drinking countries. While milk carries plenty of calcium; its relatively high protein content,

Are those the main problems with milk?

Unfortunately there are more.

● The incidence of coronary heart disease in North America is much higher than in non-milk-drinking cultures. Whole milk, with its saturated fat and cholesterol, contributes to heart disease.

● Certain proteins raise blood cholesterol levels, and casein, a common milk protein, is one of the worst.

● Each animal's milk is designed to fit the growth rates of its own young. Human babies develop very slowly, and the composition of human milk reflects that difference. Animal milks may contribute to the earlier maturation noted in many of today's children.

● After weaning, humans have a high percentage of

107

...ut shouldn't adults be leaning toward weaning?

How about calcium? Isn't milk needed for its calcium content to prevent osteoporosis?

It's true that milk is high in calcium, but that isn't the whole story. The dairy industry capitalizes on the concern about osteoporosis and pushes its

when added to the large amounts of protein consumed in the form of meat, fowl, and fish, actually leaches calcium from the bones as it is being metabolized (see pages 56-59).

● Only 25 to 30 percent of the calcium in milk is absorbed by the human body.

Humans are the only mammals who drink milk after the weaning period.

Mom's Own Milk

Infantile colic symptoms disappeared in one third of breast-fed infants when the mother stopped drinking cow's milk.

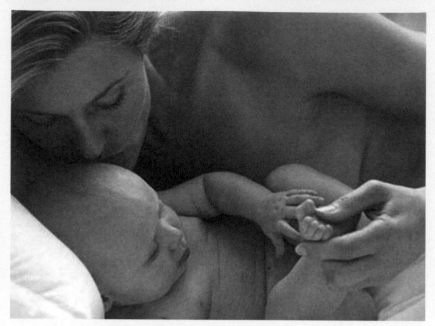

lactose intolerance (inability to digest milk sugar properly). This is evidenced by excessive gas, cramps, and diarrhea. Roughly 75 percent of the world's population has this problem.

❖ Milk is the most common cause of food allergies. More than 100 antigens (perpetuators of allergies) may be released by the normal digestion of cow's milk. Many people with diseases such as asthma, rheumatoid arthritis, hay fever, and digestive disorders do better when they stop drinking milk.

❖ Several studies have implicated milk and other dairy products as probable contributors to breast cancer. In men who regularly drank more than two glasses of milk per day, prostate cancer risk jumped 400 percent (see pages 48-51).

❖ Infectious agents can be effectively transmitted through milk, ice cream, and cheese. Hormones, antibiotic residues, viruses, pesticides, industrial chemicals, and other contaminants can also find their way into milk.

❖ Just as some bacteria can survive the pasteurization process, so do many viruses, including certain leukemia and sarcoma viruses. Another worry is that prions, which come from cattle with mad cow disease, could taint milk. Not even boiling will inactivate these disease-causing prions.

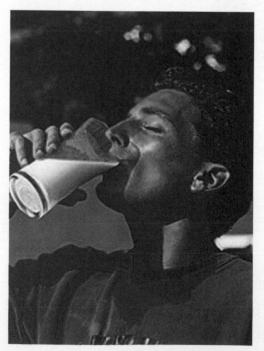

Are you implying that adult humans don't need milk?

Many people live their whole lives in good health without drinking milk or using other dairy products. If used, milk should be consumed—preferably in nonfat form—in small quantities, such as in cooking or on breakfast cereal.

Many concerned people are choosing other sources of calcium, such as grains, legumes, vegetable greens, and, if needed, supplements.

Moreover, an abundance of milk-like products is now available that are suitable substitutes for animal milks. Most food stores have liberal supplies of various kinds of soy milk products, or "milks" made from rice, oatmeal, potato, and almond.

All the nutrients we need for maximum health can be obtained without resorting to dairy foods. And there is a bonus: we can also avoid a host of "problems" by shunning these harmful substances.

Remember—every creature's milk is a health food only for its own offspring.

Application

Milk is a concentrated protein and high-fat food. If used at all, it should be used sparingly in nonfat form. Many types of soy or tofu milks are now commercially available. They make excellent milk substitutes.

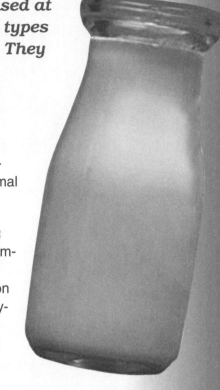

The Optimal Diet

Research on nutrition has clearly demonstrated a unitary dietary principle in dealing with our Western killer diseases. There isn't one diet for treating heart disease, and another for overweight, and yet another for hypertension and diabetes.

Instead, there is one optimal diet consisting of a wide variety of plant foods, freely eaten "as grown," prepared with sparing use of fats, oils, sugars, and salt, and almost devoid of refined or processed foods. If animal products are eaten, they are used like a seasoning and not as the focus of the meal.

Take a look at how the standard American diet compares with the optimal diet.

Your Challenge:

Pick up some samples of milk substitutes and embark on a new habit of dairy-free living. And observe the impact on your health.

COMPARISON		
	Standard American Diet/day	Optimal Diet/day
Fats and Oils	35-40%*	10-20%*
Complex Carbohydrates	22%	60-70%
Refined Sugar	21%	minimal
Cholesterol/Day	400 mg	under 50 mg
Salt/Day	10-15 gm	under 4 gm
Fiber/Day	10 gm	40 gm
Water (Fluids)/Day	minimal	8 glasses

of total calories

COMPARISON OF MILKS OF DIFFERENT SPECIES		
Milk of	Mean values for protein content	Time required to double birth weight
HUMAN	1.2%	180 days
MARE	2.4%	60 days
COW	3.3%	47 days
GOAT	4.1%	19 days
DOG	7.1%	8 days
CAT	9.5%	7 days

Current U.S. Public Health Service regulations state that milk, after pasteurization, should contain no more than 20,000 bacteria/milliliters of milk and no more than 10 coliform bacteria/milliliters (about 1/4 teaspoon). This means that a glass of milk with up to 5 million bacteria is still acceptable. It also means that 2,500 of these coliform bacteria are allowed per eight ounces of milk.

MEAT

Looking for the Real Food

R eal food! In fact, Real food for real people! What an attractive thought! What an exciting promise!

Real Food? Are you talking about those old commercials?

The commercials may be history, but the sound bite is brilliant. The real food turns out to be beef—and a beautiful girl croons that she's not sure she wants to know anyone who doesn't eat it. A macho actor complains that vegetables fall off his shish kebob. An authoritative voice informs us that three ounces of the new, leaner cuts of beef contain no more cholesterol than is found in three ounces of chicken.

What that voice didn't tell you is that lean beef, while comparable to chicken in cholesterol content, contains three to six times more dangerous, cholesterol-raising saturated fat. Besides, who eats three-ounce portions? The average hamburger weighs close to five ounces, and an average-size steak weighs in at six ounces.

But isn't meat an important source of protein?

Meat is a nutritious source of protein, but it carries along a number of problems:

For one thing, most people overestimate their protein needs. The recommended daily allowance (RDA) for protein is a generously adequate 45 to 60 grams. Most Westerners, however, consume two to three times this much. These excessive amounts of protein are hard on the kidneys, promote gout, and cause calcium to be leached from the bones.

An even bigger problem is the hefty dose of fat (mostly saturated) and cholesterol. Scientific research has overwhelmingly implicated a rich diet as the major culprit in today's Western diseases. And the rich foods that are doing us in are mostly animal products, such as meat, eggs, and dairy products.

In a lifetime, the average American meateater subsidizes the killing of 2,480 chickens, 98 turkeys, 32 pigs and sheep, and 12 cows.

> Eating a quarter-pound hamburger, a serving of French fries, and a milk shake presents the body with an artery-clogging 15 teaspoons of grease. Americans are increasingly being presented with meals that promote life-threatening diseases.

"A total vegetarian diet can prevent up to 97 percent of our heart attacks."
Journal of the American Medical Association

The trouble is, while the human body is able to nourish itself on animal foods, it lacks protection against large amounts of fat and cholesterol. Excessive fat and cholesterol stack up in the bloodstream and begin attaching themselves to the linings of blood vessels. Gradually, over time, arteries thicken and narrow, plaque forms, and atherosclerosis has established itself.

As a result, blood supplies to vital organs diminish or get cut off, and the stage is set for many of today's killer diseases, such as heart disease, hypertension, stroke, diabetes, and several types of cancer.

Americans have always eaten meat. Why all these problems now?

● Let's look at the turn of the century. We didn't have many of these atherosclerosis-related diseases because in 1900 we didn't eat meat two or three times a day as we do now. Some 70 percent of our protein then came from plant foods. Today we get 70 percent from animal products loaded with saturated fat and cholesterol.

● We also raised our animals differently then. Chickens scratch in barnyards and pigs loaf around in mudholes. These idyllic, happy farms, however, have been replaced by today's factory farms. The greatest possible number of animals are raised in the smallest possible space at the lowest possible cost. Most food animals today are raised on feedlots or contained in cages, with practically no exercise. The meat from these animals may contain up to twice as much fat as the meat from range-fed and free farm animals.

● Animals ingest and store chemicals in their bodies from the fertilizers and pesticides used on their food. Hormones, antibiotics, and other chemicals are routinely administered to animals in intensive confinement systems to mask stress and disease and to speed growth. Residues of these contaminants find their way into the food chain.

To those willing to look at the evidence, the bulk of the scientific literature implicates a rich diet as the major culprit in today's health problems. Those culprits are mainly animal foods.

The message, however, is slowly getting through: Americans today consume considerably less beef, eggs, whole milk, and butter than they did 10 years ago.

Are you suggesting that a meatless lifestyle is better?

Billions of people around the world are getting along just fine on plant protein diets. Here are some of the advantages:

HEALTH ADVANTAGES
People who don't eat animal products have:

✓ greater longevity;

✓ fewer heart attacks and strokes;

✓ fewer weight problems;

✓ lower cholesterol;

✓ lower blood pressure;

✓ less diabetes;

✓ fewer hemorrhoids, less diverticular disease, and good regularity;

✓ less cancer of the breast, prostate, and colon;

✓ stronger bones, less osteoporosis;

✓ fewer stones of the kidney and gallbladder, and less kidney disease, gouty arthritis.

In addition, such a diet is fun, rewarding, and cost-effective.

USDA STUDIES SHOW that more than one third of broiler chicken carcasses on the market are contaminated with illness-causing bacteria.

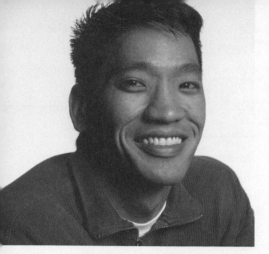

The food fanatics of yesteryear have become today's trendsetters. Whether CEO, lawyer, tennis champion, or housewife, vegetarians are now widely respected. Today, vegetarianism is increasingly viewed as being smart, healthy, caring, and a responsible choice.

ENVIRONMENTAL PROTECTION

Animal agriculture is the single most environmentally destructive industry in the world. Switching to a meatless diet would—

- **Conserve water:** Some 25 gallons are needed to produce one pound of wheat, whereas 2,500 gallons are needed to produce one pound of beef.
- **Protect rain forests:** Producing a single pound of hamburger in Costa Rico involves the destruction of 55 square feet of rain forest to grow the needed animal food.
- **Preserve topsoil:** Every year 5 billion tons of topsoil are lost in the U.S. largely because of overgrazing of livestock and unsustainable methods of growing animal feed.
- **Save trees:** Forests are cleared to raise crops for animal feed. Each meat eater who switches will save an acre of trees per year.
- **Keep water clean:** Every year American feedlot operations alone produce 1 billion tons of animal wastes—a significant source of water pollution.

INCREASED WORLD FOOD SUPPLIES

About 85 percent of American-grown grain is fed to animals. If Americans would cut their meat consumption in half, the land, water, grain, and soybeans saved could feed the entire developing world.

That's pretty impressive!

The evidence against meat and other animal products is stacking up as nutritional research confirms that a diet built around whole plant food is not only adequate, but it is superior.

Humans don't have the instinct to kill.

We are more apt to salivate over a bunch of cold grapes than a piece of raw meat. It's comforting to know that a diet of fruit, vegetables, legumes, and grains is perfectly suited to our needs— anatomically, physiologically, and instinctively.

It's not easy, however, to examine our lifelong eating habits and to find them wanting. But the wise among us will examine. And the wise among us will not look to the slaughterhouses or to the factories to find real food. The wise among us will find the real food in the gardens and farms of our land.

SUMMARY

- Raising of animals for food wastes foodstuffs that should be used to feed the world's hungry people and depletes drastically our irreplaceable food production resources, such as topsoil and groundwater.

- Raising of animals for food devastates forests and other wildlife habitats and dumps more pollutants into our lakes and streams than all other human activities combined.

- Raising of animals for food on today's "factory farms" involves the confinement, crowding, deprivation, mutilation, and other gross abuse and slaughter of nearly nine billion feeling, innocent animals.

- Consumption of animal fat and meat has been linked conclusively with a high incidence of heart disease, stroke, cancer, and other chronic diseases that cripple and kill 1.5 million Americans each year.

Application

The evidence keeps mounting that a diet built around whole-plant foods is superior to a meat-based diet. Meat is high in fat and cholesterol. It also lacks the fiber found in grown foods. In populations around the world vegetarians have better health, are thinner, and live longer.

Kicking the Meat Habit

Many who have made meat and dairy products the center of their meals feel at a loss when trying to plan a meatless menu. For a while their meals seem incomplete without flesh foods.

You can satisfy your appetite on a meat-free diet. It may take a while to adjust, but eventually this way of eating becomes acceptable, and then preferable. Here is a sample menu to get you started planning delicious meat-free meals:

Sample Menu
Breakfast:
- Cooked cereal (seven-grain cereal) or cold cereal (Shredded Wheat, Nutrigrain) with skim milk or milk substitute, and half of a banana or other fresh fruit sliced on top.
- Citrus fruit: orange or grapefruit—peel and eat the whole fruit.
- Three slices of whole-wheat toast with "mashed" banana topped with pineapple ring or slice of kiwi.
- Herbal tea.

Lunch:
- Two whole-wheat pita (pocket) breads stuffed with lettuce, sprouts, cucumbers, tomatoes, radishes and some low-fat cottage cheese or its tofu equivalent.
- Split-pea soup with pearl barley or rice.
- Fresh fruit such as papaya, pear, apple, or mango.

Dinner:
- Whole-wheat spaghetti and tomato sauce.
- Tossed salad with a low-calorie Italian dressing.
- Slice of whole-grain bread
- For dessert: baked apple (microwaved) with date and a walnut.

Food Selection

Develop your own one-day menu. Use the guidelines provided. Enjoy!

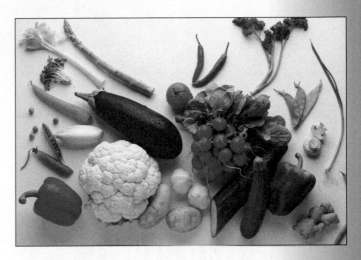

Your Challenge:

As you are planning a more natural dietary program, build your meals around the food categories listed below.

Selection Suggestions

Optimal Foods

Fruit: all fresh fruit (avocados and olives sparingly).

Vegetables: vegetables, greens, herbs, and squash.

Legumes: all beans, peas, lentils, garbanzos.

Tubers: potatoes, yams, sweet potatoes.

Grains: all whole grains, bread, pasta.

Nuts: eat sparingly only.

Optional Foods *(if you feel you must use them)*

Dairy: nonfat milk, plain yogurt, skim milk cheeses, buttermilk, and low-fat cottage cheese in moderation.

Eggs: whites only—or replace with Ener-G powder for binding.

Meats: small amounts *if you insist.* Skinless fowl, fish fillet, lean beef.

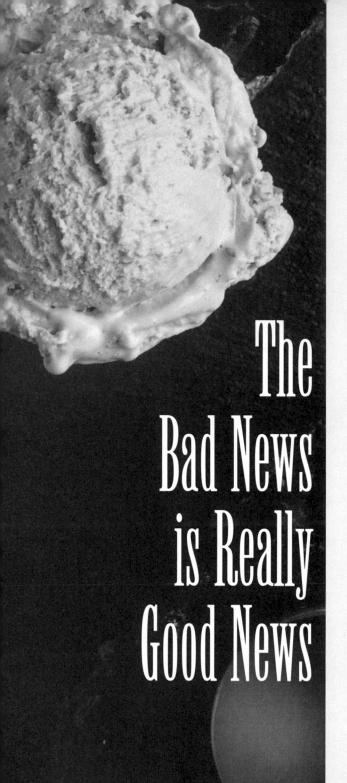

The Bad News is Really Good News

FAT

An insidious villain is at work in our country quietly disabling and killing more Americans each year than all the wars in this century. *That villain is the fat in our food!*

Are you saying that eating fat can kill us?

The excess fat in food is being singled out as the most damaging component of the Western diet. That deadly duo—the high-fat, low-fiber diet—is now linked to such diverse problems as coronary artery (heart) disease; obesity; gallstones; appendicitis; cancers of the colon; breast, and prostate; strokes; constipation; and diverticulitis, to name a few. And the list continues to grow.

Don't we need fat to be healthy?

Fat is a vital part of every living cell. Fat is also the body's backup fuel system. We could not be optimally healthy without fat in our diets.

Problems occur because most of us eat too much fat, often in forms the body cannot easily handle. We understand that a car runs best with its specified fuel. We might get a car to run on kerosene, but it would be disastrous to its engine. Improper fuel damages the body motor also, though it's not as readily seen because a healthy body has great reserves. Up to 80 percent of the liver and kidneys can be destroyed before the organs go into failure. By the time the first anginal pain or heart attack is experienced, the diameter of coronary arteries in important locations may already be reduced by 80 percent.

How does fat damage the body?

An excessive amount of fat in the diet sets up conditions for the development of atherosclerosis—a hardening and narrowing of vital arteries that supply food and oxygen to the body. Excess fat makes the blood thick and sticky, slowing circulation and causing red blood cells to adhere to each other in bunches. These clumped blood cells cannot carry their full load of oxygen, and they are unable to navigate tiny capillaries. Deprived of oxygen and nutrients, body cells become susceptible to injury, disease, and death.

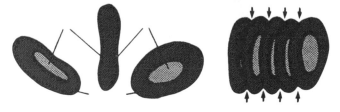

Design of Red Blood Cell (RBC) maximizes surface area and minimizes volume. Oxygen is carried on the RBC surfaces, which become greatly reduced when RBCs clump in response to a high-fat diet.

Get the "Fat Tooth" Pulled!

We eat two to three times more fat, oil, and grease than appears ideal. The average North American diet contains 36 to 40 percent of calories as fat. Researchers feel it ought to be around 15 percent or less.

Most high-fat foods are loaded with cholesterol, which injures the linings of arteries. The body responds by sealing off these damaged spots with extra cells. In the presence of excess fat and cholesterol more and more band-aids are added, one on top of the other, until plaques are formed. When plaques grow large enough to narrow and obstruct coronary arteries, heart attacks occur. When it happens in arteries feeding the brain, a stroke takes place.

Some of the by-products of fat digestion appear to be involved in the promotion of certain cancers. These substances often cause irritation and inflammation of bowel walls, and may be a factor in colitis and colon cancer. When adequate fiber is present, however, feces move along quickly, leaving less time for toxic carcinogens to act on bowel walls.

On another front, excess fat in the bloodstream is one of the factors that depresses immune cell production.

High-fat diets have been shown to impair the efficiency of the body's insulin mechanism, which may lead to diabetes. The amount of saturated fat in the diet also powerfully affects blood cholesterol levels.

What can we do to protect ourselves?

It's crucial that we cut down on the fat in our diets. Butter, margarine, shortening, and cooking and salad oils are nearly 100 percent fat. Meats, cheeses, eggs, and whole milk

WHERE IS THE FAT?		
Foods	Percent Fat Calories	Total Calories Per Cup (8 oz.)
Visible Fats		
Butter, Margarine, Shortening, Lard	100	1900
Invisible Fats		
Peanut Butter	80	1500
Nuts	75-92	800
Pork, Beef	65-80	500-800
Double Beef Whopper (Burger King)	60	970
Whole Milk	50	160
Ice Cream	70-80	350
Processed Cheese	60-85	450
Cream Cheese	90	850

BEWARE!

Of meats and cheeses—

They are very calorie-dense foods (fattening), and they have no fiber.

Of trans fats—

Formed when oils are partially hydrogenated to make them spreadable (like margarine and shortening). These fats raise blood cholesterol levels about as much as saturated fat.

Of saturated fats—

They raise cholesterol levels in the blood, increasing the risk of heart disease and colon and prostate cancer. So keep meat, cheese, pizza, ice cream, whole milk, butter. and most pies, cakes, and pastries in the doghouse.

Of Olestra—

Not absorbed by the body, this fat can cause diarrhea and snare important fat-soluable vitamins and drag them out of the body.

Of fat-free foods—

Many people feel safe in eating large amounts—but these foods may still be high in calories, especially from sugar.

115

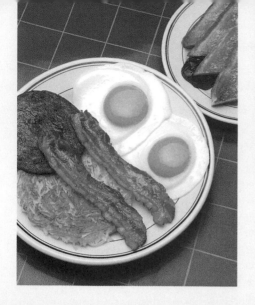

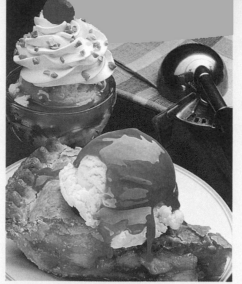

average 50 to 80 percent of calories as fat.

Furthermore, we need a big increase in fiber intake. Fruits, vegetables, whole grains, and legumes are gaining in popularity. Because these plant foods are high in fiber, low in fat, and free of cholesterol, they are the ideal way to go.

The Western diet, bloated with fat, is slowly killing us. We know now that the situation can be turned around by replacing most of the fat calories we eat with unrefined plant foods.

The good news is that a diet balanced in this manner will prevent many Western-type diseases and help reverse coronary heart disease and most adult diabetes. And there is more. You will enjoy better health and feel more energetic. You can also eat a higher volume of food and lose weight, too!

> *More than 30 percent of cancers in the Westernized countries are directly related to overnutrition, particularly the high intake of fat. To cut the risk of cancer, heart disease, and stroke, people need to eat more protective fruits and vegetables, and much less fat, especially animal fat.*

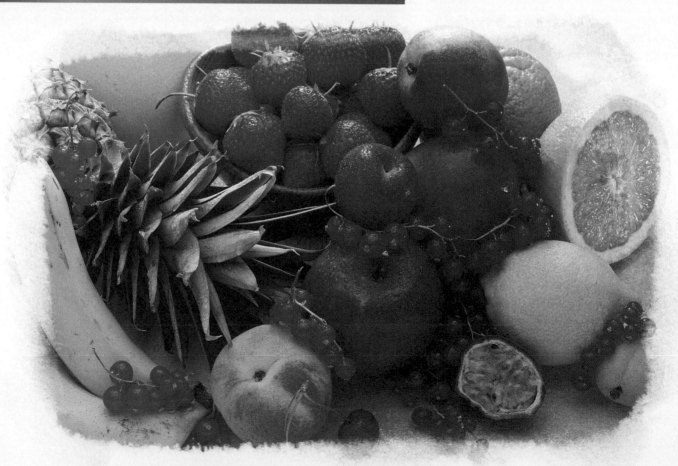

Application

Excess fat in foods is probably the most damaging component of the Western diet. Reducing the amount of fat we eat is essential. Butter, margarine, cooking and salad oils, meats, cheeses, eggs, and whole milk all must be limited.

The Old Four Food Groups

Do you remember the Four Food Groups? That model of the "proper" diet issued by the U.S. Department of Agriculture in 1956? We've discovered a lot about nutrition since then. One of the things we've learned is that the emphasis on meat and dairy products made the Four Food Groups high in fat, protein, and cholesterol, and low in fiber. Study after study has linked this diet to increased rates of cancer, heart disease, obesity, and diabetes. Clearly a big change is needed: Enter the *New* Four Food Groups.

The New Four Food Groups
Recommended by the Physicians' Committee for Responsible Medicine

Food Group	Servings Per Day	Serving Size
Whole Grains	five or more	1/2 cup of hot cereal; one ounce dry cereal; one slice of bread
Vegetables	three or more	one cup raw; 1/2 cup cooked.
Legumes	two to three	1/2 cup cooked beans; four ounces tofu
Fruits	three or more	one or two medium pieces of fruit; 1/2 cup cooked or 1/4 cup dried fruit

Slimming Your Salad Down

One of the best places to cut the fat is on your salad. Too many people take nutritious greens and turn them into a high-fat nightmare by adding thick, oily dressings. Restaurants are notorious for this. At most of them you don't get a little dressing to go with your salad—you get a little salad to go with your dressing.

Next time your waiter hands you a menu, order your salad with a low-calorie dressing on the side. Better yet, ask for lemon wedges and squeeze the juice on yourself. It's a good low-calorie, no-fat alternative.

Your List

Below are the categories from the New Four Food Groups. Under each heading, list foods from that category that you currently eat or would like to try. Chances are you will find that you already eat many foods from the New Four Food Groups.

Whole Grains

_____

_____

_____

Vegetables

_____

_____

_____

Fruits

_____

_____

_____

Legumes

_____

_____

_____

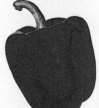

Your Challenge:

Make the New Four Food Groups the foundation of your diet by eating more of the foods you listed above.

CHOLESTEROL

You Need It, but...

W hat can turn a normal, needed, healthful substance into a dangerous killer? How can something that makes sex hormones, helps build strong bones, and balances the body's stress response also choke off oxygen and damage vital organs and tissues?

Cholesterol is both hero and villain. While we cannot live without it, in excessive amounts it can kill us.

The blood cholesterol level is the single most important factor in determining a person's risk for heart disease, the nation's number one killer. For instance, a person with a total blood cholesterol level of 260 mg% (6.8 mmol/L) is four times more likely to have a fatal heart attack than is a person with a cholesterol of less than 220 mg% (5.6 mmol/L). And 220 is far from ideal! Every 10 percent rise in blood cholesterol is accompanied by a 30 percent rise in heart attack risk.

Doesn't heredity determine cholesterol level?

Very few people have genetic cholesterol disorders. The vast majority of blood cholesterol levels are determined by dietary factors. Depending on what we eat, cholesterol levels can go up or down substantially even within a couple weeks.

How does high cholesterol cause heart attacks?

It does it by gradually plugging up the vital heart-nourishing arteries through a process called atherosclerosis.

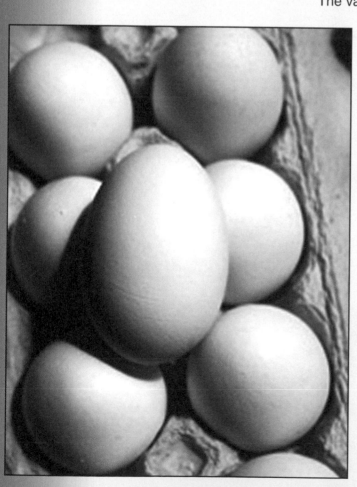

Most heart attacks are related to plaques, which are made up mostly of cholesterol and fat. Plaques are like tire patches. They are the body's response to damaged areas in arterial walls which may be caused by free radicals, especially those found in oxidized cholesterol. The body responds to the irritation by adding more and more "patches" to *protect* the area, causing the plaque to slowly enlarge. But in doing so it also chokes off the blood flow and may eventually obstruct the artery completely.

When blood cholesterol levels are under 150 mg% (3.8 mmol/L), initial arterial damage usually heals quickly and the scars shrink. But when cholesterol levels edge past 180 (4.6 mmol/L), LDL-cholesterol begins to attach itself to the vessel walls, causing atherosclerosis

Animal products are the largest source of fat in the diet and the only source of cholesterol.

(thickening, stiffening, narrowing, and plaque formation).

Massive studies of world populations have documented the fact that blood cholesterol levels are the most dependable predictor of arterial obstructions resulting from plaque formation. Research on migrant groups of people confirms that this is not so much a disease of genetics as of lifestyle. When people who have been protected by a simple diet move into a Westernized culture with its dietary excesses, their blood cholesterol levels go up and soon they begin developing the same arterial diseases as Westerners.

But doesn't the body need cholesterol?

Yes, but we don't have to eat it. The liver manufactures all the cholesterol the body needs. But most Westerners eat an additional 400 milligrams of cholesterol a day. It's this extra dietary cholesterol that causes a considerable part of the problem.

What foods contain cholesterol?

Cholesterol is found *only* in animal foods. Plant foods do not contain cholesterol. It's as simple as that.

What is a safe blood cholesterol level?

Many heart researchers suggest that cholesterol levels under 150 mg% (3.8 mmol/L) will protect people from atherosclerosis.

Aren't there several kinds of cholesterol in the blood?

Cholesterol never travels alone—in the blood it has different carriers. The heaviest carrier is HDL (high-density lipoprotein), known as the "healthy" cholesterol. HDL is protective because it removes cholesterol from arteries and takes it to the liver, where it is made into bile. The higher the HDL in the blood, the better the protection. Men with HDL over 75 mg% (1.9 mmol/L) are protected from heart attacks.

A simple way to estimate heart attack risk is to divide the total cholesterol by the HDL. Ideally it should be under 4.0.

A lighter cholesterol carrier, the LDL (low-density lipoprotein), is the

Risk	Blood levels (mg%) for Cholesterol	LDL-chol.
Ideal	100 plus age	under 90
Elevated	161-180	90-110
High	181-220	111-150
Very High	221-260	151-190
Dangerous	above 260	above 190

"lethal" one. LDL basically determines the rate at which cholesterol is deposited on artery walls. To be safe, LDL cholesterol should be under 90 mg% (2.3 mmol/L).

While there are several kinds of cholesterol carriers, these two—the HDL and LDL—are the most important ones.

Would you explain "oxidized" cholesterol?

When cholesterol is exposed to air, it can become oxidized by combining with oxygen. Even a small amount of this substance can be quite toxic (damaging) to the lining of our arteries. Damaged arterial linings initiate atherosclerosis. Known sources of this most harmful cholesterol include pancake and custard mixes, parmesan cheese, lard, and ice cream. Eating foods high in antioxidants (plant foods) helps neutralize these kinds of dangerous free radicals.

What are some practical ways to lower cholesterol?

Blood cholesterol levels are largely determined by what we eat. If you are serious about lowering your cholesterol, follow these guidelines:

119

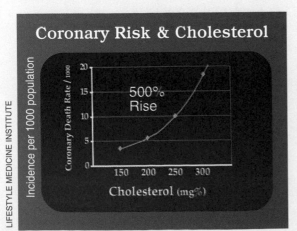

Coronary Risk & Cholesterol

500% Rise

Coronary Death Rate / 1000

Incidence per 1000 population

Cholesterol (mg%)

- **Eat less cholesterol.** Reduce the usual amount of 400 milligrams of cholesterol eaten to less than 50 milligrams a day, or better yet, to zero. Markedly reduce meat, especially organ meats and sausages, egg yolks and most dairy products; ideally, stop them altogether.

- **Eat much less fat.** Saturated fats and trans fats push the liver into overdrive in making cholesterol. These fats are more potent in raising blood cholesterol levels than the cholesterol we eat.

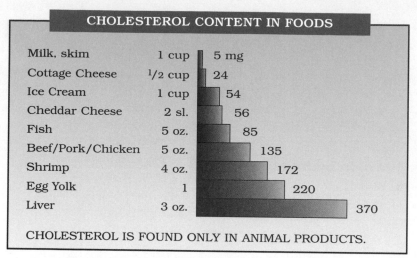

CHOLESTEROL CONTENT IN FOODS

Food	Amount	mg
Milk, skim	1 cup	5 mg
Cottage Cheese	1/2 cup	24
Ice Cream	1 cup	54
Cheddar Cheese	2 sl.	56
Fish	5 oz.	85
Beef/Pork/Chicken	5 oz.	135
Shrimp	4 oz.	172
Egg Yolk	1	220
Liver	3 oz.	370

CHOLESTEROL IS FOUND ONLY IN ANIMAL PRODUCTS.

✔ Saturated fats are solid at room temperature (butter, lard) and are prominently found in animal products.

✔ Trans fats are formed when oils are partially hydrogenated to make them more "spreadable." They are found in margarines, most peanut butters, and many other processed foods.

✔ Polyunsaturated (liquid) fats don't directly raise blood cholesterol levels, but they relate to certain adult cancers and overweight.

- **Eat less animal protein.** Homocysteine levels rise after a meal rich in animal protein, and these elevated levels have been associated with increased cholesterol and an increased risk of coronary heart disease.

- **Eat more fiber.** Soluble fibers, plentifully found in oats, beans, and fruits, bind to cholesterol and bile acids in the intestines and prevent them from being reabsorbed into the bloodstream. Eating more of these fiber-rich foods can lower blood cholesterol levels as much as 10 percent.

- **Medications.** While the optimal diet will reduce your blood cholesterol by an average 15 to 30 percent within four to eight weeks, cholesterol-lowering medications may be needed for a few who may not respond to the lifestyle measures. Be sure to check this with your physician.

Will these measures help raise HDL, the good cholesterol?

They will lower the cholesterol/HDL ratios, which then will decrease cardiovascular risk. Here are some ways to raise HDL:

- **If you smoke, stop**!

- **Lose excess weight.** Cutting down on highly refined empty-calorie foods, such as visible fats and oils, sugar and alcohol, helps here.

- **Exercise daily.** Active aerobic exercise, such as brisk walking, is absolutely essential.

- **Eat foods high in antioxidants (plant foods) and very low in saturated (animal foods) and trans fats.** Garlic, onions, and brewer's yeast may also boost HDL levels.

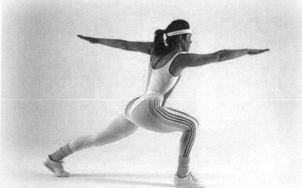

Just remember, blood cholesterol is directly affected by the richness of the diet. A diet very low in fat (under 15 percent of calories) and high in fiber has been shown to lower most blood cholesterol levels by 20 to 30 percent in 30 days.

If you don't know what your blood cholesterol is, *run,* don't walk, to the nearest checkpoint. If the result is over 160 mg% (4.1 mmol/L), it's time to get serious!

Application

Blood cholesterol level is the most important factor in determining a person's risk for developing cardiovascular disease. A diet high in fat and animal products raises cholesterol levels. The opposite is true also. A diet very low in fat and cholesterol and high in fiber has been shown to lower blood cholesterol levels as much as 20 to 30 percent in 30 days.

Blood Cholesterol Level

All too often the first sign of heart disease is sudden death. The best way to assess the risk of heart disease before disaster strikes is by looking at blood cholesterol levels. This is the single most important predictor of heart disease.

Do you know your blood cholesterol level? If you don't, make an appointment with your doctor to find out. The procedure is simple. But more important, what you learn could save your life.

What is your blood cholesterol level? _____

Take Aggressive Action

If you don't find yourself inside the safety zone with a blood cholesterol level below 160 mg% (4.1mmol/L), don't despair. It is time to take aggressive action. You can lower your cholesterol level by making important lifestyle changes.

Six Ways to Lower Cholesterol Levels

Here are six prescriptions that will help lower your cholesterol level. Put a checkmark by the ones you are already working on. Below each item, write ways you might achieve that objective. After you're done, review this chapter to see how your answers match.

Eat Less Cholesterol: _____

_____

_____

Eat Less Fat: _____

_____

_____

Lose Excess Weight: _____

_____

_____

Eat More Fiber: _____

_____

_____

Exercise More: _____

_____

_____

Medications (if necessary): _____

_____

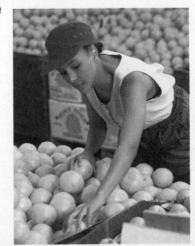

Your Challenge:
Review your list of things you can do to lower your blood cholesterol level and begin acting on these strategies.

It used to be that no self-respecting food lover would be caught dead caring about fat grams and food groups. No more. Today's true gourmets are showing America how delicious healthy cooking can be.

How many of these chemicals have been discovered so far?

When you hear reports about every carrot and every tomato containing hundreds of these compounds, you'll get some idea of the complexity of these findings. They are opening up a whole new dimension in our understanding of nutrition.

How much can a person expect to reduce the risk of cancer by eating more fruits and vegetables?

Actually quite a bit. More than 200 major scientific studies over the past 25 years have consistently shown that high plant food eaters are about half as likely to have cancer as those who eat few plant foods. This is also true for heart disease, adult diabetes, and certain other lifestyle diseases.

Do we know how phytochemicals protect against cancer?

Researchers suggest that phytochemicals usually work either as blocking agents or suppressing agents.

Phytochemicals and anti-oxidants appear to interact with every step in the cancer-producing process — by slowing, stopping, or reversing the reactions.

● Blocking agents work on the carcinogens (cancer-causing compounds). They prevent them from affecting the body's cells. For example:

✔ Indoles found in cruciferous vegetables (cabbage, cauliflower, broccoli) work as blocking agents by increasing colon enzymes that can deactivate some of these carcinogens.

✔ Others block the ability of bacteria to attach themselves to the surface of the cell.

● Suppressing agents work on the body's own cells, combating malignant changes that have been started by free radicals or carcinogens.

✔ They can slow tumor growth by suppressing the cancer cells' ability to reproduce.

✔ They can suppress certain enzymes that cancer cells need in order to grow.

Do some fruits and vegetables contain more potent cancer-fighters than others?

Some of them do seem to stand out, although this probably reflects the fact that these foods have been studied more extensively than others.

● For colon cancers, it's the cruciferous vegetables.

● A high fruit and carrot intake appears to decrease the risk of lung cancers significantly.

● Research subjects eating one or more onions a day were found to have only half the stomach cancer risk of those who never ate onions.

● Soy, a more recent star on the food scene, is a veritable gold mine of cancer-protective phytochemicals. Studies suggest that soy foods decrease cancer risk at many sites, including breast, colon, rectum, lung, and stomach.

Despite such findings, most scientists feel that the lower cancer risk is really associated with eating a wide variety of fruits and vegetables rather than isolating certain ones.

How many fruits and vegetables should we be eating to make a substantial difference?

The National Cancer Institute advocates a minimum of five servings a day; most researchers tell their people to eat up to eight servings a day.

This is pretty radical considering how few fruits and veg-

Do Americans Eat Their Disease-Prevention Foods?

- *80 percent do not eat fruits or vegetables rich in carotenoids (an anti-oxidant).*
- *82 percent do not eat cruciferous vegetables.*
- *41 percent do not eat any fruits.*
- *72 percent do not eat fruits or vegetables rich in vitamin C.*
- *84 percent do not eat high-fiber grain food, like bread or cereal.*

Your body has the ability to prevent many diseases . . . if you provide it with whole-food nutrition.

etables most people in North America actually eat. Some don't eat any at all!

Some good news about phytochemicals is that you don't have to eat the foods raw to get the benefits. While a few of these compounds lose a fraction of their effect when cooked, most are heat-stable. In some instances cooking actually frees up some of the compounds, making them more effective. Also, it doesn't seem to matter whether the vegetables are canned, frozen, juiced, or peeled. Most survive boiling, microwaving, baking, pickling, and drying.

What about antioxidants? How do they differ from phytochemicals?

Like phytochemicals, antioxidants are also natural chemicals found in food, but they are not limited to plant foods. The term *antioxidant* refers to a specific function they perform—they help the body dispose of free radicals that can genetically damage normal cells and set the stage for cancer.

All matter is made up of molecules, including every cell in our bodies. Normally every molecule has electrons in orbit around its nucleus. These electrons normally come in pairs. This makes the molecule stable.

Some molecules, however, have electrons that are not in pairs, leaving them extremely unstable. These molecules are called *free radicals*, and they have a powerful drive to acquire a partner. A free radical will grab an electron from a neighboring compound, causing it to become "oxidized." This newly "oxidized" compound has now become a free radical itself, which, in turn, looks for another electron to steal. The result is a chain reaction where oxidation and damage can spread from one molecule to the next until something stops the process. *Substances that can stop this chain reaction are called antioxidants.*

Can we do something to prevent our bodies from forming free radicals?

Free radicals are not all bad. For example, one of the ways the body destroys poisons is through a system which uses oxidation reactions and free radicals. Free radicals are also essential for effective destruction of germs by the body's white blood cells.

However, free radicals can be extremely dangerous when present outside these functions. They have been found to have a role in at least 50 diseases. They have been observed to damage DNA and are linked to cancer. Because all living creatures produce free radicals—we cannot avoid them—it is important to strengthen our body's antioxidant defenses.

We hear so much about the vitamins A, C, and E as antioxidants. Are there others?

There are many more. The natural body hormone melatonin, for example, is a very active antioxidant. Many of the phytochemicals are also antioxidants. Some caution, however, should be kept in mind when dealing with antioxidants.

- Too large a dose of one antioxidant can suppress the action of another. For example, high doses of beta-carotene pills can deplete the body's supply of needed vitamin E.
- When taken alone, in high dosages, some antioxidants can become free radicals.
- Preformed vitamin A is toxic in large doses, whereas beta-carotene and its relatives, the carotenoids, can be converted to vitamin A whenever the body needs it.
- Supplements do not furnish the same protection as does eating the foods. For example, beta-carotene tablets do not contain the many other carotenoids the body uses. The vitamin E commonly found in supplements is the wrong kind for some body needs.
- Research on antioxidants is done with foods, not supplements.
- The Federal Drug Administration is not allowed to test supplements, because they are considered foods. So we do not know for sure the toxic range, side effects, efficacy, or even that the supplement contains what it is advertised to contain.

Are you saying we shouldn't use supplements?

No, just that we must be very careful about how we use them. If used, they should be taken in modest doses. More of a good thing is not always a good thing. Besides, with so many different compounds having so many different actions, increasing the intake of certain ones over others can upset the balance of the system, and possibly suppress the effectiveness of compounds not yet discovered.

Perhaps, someday, Americans will realize that swallowing pills instead of eating the food is sheer nutritional madness—and slow suicide. But as long as hope persists that a special pill, a magic bullet, will appear someday to take care of everything, we will continue to be bombarded by every new "discovery" that comes along.

This is a relatively new field with seemingly endless challenges. We will continue to learn about these wondrous substances for years to come.

Application

Unrefined plant foods are found to contain substances that protect the body from cancer and other diseases. The best way to take advantage of this protection is to eat a wide variety of fruits, vegetables and grains.

Plant sources of nutrition are generally modest in protein and reasonable in fat content; furthermore, they never contain any cholesterol. With our growing understanding of protein physiology, a plant-based diet has emerged as the optimum way to eat for those interested in longevity and the quality of living.

—*Proof Positive, p. 167*

Following are lists of fruits and vegetables known to be especially high in phytochemicals and antioxidants. Check those that you eat fairly regularly.

The New Basic Four Food Plan

Legumes Seeds & Nuts	Fruits
Vegetables	Whole Grains

1 3 7

Fruit
___ Cantaloupe
___ Strawberry
___ Plum
___ Orange
___ Red grapes
___ Kiwi
___ Pink grapefruit
___ White grapes
___ Bananas
___ Apple
___ Tomato

Vegetables
___ Soybeans
___ Garlic
___ Kale
___ Spinach
___ Brussel sprouts
___ Alfalfa sprouts
___ Broccoli
___ Beets
___ Red bell pepper
___ Onion
___ Corn

List below some new plant foods you would like to try this week:

_____
_____
_____
_____

A GOOD RULE OF THUMB

Eat at least three different colors of fruits and vegetables every day.

In one year a typical American diet yields 270,000 fat calories. A starch-based diet will cut that figure to 73,000. As a result, you can eat more and not gain weight! Even five to 10 pounds of extra weight is associated with higher mortality rates. Almost any degree of overweight has an adverse effect on health and longevity.

WEIGHT CONTROL

- Ads and Fads
- Diets
- Soft Drinks
- Snacks
- Fat-Burner
- Calories
- Children
- Ideal Weight
- Breakfast
- Fail-safe Formula

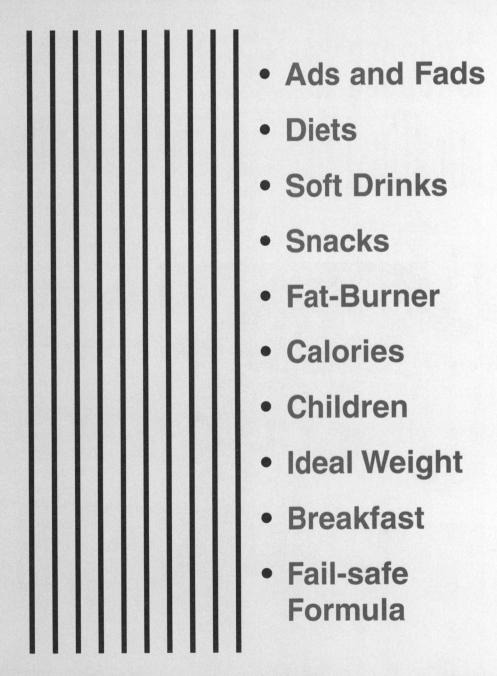

139

AS BEFITS A COUNTRY WITH 150,000 FAST-FOOD RESTAURANTS AND 4 MILLION FOOD-VENDING MACHINES, AMERICA IS STOMACH AND HIPS AHEAD OF THE REST OF THE WORLD.

ADS AND FADS

When Success Is an Illusion

The appeal is irresistible. "LOSE 10 POUNDS IN 10 DAYS—*with a new, scientifically proven formula!*" The struggling, discouraged, and overweight grasp at another straw. They need to believe.

Weight loss is weight loss, isn't it? Does it matter how a person loses it?

Most people who lose weight believe they are losing fat; in reality they may be losing mostly water plus muscle and other vital tissues.

People long for a safe diet pill, but so far this route has been anything but safe. Results are inconsistent and mostly disappointing. Some diet pills have caused permanent health damage, and a few have proved to be deadly.

Many diet plans include a diuretic (water pill). Since the body is about 70 percent water, it is relatively easy for such pills to remove several pounds of water quickly. The scales look good—for a few days. But gradually the body balances itself by replacing the water, and there goes the weight loss.

An overdose of protein will accomplish basically the same thing. The liver changes excess protein into blood urea nitrogen (BUN), which causes the kidneys to force water from the body. It takes much more water to wash out the products of excess protein metabolism than it does to take care of the breakdown products of either carbohydrates or fats.

Some quick weight-loss diets take advantage of the fact that a high-protein intake can cause spectacular weight loss in a short time. This is a dangerous practice, however. That's why such diets

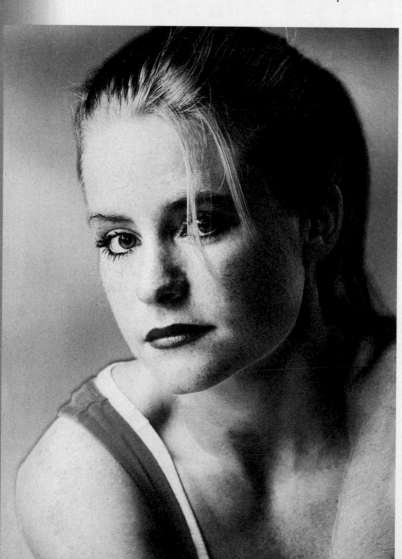

Losing Weight can prove lifesaving, especially for people with diabetes, high blood pressure and coronary heart disease.

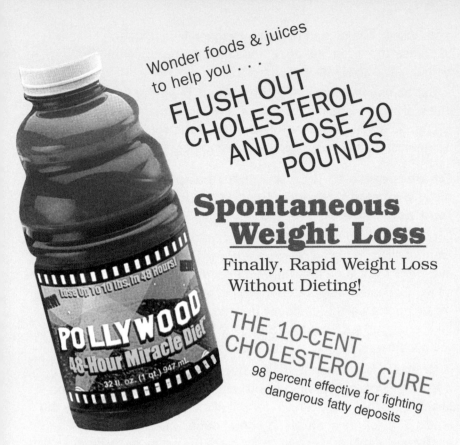

Wonder foods & juices
to help you . . .

FLUSH OUT CHOLESTEROL AND LOSE 20 POUNDS

Spontaneous Weight Loss

Finally, Rapid Weight Loss Without Dieting!

THE 10-CENT CHOLESTEROL CURE

98 percent effective for fighting dangerous fatty deposits

Lose Up To 10 lbs. In 48 Hours!

POLLYWOOD
48-Hour Miracle Diet
32 fl. oz. (1 qt.) 947 mL.

---

of fat, one pound of protein tissue (muscle) and eight pounds of water.

If you feel you need to go on a diet, make sure that you get enough calories from protein and carbohydrates to prevent muscle tissue loss. For an average person this means at least 200 calories of protein (50 grams) and at least 600 calories of carbohydrate a day.

Can I really lose weight on such a gradual diet?

Moderately overweight people usually lose one to two pounds a week on a well-balanced diet; seriously overweight persons may lose a little more. Slow, steady weight loss has many advantages over the radical diets: it does not throw the body into the mode of starvation

Diet Failure

Twenty years of a nation-wide struggle against obesity have failed. In spite of a plethora of weight-loss programs, more than 90 percent regain the weight they lost within a year.

141

---

are usually physician-supervised and limited to short periods of time, normally about two weeks. The scales show gratifyingly low numbers, but most of the weight returns in a short time as the body replaces lost water.

What other possible problems can such diets cause?

Many of the quickie diets drop daily intake of 1,800 to 2,500 calories to less than 500 calories a day. Some of these starvation diets may go as low as 300 to 400 calories. The body misreads this dramatic calorie drop as acute starvation and actually

begins to digest its own protein (usually in the form of muscle) in an effort to protect more vital tissues. Careful testing has shown that weight loss on these diets can come from both fat and muscle tissues.

So beware! When you think you are losing 14 pounds of fat, for example, you could actually be losing five pounds

CORBIS

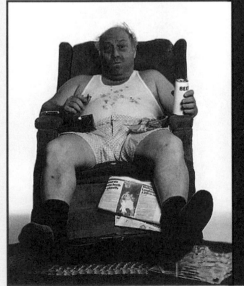

Looking at statistics and waistlines—we are the butt of jokes around the world. Some reasons:

- Portion sizes border on the obscene—
  - ✔ doughnuts the size of pie plates
  - ✔ monster muffins
  - ✔ 64-ounce soft drinks
  - ✔ one-pound burritos
  - ✔ McDonald's "original" 3.7-ounce burger is now the 9-ounce Arch Deluxe Burger.
  - ✔ it takes seven Euro candy bars to beat the Butterfinger Beast.
- Americans are sedentary: 4.4 hours of daily TV, plus Internet use.
- Our food isn't served—it's shoveled!

When you lose weight, you gain:

Energy, Sex Drive, Happiness . . . Life

metabolism; binges and failures are much less frequent; hunger becomes more manageable; and chances are good that the weight lost is really fat.

But perhaps the most important aspect of slower weight loss is that it allows time to establish new and more healthful habits of eating. A person must develop a better, healthier lifestyle for weight loss to have any chance of being permanent.

I'm desperate to lose weight; I have no patience with slow programs. Wouldn't quick weight loss be better than none at all?

Losing and regaining weight over and over is one of the most harmful things you can do to your body. The truth is that remaining overweight would be less harmful to overall health than this yo-yo effect. Repeated weight loss through crash diets, followed by regaining the weight, gradually depletes muscle tissue and adds fat tissue. And because muscle tissue is where fat is burned, you will become increasingly unable to lose weight.

Of even more concern are the psychological consequences. Enduring years of repeated failure and humiliation produces emotional scars that often remain for a lifetime. People seduced by the magic of quick weight loss, do shed pounds initially; but they almost invariably end up weighing more than they did before.

This is not to minimize the fact that overweight persons carry increased health risks. They have more heart disease, hypertension, diabetes, gallbladder disease, and cancer than do people of normal weight. They also die sooner.

Don't become a slave to the scale, checking it daily for immediate results to problems that took years to develop. Get started on a healthful program. And be patient. It's the long haul that matters. The illusions will fade, but the eventual rewards will be solid and lasting.

THE SKINNY ON CELLULITE

- Thigh creams haven't produced lasting results.

- There are no miracle pills. They only slim down your pocketbook.

- Liposuction is expensive. The fat goes, but not the dimpled skin.

- Massages, wraps and such—save your money!

- With a low-fat, reduced-calorie diet you'll lose one to two pounds a week, and reshape your cellulite.

- Best bet: low-fat optimal diet plus regular active exercise.

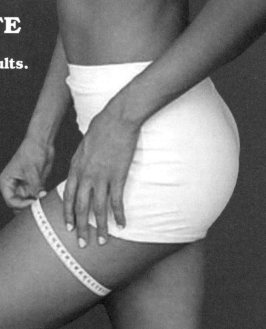

Application

Diets that promise to help you lose weight quickly are suspect. They use tricks that make you weigh less, but often have no lasting effect. Overweight people can usually lose one to two pounds a week on a well-balanced program of healthy eating and exercise. That's the wise way to take (and keep) weight off.

The Wrong Way to Lose Weight

This chapter lists three wrong ways to lose weight. Look them up, then explain what's wrong with them.

1. Diuretics (water pills) _____

_____

2. Extra protein _____

_____

3. Starvation diets _____

_____

The Right Way to Lose Weight

By switching to the optimal diet plus some walking, you can lose one to two pounds a week. That might not get you slim in time for summer, but it is a sensible health-conscious approach to long-term weight management. Read on until you get to page 176; you'll be amazed!

How Fiber Helps

One of the many virtues of fiber is that it acts as a safety mechanism to keep you from overeating. It helps you feel full before you can eat too many calories.

Fiberless foods lack this automatic shutoff. By the time you feel full, you've eaten enough calories for a family of five. Willpower is the only thing that stands between you and obesity—and we all know how effective that is!

Low-Fiber Foods

All animal products lack fiber. That includes meat, milk, eggs, and cheese.

In addition, modern food-processing mills take the fiber out of many foods that used to have it. Sugar, white flour, oils, and most packaged foods fall into this category.

Corn oil is a good example of this process. It takes 14 ears of corn to make one tablespoon of oil. Imagine trying to eat 14 ears of corn at one sitting. Impossible! Yet it's easy to sit down and eat several tablespoons of oil in the form of salad dressings and fried foods.

Your Challenge:

Fruits, vegetables, whole grains, and legumes are high in fiber. Eat them in abundance. Start with this low-fat, high-fiber soup. Serve it with hearty whole-wheat bread and a salad. Eat all you want. You'll fill up long before you'll fatten up.

Eat whole fruits, with all their fiber, instead of drinking the juice.

143

Split-Pea Soup (for six)

1 c. split peas	6 c. water
1 c. onions	1/4 c. barley
1 bay leaf	1 potato, chopped
1/2 tsp. thyme	1 carrot, chopped
1 celery stalk, chopped	1/2 tbs. sweet basil

Add peas, water, onions, barley, and bay leaf to Crockpot and cook until "almost" tender. Add remaining ingredients and cook another 45 to 60 minutes. Add water if necessary. Leftovers can be used as a spread for bread or as a topping on baked potatoes.

DIETS

Quick-Fix Traps

We spend billions of dollars every year on diets and weight control paraphernalia, yet the results are dismal. For many, permanent, successful weight control is more difficult to achieve than victory over drugs, tobacco, or alcohol.

Would it be better to stop trying? Just to stay fat?

Yes, it would be safer to remain obese than to jump from one diet fad to another, lose pounds now, and gain them back later. Research shows that this yo-yo effect gradually depletes important body tissues such as muscle and bone. Eventually it weakens the body so that it becomes more susceptible to disease and less able to shed excess fat.

But isn't it dangerous to remain overweight?

Being fat isn't healthful. Excess weight impairs health and shortens life. As little as 10 to 15 pounds of extra weight produces measurable changes that can lay the foundation for degenerative disease. And for every 10 pounds of overweight, the life span can be shortened by as much as a year.

So what is the answer?

People who are overweight need major revisions in thinking and attitudes. The scenario played out in millions of lives goes something like this: a few weeks on the latest wonder diet; have the jaws wired; take a series of shots or pills; have the stomach stapled; get an

PHOTODISC, INC.   PHOTODISC, INC.

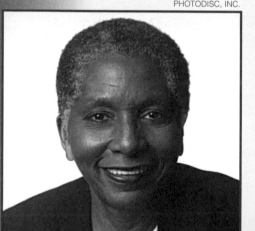 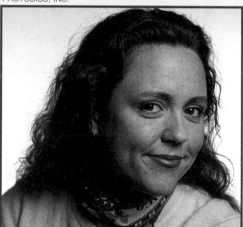

Surveys reveal that at any one time 40 to 50 percent of Americans between 35 and 59 years old are on a diet.

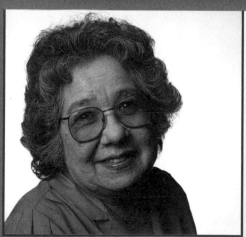 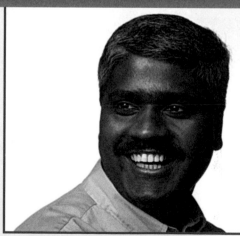

PHOTODISC, INC.   PHOTODISC, INC.

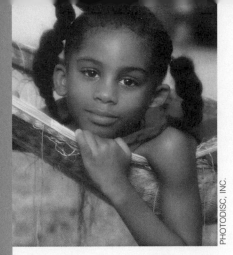

PHOTODISC, INC.

Begin early in a child's life to shape healthful attitudes toward food. Don't use favorite foods as a bribe or withhold them as punishment. When food is linked to behavior, the food takes on a far greater meaning than it should in a child's life.

intestinal bypass; check into a fat farm. And presto, down goes the weight! Celebration! New clothes!

But within days these people resume their former eating patterns and lifestyle. In a few weeks or months their lost pounds are back, often with a bonus.

Weight-control programs usually fail because they are short-term fixes for long-term problems. It's time to face the reality that obesity can be a serious and life-threatening condition.

OK, I'm convinced. What must I do?

Managing obesity is much more than a dietary problem. Like diabetes, hypertension, alcoholism, or smoking, obesity requires a comprehensive approach to lifestyle changes.

● *First,* you have to have a long-term commitment to better health, a commitment that does not change when binges or other lapses occur. With this kind of commitment you can get up when you fall, start again, and persevere.

● *Second,* you need to identify and change habits that cause obesity. This may be as simple as eliminating soft drinks or cutting back on fats and oils. Or it may require you to re-structure your eating patterns and your lifestyle completely.

Changing lifelong habits is among the most difficult things a person can do. For many people the process can be very threatening. Faithful, regular meetings with a support group greatly increase the chances of success. This kind of team effort is almost

a *must* for those more than 30 pounds overweight, or who have had problems for several years.

● *Third,* attitudes often need radical surgery. *Willingness* to change is critically important. Read books, attend seminars, join fitness groups, and make friends with health-minded people. Weight control is not a

You don't need a new "diet"— you need a new dietary lifestyle!

1
4
5

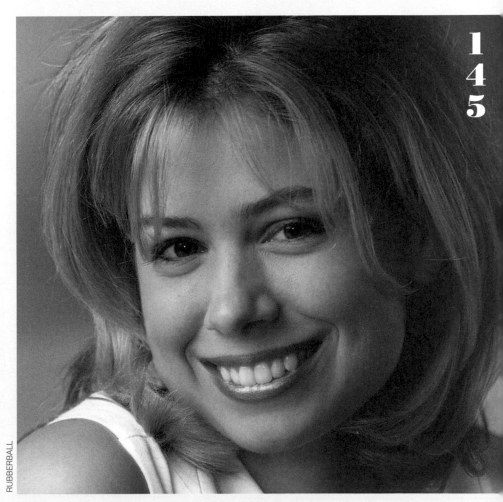

RUBBERBALL

Real Women Forget Diets

To Your Good Health!

The dream of many people is a magic pill taken before each meal that will remove all the calories.

In the absence of such a magic pill, we continue to try dozens of diets, spend a fortune on exercise equipment and health club memberships, and even hire trainers who will come to our homes and work out with us.

We read so much about what is good for us and what is bad that the picture has become muddled. Advertising nowadays is so slick that we often don't know what to believe anymore. To help you, here are some hard facts you can depend on. To accomplish weight loss in a healthy way:

- Always have a breakfast. In a hurry? Try a bagel, toast, or dry cereal.

- Carry your lunch to avoid fast food. Stay away from vending machines.

- Go outdoors for a brisk walk during lunch. Join a health club.

- Try new low-fat, easy-to-prepare recipes for dinner.

- Eat before you go to a party at which dietary dangers abound.

- Find a support partner to collaborate in weight and exercise goals.

vanity trip. Keep the focus on improved health, and the weight will take care of itself.

Finally, look for a weight-control plan that is consistent with a lifetime of good health. This will include a low-fat, high-fiber diet, regular exercise, and a physical, mental, and psychological outlook that meets your needs. Weight control should be only part of a full and fulfilling life—not its main preoccupation.

Such a workable life plan is possible. Many have succeeded. Put your heart into it and keep it there.

THE 10 PRINCIPLES OF LOSING WEIGHT

1. *Think long-term.* Shortcuts and quickie plans never last.

2. *Do it for yourself.* Improving your health and energy are better motivations than a coming class reunion.

3. *Prepare the way.* Don't rush into a diet before you are ready for long-term changes. Keeping a diet journal will help you become more aware of what you eat and why.

4. *Think fruits, grains, legumes, and vegetables.* In the standard American diet more than 50 percent of calories come from fat, sugar and alcohol.

5. *Control portion sizes.* Use a smaller plate. Serve yourself smaller portions and put away leftovers *before* you eat. At restaurants, ask for a doggie bag instead of cleaning your plate.

6. *Eat three meals a day.* Eating at regular intervals will not send your body into a deprivation (starvation) mode, which may cause you to eat and binge more.

7. *Maintain your program.* Successful weight-loss managers realize that they are not on a temporary diet—they are starting a permanent new lifestyle.

8. *Exercise.* It's fun and keeps you flexible. Activity is the key to successful weight control, particularly in middle age.

9. *Don't overdo it.* Don't push yourself to the higher end of the target range. A brisk one-hour walk a day is a terrific goal for steady, healthy weight management.

10. *When you think activity— think "play."* Walking the dog, gardening, yardwork, household chores, sports, bicycling, and playing with kids are all productive activities. How do kids exercise? They play! You can have fun too.

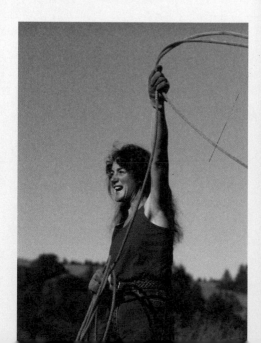

Application

Diets are quick-fix traps that don't last. Many people skip from one to the next, losing weight now and gaining it back later. This cycle is discouraging, defeating, and often dangerous. A lifetime commitment to good health practices is the only safe path to permanent weight control.

Take the Long-term Approach

It's virtually impossible to lose weight and keep it off if you don't modify your lifestyle. Diets are a short-term solution to a long-term problem. That is why most dieters regain their lost weight within a year.

Make eating the right foods a permanent part of your daily life. This is the solution to weight control. You can beat the bulge and live a happier, healthier life. Here's how:

Basic Guidelines for Good Eating

Turn to the summary on page 246. You can have fun too. Read each item carefully, imagining how you could incorporate it into your way of living.

Can You Make the Commitment?

Turn inward for a moment. Can you make a long-term commitment to this style of eating? Are you willing to bypass the seductive offers of diets that claim to "melt the pounds off" in favor of a focus on good health?

Take a few minutes to think it through. Then answer the following question: "How do I feel about making a lifelong switch to this way of eating?" Be honest with yourself. Give the part of you that wants to eat only chocolate as much of a voice as the part that promises never to eat anything "bad" again. Recognize that each voice

is an extreme that exists in all of us. Lasting change happens somewhere in the middle, and it does not happen overnight. It is a growth process in which new behaviors and values gradually replace old ones. Now go back to the question and answer it. Use an extra sheet of paper if necessary.

_____

_____

_____

_____

_____

_____

_____

_____

_____

Your Challenge:

Read the Optimal Diet outline on page 246. Study the 10 principles until you know them well. Start putting them into practice. The reward is worth every effort.

The REAL RISK comes when people cut back on fat and load up on sweets and other refined foods and snacks instead of eating more real foods, such as potatoes, rice, fruits, and vegetables.

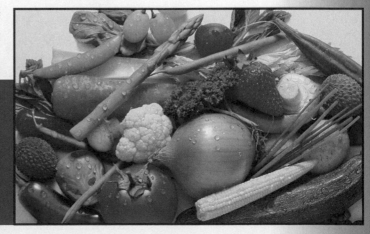

SOFT DRINKS

The Carbonated Generation

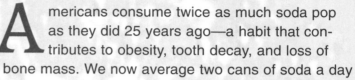

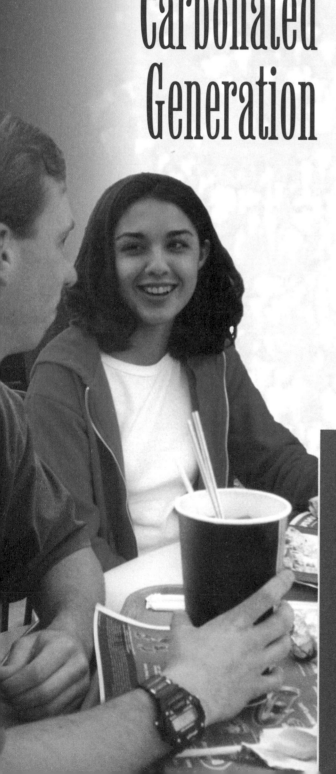

Americans consume twice as much soda pop as they did 25 years ago—a habit that contributes to obesity, tooth decay, and loss of bone mass. We now average two cans of soda a day for every man, woman, and child in this country.

Aren't soft drinks a good way to help people drink more fluids?

Take one glass of water, add eight to 12 teaspoons of sugar, mix in a dose of chemicals—and you'll get a soft drink.

The extra sugar intake from soft drinks produces at least five undesirable side effects:

1. *Unbalanced nutrition.* Most soft drinks contain 120 to 180 calories of sugar, but no needed nutrients. A typical sedentary woman requires only about 1,200 to 1,600 total calories a day to maintain optimal weight and good health. Two or three soft drinks can considerably reduce her daily food allotment and thus also her nutrient supply. Over time this imbalance could cause her nutritional status to become marginal.

The same applies to sedentary men, who may need about 1,800 to 2,400 calories a day.

2. *Extra fat storage.* If the soft drink calories are added to the food calories, the

SODA POP is the number one source of refined sugar in the U.S. diet, providing the average person with one third of their sugar intake. Teenage boys get 44 percent of their 34 teaspoons of sugar a day from soft drinks; girls, 40 percent of their 24 teaspoons.

BIGGER serving sizes spur consumption. In the 1950s Coca-Cola was sold as a 6 ½-ounce bottle. That grew to a 12-ounce can, which was soon augmented by 20-ounce bottles.

And now there's the 64-ounce, 600-calorie "Double Gulp"—the Pop Belly Special!

excess will be stored as fat.

3. *Uneven blood sugar.* Sugar calories lack fiber and rapidly enter the bloodstream, raising blood sugar levels and providing a temporary boost of energy. When the blood sugar level goes up, insulin enters the bloodstream to pull the raised blood sugar back down, and energy levels drop. This sequence promotes the cycle of reaching for another, and yet another, soft drink or other sugary snack.

4. *Delayed digestion.* When a sugared drink arrives in a stomach that is processing other food, digestion slows down until the new calories can be handled. An occasional drink probably wouldn't make much difference, but if it happens several times a day it can prolong digestion and stress the stomach.

5. *Acid rebound.* Most beverages, including sodas, increase acid secretion in the stomach. This increase usually occurs after the beverage leaves the stomach, producing a rebound effect.

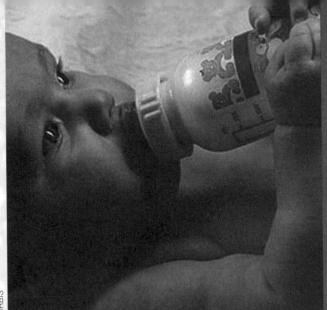

CORBIS

Several soft drink manufacturers encourage feeding soft drinks to toddlers by licensing their logos to makers of baby bottles. Infants and toddlers are four times likelier to be fed soda pop out of these bottles than out of regular baby bottles.

No wonder diet drinks have become so popular! Is this a good solution?

Diet drinks solve the sugar problem, but that's not the whole story. Most beverages, sugared or not, contain preservatives, flavorings, colorings, and many other chemicals. Some of these need to be detoxified and eliminated from the body. Some may also irritate sensitive stomach linings.

Many soft drinks, whether diet or not, contain phosphoric acid, a powerful chemical used to etch glass. Americans already consume too much phosphorus, which the body eliminates through the kidneys by combining it with calcium. With today's worries about osteoporosis, the bone-thinning disease, the fact that each phosphorus-containing soft drink takes some calcium from the bones could be a greater risk than many want to take.

149

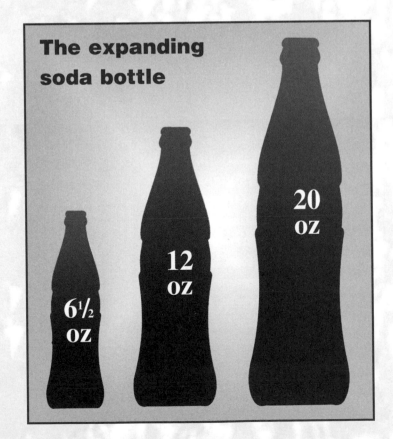

The expanding soda bottle

6½ OZ

12 OZ

20 OZ

How Many Calories Do You Drink in a Day?

Drink	Serving Size	Cal.	Number of Servings	Total Calories
Coffee, cream, and sugar ......1 cup		75	____	____
Orange juice ....1 cup		110	____	____
Soft drinks, juice, punch ....12 oz.		140	____	____
Diet soft drinks ....12 oz.		0	____	____
Nonfat milk...........................1 cup		90	____	____
Whole milk............................1 cup		160	____	____
Milk shake.............................12 oz.		425	____	____
Beer ....12 oz.		150	____	____
Cocktail 1		150	____	____
Mineral water/Water..............12 oz.		0	____	____

Your Grand Total ▢

TIRED? Drink More Water

People by and large know they should down eight glasses of water a day, and most end up getting about that much from water, milk, and juice. But according to a survey by Cornell Medical Center, they also imbibe a daily average of five cups of caffeinated or alcoholic beverages. Both dehydrate the body, leading to fatigue, dry skin, indigestion, and headaches. The solution? For every alcoholic drink and for every cup of coffee or cola, drink an extra glass of water.

What, then, is the safest way to meet body fluid needs?

Water is the perfect beverage. It has no calories, requires no digestion, does not irritate, and is exactly what the body needs to carry on the life processes. How much should we drink? We should drink enough to keep the urine pale—about six to eight glasses of water a day.

ORANGE JUICE may be nutritious, but it's not as good as the original orange. Orange juice, after all, is defibered orange. The whole fruit, when compared to juice, requires less insulin to assimilate, lowers cholesterol more effectively, provides smoother digestion with longer appetite satisfaction, and has fewer calories.

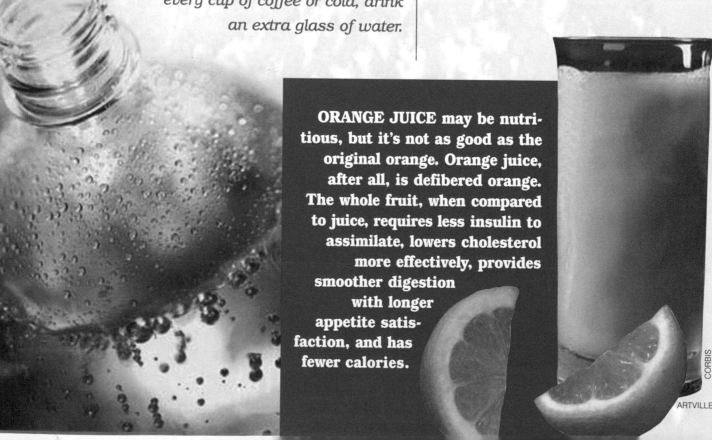

CORBIS

ARTVILLE

Application

North Americans, on average, drink more soft drinks than water. That means they are getting a lot of calories but not much nutrition. Drinking calorie-loaded beverages is one sure recipe for gaining weight. Switch to water—it's the slender person's drink of choice.

An Inventory

What are you drinking? Sometimes it's eye-opening to find out. Listed on the opposite page are some popular beverages. How many of each do you drink on a typical day? Then, for each type of beverage, multiply the number consumed by the number of calories. Write this in the Total Calories column. When you're done, add all the totals to get your Grand Total.

Drinking It On

It takes 3,500 excess calories to make a pound of fat. Assuming you eat enough to maintain your weight, how many days would it take you to drink on an extra pound?

You can calculate this by dividing 3,500 by the number of calories you get from beverages each day. For example, if you drank a beer and two coffees, the calculation would be:

Total calories for a beer and two coffees = 300.
3,500/300 = 11.6 days

In other words, it would take just under 12 days to add an extra pound of fat. At that rate you could gain 30 pounds a year just from what you drink!

Now it's your turn. Take your Grand Total from the previous exercise and divide it into 3,500 to see how long it takes you to drink an extra pound's worth of calories. Fill in the blanks below.

Water Is the Way to Go

If you are serious about controlling your weight, it would be wise to eliminate those sneaky liquid calories. Stop the sodas, lose the liquor, shelve the shakes. Water is what your body needs and craves.

Your Challenge:

Cut calories by drinking more water and fewer high-calorie beverages. If you don't like the taste of tap water, add a twist of lemon or buy bottled water. The more water you drink, the less likely you are to reach for other beverages. That alone will cut calories and help stabilize your weight.

No Energy?

You may be dehydrated. Your body needs six to eight glasses of water besides other beverages. In fact, since caffeine pulls water out of your system, every time you have a caffeinated drink you need to back it up with extra water. Keep your body hydrated, and it may chase away that tired feeling.

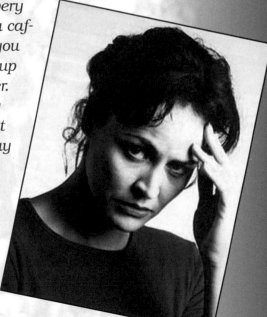

151

Number of days to drink 3,500 calories

3,500 ÷ calories you drink _____ = _____ days

SNACKS

A Nation of Grazers

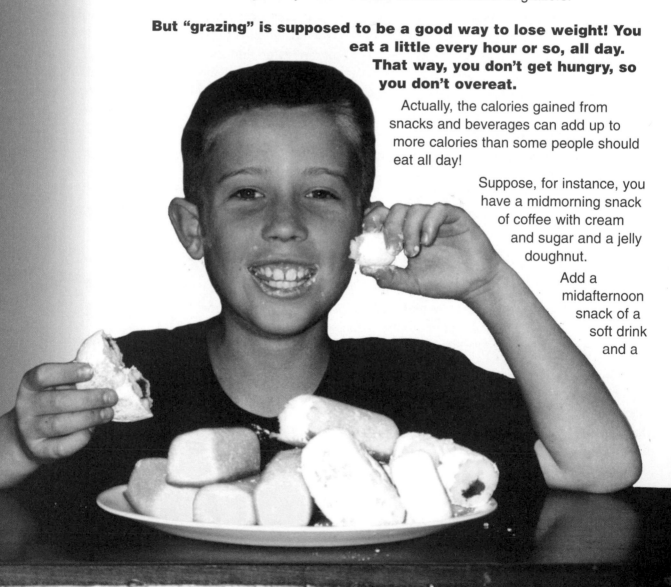

Americans spend $10 billion a year on salted snack foods such as potato chips, pork rinds, popcorn, and the like. And we spend at least that much more on sweet snacks.

We need snacks, don't we? I read somewhere that it's difficult to get all the nutrients a person needs without snacks.

That bit of wisdom came out of a study done on children. It holds up only when children don't get nourishing, well-balanced meals, or when they aren't hungry enough at mealtime to eat the calories they need.

Most Americans, children or adults, have no real idea what it's like to be hungry. From birth kids are fed almost constantly. The habit carries on through the years. We have become a nation of grazers.

But "grazing" is supposed to be a good way to lose weight! You eat a little every hour or so, all day. That way, you don't get hungry, so you don't overeat.

Actually, the calories gained from snacks and beverages can add up to more calories than some people should eat all day!

Suppose, for instance, you have a midmorning snack of coffee with cream and sugar and a jelly doughnut.

Add a midafternoon snack of a soft drink and a

Commercials push the idea that we need some kind of energy lift between meals. Yet most snacks are junk food—coffee, colas, cheese, soda pop, popcorn, cookies, salami, milk chocolate, chocolate-chip cookies, chips, crackers, doughnuts, candy bars, etc.

candy bar, plus a late-afternoon snack of a cup of coffee with cream and sugar and three cookies.

Top it off in the evening with a typical TV snack: a soft drink, 10 potato chips, and five cheese crackers. If this sounds familiar, you'd better watch out—all that snacking added approximately 1,500 calories to your day! Now you know why the old saying is still true: *The bigger the snacks, the bigger the slacks.* Many people, as a matter of fact, have gained control of their weight simply by cutting out snacking.

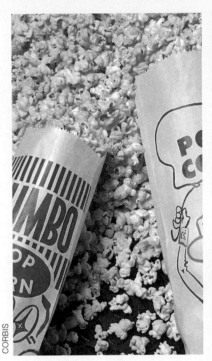

CORBIS

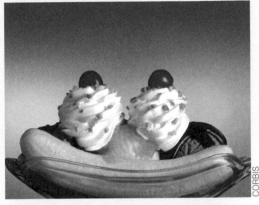

CORBIS

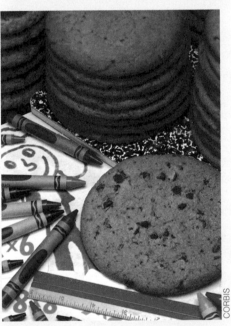

CORBIS

153

But a lot of people can't get through the day without those "pick-me-up" snacks!

That's because they eat refined, fiber-poor, sugar-rich meals, without enough complex carbohydrates (starches) and fiber. A breakfast of pre-sweetened dry cereal and orange juice, for instance (or coffee and doughnut), is quickly digested. The sugars rush into the bloodstream, push up the blood sugar, and provide a temporary high.

But it doesn't hold for long, and when the blood sugar

CALORIES FROM SNACKS AND BEVERAGES		
Mid-Morning	Coffee with cream and sugar	75
	Jelly doughnut	255
Mid-Afternoon	Soft drink	140
	Candy bar	295
Late Afternoon	Coffee with cream and sugar	75
	Cookies (3)	350
TV Snack	Soft drink	140
	Potato chips (10)	125
	Cheese crackers (5)	90
Calories from snacks and beverages		**1,545**

The bigger the snacks, the bigger the slacks.

Don't be enslaved to the first inch of your tongue!

drops, there is that weak, all-gone feeling that cries to be relieved by a beverage or snack. And the cycle repeats itself.

A breakfast of whole-grain cooked cereal, whole-wheat bread, and a couple whole fresh fruits, on the other hand, will furnish plenty of steady energy all morning long. A similarly high-complex-carbohydrate, high-fiber lunch will do the same for the afternoon.

In a study of 10-year-olds, 70% of their total daily calories came from snacks.

Are you saying that we don't need snacks?

The snack habit is just that, *a habit.* With regular, adequate meals there will be much less need for snacks.

What's more, people have fewer digestive problems when they eat simple meals of mostly high-fiber plant foods and then allow their stomachs to rest for a while. Ideally, meals should be spaced about four to five hours apart.

If you suffer from indigestion, heartburn, irritability, insomnia, mental dullness, gas, or weight gain, it could be because of between-meal snacking. A pattern of three meals a day with no snacking could solve many of these problems.

Any suggestions for a "must have a snack" attack?

Drink a big glass of water. It has no calories and requires no digestion. It passes right through, giving everything a good rinse.

If you must have more, eat a piece of fresh fruit or a handful of raw veggies.

The best way to fight off a *snack attack,* however, is to remember that the calories you save by shunning those snacks will gradually melt off unwanted bulges.

While it may not always be true that *once on the lips, forever on the hips,* there's no more doubting the fact that *the bigger the snacks, the bigger the slacks.*

A Snack Study

At a large university a group of students received a breakfast of cereal, toast, fruit and an egg. Within four hours, their stomachs were empty.

A few days later, the same students ate the same breakfast, but two hours later were given either a peanut butter sandwich, or a piece of pumpkin pie with a glass of milk. Six to nine hours later a part of that breakfast was still in their stomachs.

One person received a little chocolate twice in the morning and twice during the afternoon. Some 13 hours after breakfast, more than half the breakfast was still in the stomach.

Application

The calories you get from snacking can add up to an extra meal—a big one at that. Many people are able to control their weight just by kicking the snack habit. You can too, by eating adequate meals high in complex carbohydrates and fiber. These meals will provide you with the steady energy you need to make it from one meal to the next.

WARNING: Snacking Can Be Hazardous

Stop for a moment and think of the foods you snack on. Do you reach for a juicy apple, or do you unwrap a candy bar? Do you munch raw vegetables, or tear into a sack of chips? Most people opt for high-sugar, high-fat, high-salt goodies to get them from one meal to the next. The extra pounds they wear testify to their devotion.

If you want to lose weight, you must deal with that snack habit. Here are some hints to help you make the change:

Don't Snack for the Wrong Reasons

People snack for many reasons besides hunger. Some people use it as a way to release stress. Others feel guilty taking a break. To them, eating something is a way to legitimize a needed rest.

Do you snack only when you're hungry, or do you use snacks to meet other needs? Think about this, then write down some of your reasons for snacking.

Start With a Good Breakfast

Beating the snack habit begins with a hearty breakfast. It should provide plenty of complex carbohydrates for lasting energy. Let whole grains, which are high in these carbohydrates, form the core of the meal.

Watch out for Triggers

Many habits, snacking included, are linked to signals from your environment. For example, you might get the urge for a candy bar whenever you pass that vending machine at work. Or there might be a certain television commercial that makes you want to open a bag of chips. What triggers *your* urge to snack?

Develop Alternate Behaviors

How do you fight a snack attack? By doing other things to disrupt the pattern. If you are bogged down in your work and need a boost, go for a quick walk to the corner and back. Drink a glass of water rather than the usual soda. If you must eat something, try a piece of fruit or some raw vegetables.

Your Challenge:

Break the night's fast and start your mornings with a hearty breakfast, and skip the midmorning goodies. Together these habits will help you look good and feel better.

Building a Hearty Breakfast

Cereals—cooked cereal, waffles, low-fat granola topped with banana, peaches, berries, etc.

Fresh Whole Fruit—all types, especially citrus and melon

Additional fruit—fresh or frozen without sugar

Bread—whole-wheat or multigrain bread

Protein—tofu, legumes, or a little nut butter

REMEMBER:

Every extra pound shaves off about one month from your life span. Sixty pounds can cost you five years of life!

155

FAT-BURNER

Walk Out of Obesity

In America today, fitness is *in. Strut your sweat. Lace up your Reeboks. Flaunt your leotards.* The majority of Americans, woefully unfit, are feeling out of step.

When I hear that a person has to run 10 miles to work off an ice-cream sundae, I feel like—"What's the use!"

There are other choices. You can burn the calories by sleeping for 15 hours or by watching TV for 12 hours. The problem, of course, is that there aren't enough hours in the day to sleep away an ice-cream sundae along with your other meals. That's why exercise is so important. It helps your body burn calories faster.

The body is a motor that runs all the time. The rate at which the body motor idles is called its basal metabolic

We can no longer afford to be complacent about the epidemic of obesity in America. Overweight kills primarily by promoting heart disease, stroke, and many cancers. Obesity increases the risk of diabetes in adults by 10 times and contributes heavily to chronic disease and disability.

—*Harvard University Nurses' Health Study*

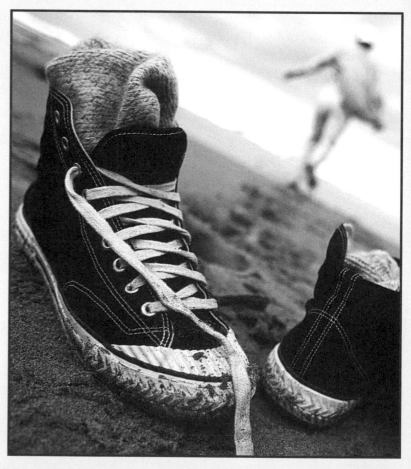

EXERCISE FOR VIGOR: *"Action is a law of our being. Every organ of the body has its appointed work, upon the performance of which its development and strength depend. The normal action of all the organs gives strength and vigor, while the tendency of disuse is toward decay and death."* Ellen G. White, *The Ministry of Healing.*

rate (BMR). The faster the motor runs, the more fuel is used.

However, when fuel supplies are cut (not enough calories consumed), an inner mechanism turns down the body's idling speed. Available fuel now burns more slowly. This function is lifesaving under conditions of starvation, but it defeats the person trying to lose weight.

Can this reaction be prevented?

Activity speeds up the body's metabolic rate. Not only are more calories burned during exercise, but the effect

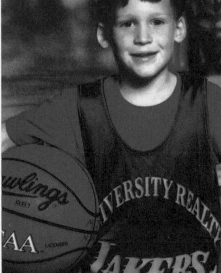

PHOTODISC, INC.

continues for several hours. That's why most people feel more energetic when they exercise. The BMR of the body reflects this. A regular exercise program promotes weight loss by pepping up the metabolism—burning calories faster.

How many calories do I need a day?

Multiplying your ideal weight by 10 approximates the daily calories you would need to maintain the status quo if you are inactive—this is your BMR. Most people use an additional 30 percent of their BMR calories for activity calories. Added

together, this figure represents the number of calories you need to eat every day to maintain your weight.

If you're fairly sedentary and weigh 150 pounds, for example, your BMR needs would be 1,500 calories, and your activity calories would be 450, for a total of 1,950 calories.

To lose weight, you need to reduce this number of calories (eat less) or increase the number of calories used (exercise more). When you develop a negative energy balance, you force your body to burn its reserve fuel—the fat.

Remember when exercise was fun?

OVERWEIGHT KIDS

Many overweight children already have higher blood pressure, insulin, lipid and "bad cholesterol" levels that make them much more susceptible to disease. Part of that has to do with less exercise.

In 1930 only 7 percent of children were bussed to school. Today more than 50 percent are bussed, and the rest are chauffeured by Mom or Dad.

Doesn't muscle tissue turn into fat as a person gets older?

Muscle tissue does not

SHELLEY SNIDER

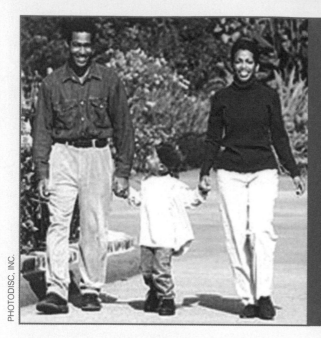

PHOTODISC, INC.

Walking has some major advantages over most other fitness activities:

- **few injuries**
- **doesn't require "stuff"—no wrist pads, goggles, knee pads, helmets, gloves, or poles.**
- **minimal cost—just the price of a pair of good walking shoes.**

turn to fat. It is physiologically impossible for this to happen.

When people become less active, however, their muscles shrink and their BMR slows down. Eating habits often are not adjusted to this lessened activity, so as excess calories accumulate, the body stores the fat in numerous places, including the spaces around the muscle fibers.

An important point to understand is that the muscles burn fat. When more muscle tissue is present, fat will burn faster and more efficiently. On the other hand, lack of exercise and a "starvation weight loss regimen" will cause the body to lose muscle. If this situation persists for a long time, it may become almost impossible to lose further weight.

Muscles are the body's furnace—that's where fat is burned. That's why men seem able to eat more and yet lose weight faster than women.

Is 30 minutes of exercise, three times a week, enough?

The best exercise program for fit people is actually done daily for 30 minutes and alternates between aerobic activity and strength training (weights, calisthenics). But people who need to lose weight must aim higher. Do an hour a day.

What is the best time to exercise?

Anytime. Do it whenever you can squeeze in some time. Or better yet: schedule your exercise. Make it part of your daily lifestyle. Some people prefer to do it first thing in the morning. Then it's done. You feel good. And you are likely to eat less and you'll stimulate your metabolism to burn more calories.

What is the best exercise?

The safest and best exercise is walking; swimming is a close second. People with higher levels of fitness may choose more strenuous exercises.

Start slowly with what you can do. How fast you go isn't the most important thing. What counts is the total distance covered and the duration of the activity. Some people must start with only five minutes at a time several times a day. A person who walks five minutes, carrying 50 pounds of extra weight, will burn more calories than a person carrying only 20 extra pounds who walks the same distance.

If you want to get in shape, put your best foot forward, begin to walk your way out of obesity, and keep going for a lifetime!

Application

A regular exercise program helps you lose weight by boosting your metabolism and strengthening your muscles. It also increases your energy and endurance and lifts your spirits. Exercise is a high-yield investment.

Important Information

Read the last two pages of this chapter; then answer these questions:

1. How much time a day should an overweight person spend exercising?

2. What is the safest and best exercise?

The answers to these questions are important because together they make up the second element of an effective weight-loss program: exercise.

Fortunately, this program can be gentle. You don't need to pump iron or run marathons. Just get yourself some comfortable walking shoes and step out the front door.

No Time to Exercise

Everyone is rushed these days. Even kids and retirees have full calendars. Squeezing in a half hour of exercise every day can seem like an impossible dream.

Many busy people get their exercise out of the way by getting up a little earlier. Some walk during their lunch hour or at break times. Others like to unwind by walking in the evening after work. Be creative, and you will find that there is always time for a high-priority activity like exercise.

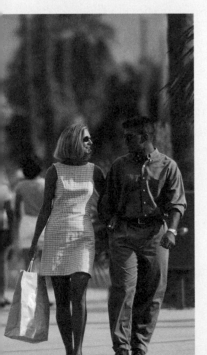

There Will Be Days

Of course there will be some days when you can't complete your whole exercise routine. When that happens, shoot for a shorter walk. A jaunt to the end of the street or around the house is better than no exercise at all.

Don't strive for perfection and then give up when you don't achieve it. Persistence is far more valuable than perfection when it comes to building a healthful lifestyle.

What are some ways you can fit a walk into your day? Write down your ideas in the space below.

_____

_____

_____

> **People who regularly walk one and a half to three miles have less heart disease, less can-cer, less diabetes, less obesity, and fewer colds.**

No Pain, No Gain?

Maybe you have heard coaches and other "exercise people" say, "No pain, no gain." Forget that advice. Walking can provide the physical activity you need and boost your metabolism. Exercise doesn't have to hurt to be good for you.

Share It With a Friend

One of the best things about walking is you don't need to do it alone. Walking with others encourages communication. Many couples find it strengthens their relationship, and friends enjoy a companionship that makes the miles fly by.

Your Challenge:

Make walking a part of each day. Start with just 10 minutes a day, and work up from there. When combined with a proper diet, walking is an effective way to keep your weight under control. But also check with the local gym or YMCA to enroll in a strength and flexibility training program to round out your overall fitness.

CALORIES

Building Caloric Bombs

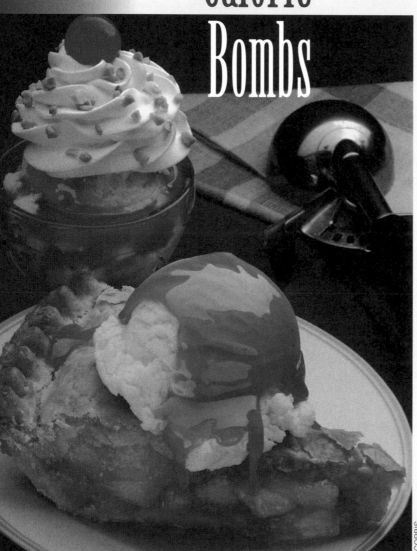

We often take healthful, nutritious foods and turn them into caloric bombs. It's easy. It's insidious. And we do it without thinking.

Take an apple, for instance. It has vitamins, minerals, fiber, and only 70 calories. If we ate apples as they come from the tree, we'd have no problem. But we love to douse them with sugar and make applesauce—doubling the calories. Or we squeeze out the juice, removing most of the fiber and concentrating the calories. Even more popular is apple pie, an American special ranked along with motherhood, the flag, and baseball. It's also a nutritional disaster—one slice *á la mode* can easily pack 500 calories.

I could eat a lot of apples for that!

That's the point. You would have to eat at least six apples to reach that caloric level. And you know you wouldn't do that. You'd feel full after two or three.

Or take the potato. By itself the lowly spud is a wonderfully nutritious food. How good is it? Well, a few years ago a scientist tried an experiment. He ate nothing but potatoes for a whole year. Surprisingly, he remained in good heath with plenty of energy.

CORBIS

Socializing with others is an important part of a healthy lifestyle. Just remember—you don't have to eat everything offered. "Note well what is before you," says the Wise Man. "Do not crave the rich man's delicacies, for that food is deceptive." Proverbs 23:1, 3

More than 4,000 times every day someone in the United States has a heart attack. Heart disease, cancer, hypertension, obesity and diabetes are epidemic in America as they are in other industrialized countries where people can afford diets rich in meat, fish, poultry, and eggs, and loaded with foods high in sugar, fat and salt.

But look at the way we eat potatoes today. A seven-ounce potato, by itself, contains about 120 calories. But who eats a plain potato? Look on the next page to see some of the ways we dress it up.

And that's just the tip of the iceberg. Fresh salads are doused with oily dressings. Most of our fruit goes into juices or pies, or is canned in heavy syrup. Even when we cook fresh vegetables we usually butter them, or add a sauce, which can double and triple the calories. No wonder people have weight problems!

How can we go about reversing this trend?

The solutions are relatively simple. Food preferences, after all, are not inborn; they are learned and cultivated. They can be changed. Substituting a good habit and repeating it over and over with persistence and determination will do the trick.

ALMOST AS BIG AS THE PENTAGON – BUT WITH CHEESE!

All told, Americans eat 90 acres of pizza every day.
–American Health

You can begin by eating more natural foods that have been simply prepared. This includes whole-grain products such as whole-wheat bread, whole-grain cereals, rice, and pasta. It also includes fresh vegetables of all kinds. Tubers like potatoes and yams, and legumes like beans, peas, and lentils, are excellent choices.

Indulge yourself with fruit. Whenever possible, eat fresh, whole fruit without added sugar. Peeling and eating an orange, for example, instead of drinking the juice, gives you more food value and fiber and it fills you up with fewer calories.

When food is eaten as grown, it is full of fiber and quite low in calories. By leaving those caloric bombs alone, at least most of the time, you can actually eat a larger quantity of food, feel full and satisfied, and still lose weight.

161

Food preferences are not inborn. They are learned and cultivated.

Food Refinement Concentrates Calories and Changes Caloric Density

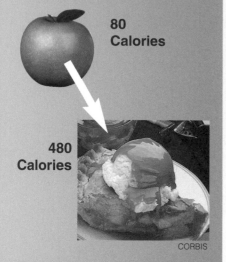

80 Calories

480 Calories

CORBIS

120 Calories

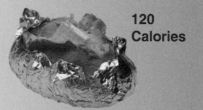

Calories

With Sour Cream and Butter	390
Hash Browns	450
French Fries	460
Potato Chips	1,000
Pringles	1,120

70 Calories

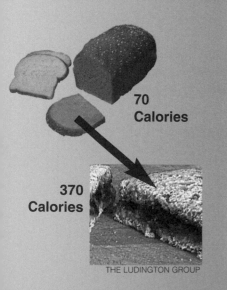

370 Calories

THE LUDINGTON GROUP

Eliminating the loved and familiar requires commitment and fortitude.

It's Time to Make a Healthy Difference

YOU CAN EAT

THIS OR THIS

The calories are the same. The volume is not!*

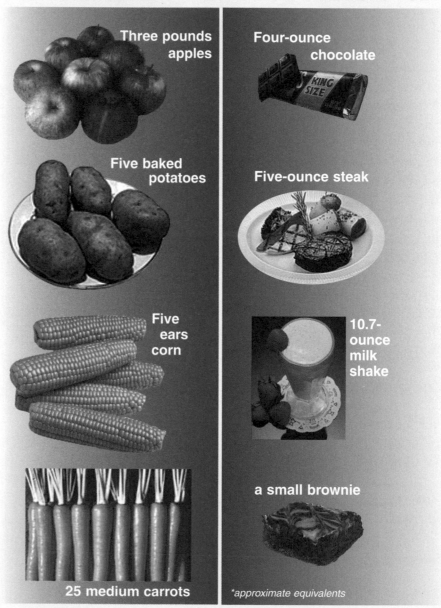

Three pounds apples

Four-ounce chocolate

KING SIZE

Five baked potatoes

Five-ounce steak

Five ears corn

10.7-ounce milk shake

a small brownie

25 medium carrots

*approximate equivalents

Valentine chocolates are always one of the great mysteries of life: How can one pound in the shape of a heart add two pounds in the shape of your bottom?

Application

We are not born with food preferences; they are habits we develop. By reeducating ourselves to avoid "caloric bombs" and to enjoy more natural, low-fat foods, we can eat more, feel full, and still lose weight.

How may calories do you need?

How many calories can you eat before your body begins storing the excess as fat? To find out, start by calculating how many calories your body needs to keep you alive over a 24-hour period.

Your basal metabolic rate (BMR for short) is the rate at which your body would burn calories if you decided to stay in bed all day. You can estimate your BMR calories by multiplying your ideal weight by 10.

BMR Calories Per Day

Ideal Weight _____ x 10 = _____ Calories

Now, if you don't have an exercise program or engage in heavy labor, you will need an additional 30 percent of your BMR calories to cover your activity calories. For example, if your BMR calories totaled 1,500, you would need an additional 450 calories to cover your activity calories. Calculate your activity calories by multiplying your BMR calories by 0.3.

Daily Activity Calories

BMR Cal. _____ x 0.3 = _____ Calories

The final step is to add your BMR and activity calories to get the number of calories you burn in a day. If you eat more than this amount, your body will deposit the excess calories as fat. If you eat less, your body uses fat from its stores and you lose weight.

Calories You Burn Daily

BMR ___ + Act. ___ = ___ Cal.

A Caloric Bomb Disaster

It would be hard to exceed your calorie limit on the optimal diet because whole foods are high in fiber and low in fat. But when you start adding fat, watch out! Look what happens to this meal:

Food	Cal.	Added Fat	Cal.	Total Cal.
Lettuce and Tomato Salad	40 +	Roquefort Dressing	160	200
Whole-Wheat Bread	65 +	Butter	70	135
Broccoli ($^1/_2$ c.)	35 +	Cheese Sauce	130	165
Vegetarian Entrée or Broiled Fish (6 $^1/_2$ oz.)	220 +	Tartar Sauce	100	320
Baked Potato with Salsa	135 +	Butter and Sour Cream	180	315
Skim Milk (1 gal.)	90	Whole Milk		160
Baked Apple With Date and Walnut	100	Apple Pie *á la mode* ($^1/_6$)		480
Total Calories	**685**	**Total Calories**		**1,775**

Your Challenge:

Avoid "caloric bombs." Work to reduce the oils, butters, dressings, and gravies you add to your food. It's time to shift the scales in your favor!

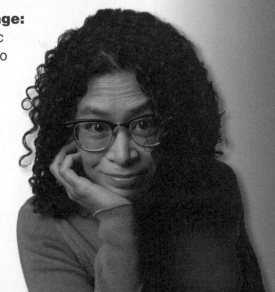

CHILDREN

Getting Fatter Faster

American children are now getting fatter faster than ever. Five million youngsters aged 5 to 11 have serious weight problems, and the number of super-fat children has tripled over the past 25 years.

That's hard to believe. Isn't our culture more health-conscious now? Aren't fitness clubs booming?

Physical fitness is a trend among adults, not children. It's grown-ups who are out running, walking, jogging, and joining fitness clubs and aerobic classes. It's the older people who flock to wellness lectures and examine menus at restaurants for healthier and leaner foods.

But don't schools have health courses, physical education, and sports activities?

Yes, but because of budget cuts, overcrowding, and teacher shortages, many schools have had to cut back on these programs in recent years. In some cases they've eliminated physical education courses and requirements altogether. Health classes are often unpopular with students, and relatively few youngsters qualify for team positions in school-sponsored sports.

Isn't obesity in children mostly inherited?

Genes do play a role in a person's weight, but they aren't the whole answer. Environment plays a critically important role—as shown by the fact that the percentage of obese Americans has increased steadily over the past 50 years. Our gene pool can't change that fast!

We now have an environment that supports obesity. Once upon a time children raced home from school to change clothes and go outside to play. They climbed

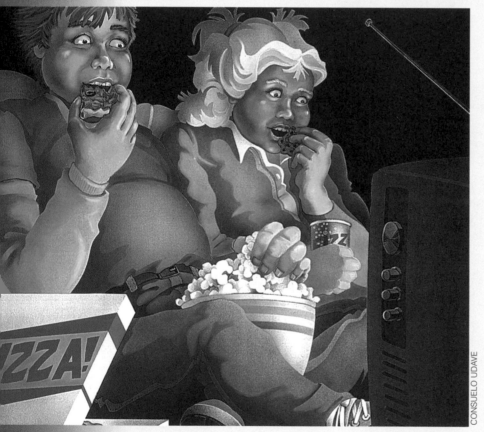

CONSUELO UDAVE

Increasingly, Type II (adult-onset) diabetes is turning up in children, and health experts fear an impending health crisis. So far, all studies have pointed to obesity as a factor.

Teen Weight Trends: Going the Wrong Way!

By age group, 22 percent of kids under age 12 are overweight, but the total goes to 57 percent for teens 13 to 17. Many parents do not perceive the problem, and more than 80 percent believe that their child is physically fit.

Thousands of school-age children have serious weight problems that affect their health, their ability to perform, and their peer acceptance.

To these children and their families, obesity is a curse. To do nothing is to sentence them to a possible lifetime of social misery, rejection, and a significantly higher risk of developing early major health problems.

Monitor your child's emotional life. Some children eat when they feel nervous or unhappy; others when they are alone or neglected. Problems may start during a divorce. Look for unmet emotional needs. ABOVE ALL—make your kids feel loved, unconditionally.

trees, rode bicycles, skated, played games, and dribbled basketballs. Today's children average five to eight hours a day watching television! Our entire culture promotes less physical activity and more eating.

CORBIS

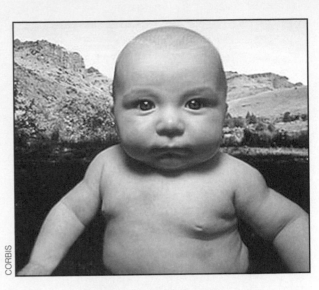

What are the chances of a fat child becoming a fat adult?

About 80 percent of overweight teenagers will remain overweight as adults. The marked increase in adolescent obesity will have serious consequences in the future. And dieting is not the answer. Some 80 percent of American girls begin a regular cycle of dieting by the time they are just 11 years old, according to William Rader, M.D.

Does obesity produce disease in childhood?

Being overweight predisposes a child to heart disease, gallstones, adult-onset diabetes, hypertension, cancer, and full-blown obesity later in life. Obese children have more orthopedic problems and upper

respiratory diseases. And that is only one side of the story. They often suffer major social and psychological problems. The rapid increase of serious depression, eating disorders, drug use, suicide, and violence among teenagers is frightening.

What can be done about this growing problem?

The major causes of obesity in children are the same as for adults—a sedentary lifestyle, TV viewing, the snack and soda habit, and the popularity and availability of highly processed and concentrated foods. Many major medical centers are developing weight-control programs for children that involve the whole family. Proper eating and lifestyle habits are a family affair, and a youngster especially needs the support of the family. Even when the rest of the family is not overweight everyone benefits from a healthier way of life.

165

PHOTODISC, INC.

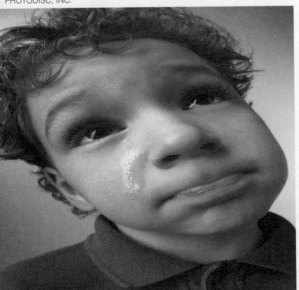

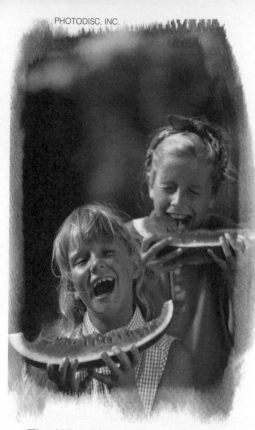

Seven Secrets for Fat-proofing Your Child

Clinical psychologists and pediatricians feel that nearly all obesity in children could be prevented if children were taught the following sensible basic habits early, before they have free access to food and become addicted to TV:

● Three meals a day at regular times with lots of whole grains, legumes, fresh fruit, and vegetables.

● Control the cupboards—get rid of tempting junk foods. Offer fruit and fresh veggies for snacks.

● Drink plenty of water. Limit sodas, juices, and other beverages.

● At least an hour of active exercise daily, preferably outdoors.

● Regular, quiet study and reading times to replace the hours spent watching TV.

● Plenty of rest. Many children are chronically tired. Put them to bed early enough so they awaken naturally, in time for a healthy breakfast.

● A wide range of interests—library visits, music lessons, arts and crafts, family outings, etc.

The Wise Man said:

"Train a child in the way he should go, and when he is old he will not turn from it." Proverbs 22:6

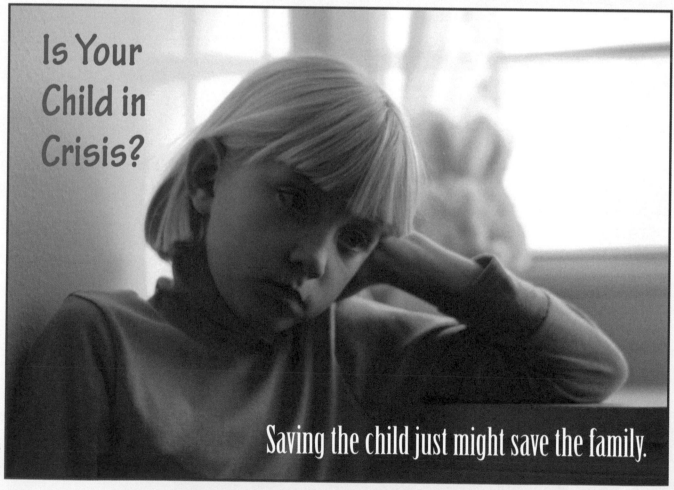

Is Your Child in Crisis?

Saving the child just might save the family.

Application

Hours of television, Nintendo, the Internet, and the easy availability of high-calorie snacks are creating a generation of super-fat children. Their obesity predisposes them to a host of lifestyle related illnesses, and has been linked to serious psychological problems. Families can help these children by adopting proper eating and lifestyle habits. Good health is a family affair.

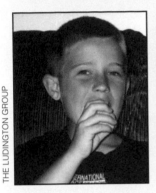 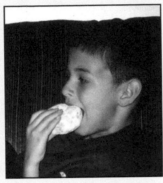

Not-So-Little Jimmy

Jimmy is overweight for an 11-year-old. The heaviest child in his class, he is often teased by the other children. Because he sees himself as slow and awkward, he resists participating in physical education and after-school sports programs. Instead Jimmy spends his afternoons at home watching television, playing video games, and snacking on pop, chips, and other goodies.

June and George, Jimmy's parents, are learning how lifestyle affects health and well-being. They're making efforts to change their own lifestyle, and also want to help their son. After some discussion, they have come up with three strategies.

1. Lead by Example

Since children learn by example, June and George committed themselves to being better role models. They decided that this means regular exercise and no snacking for either of them.

Could you be a better role model for your children and others in your family? What are some specific things you could do?

2. Create a Supportive Home Environment

To help Jimmy control his snacking, his parents stopped buying soft drinks, chips, and cookies. They replaced these high-calorie temptations with good old-fashioned fruits and vegetables. Television watching and video games were also limited.

Our environment strongly influences what we eat and how we live. Does your home environment help you achieve your lifestyle goals? What could you do to make it better?

_____

_____

_____

_____

3. Involve Family Members

Jimmy was not silent as his life was rearranged, but his howls of protest were tempered by including him in the process. June and George explained the reasons for the changes. They also listened attentively to Jimmy's concerns. Together the three of them chose new recipes to try. In the evening Jimmy rode his bike while his parents walked or jogged. The changes were difficult at first, but after a time they became routine, and eventually they actually became fun.

People tend to resist changes in those close to them. By explaining why you are making changes and enlisting the aid of others, you can turn resistance into support. How could you involve your children in the lifestyle changes you are making?

Your Challenge:

Use the ideas you came up with in this unit to make your home a place in which good eating habits can flourish. Involve your family in the changes.

IDEAL WEIGHT

The Right Weight Debate

CORBIS

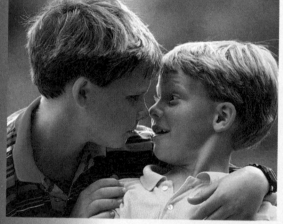

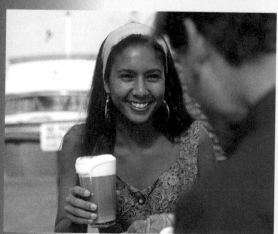

PHOTODISC, INC.

I'm not obese," said one comedian. "I'm just short for my weight!" Whether short or tall, few people are happy about what they weigh.

How can I tell if I'm FIT or FAT?

A person's weight is a highly individual thing, but here are some guidelines. By definition, obese means being 20 percent or more above one's ideal weight. A person with an ideal weight of 120 pounds would be obese at 144 pounds or more. Overweight, on the other hand, usually means being 10 to 19 percent above one's ideal weight. Our hypothetical person with an ideal weight of 120 pounds would be overweight at 132 to 143 pounds

How is your "ideal" weight determined?

Ideal weight can be set in different ways. One way is to look at the records of large life insurance companies. They are very interested in finding predictors of longevity because it affects the way they structure their premiums. They have discovered that certain ideal weight-to-height relationships correlate well with optimum life expectancy. The massive actuarial data of the

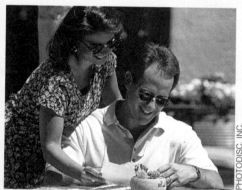

PHOTODISC, INC.

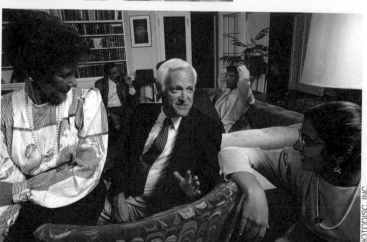

PHOTODISC, INC.

"By stupid decisions a man ruins his life; then he gets angry at God." Proverbs 19:3, Clear Word

Metropolitan Life Insurance Company formed the basis of its gender-specific Table of Ideal Weight, based on height and bone size.

How is bone size calculated?

Although most people have a pretty good idea of their frame size, wrist (and sometimes ankle) measurements provide a more reliable method. In general, a woman's wrist measurement of five and a quarter inches or less is considered small-boned, between five and a quarter to six inches is medium, and over six inches is large. For men, anything under 6 inches is small and anything over seven inches is large.

Is there a simpler way to calculate ideal weight?

Here is a time-honored rule of thumb:

Besides a shortened life span, obese people are at higher risk for painful heel syndrome, stress fractures of the pelvis and osteoarthritis of the hips and knees. Death and taxes are both inevitable, but ending life as a cripple is not inevitable. Lose that weight now!

PHOTODISC, INC.

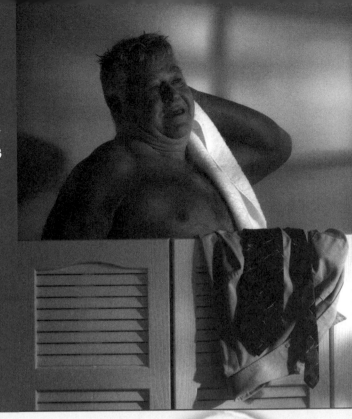

● For men—allow 100 pounds for five feet of height. For each additional inch, add six pounds. The ideal weight for a five-foot-ten-inch man would therefore be 160 pounds.

● For women—allow 106 pounds for five feet of height, but add five pounds for each additional inch. For a five-foot-five-inch woman,

that comes to 131 pounds. Large-boned men and women can add 5 pent to these figures. Small-boned can subtract 5 percent.

Some athletes I know would flunk that test!

That's right, and that's why it's only a rule of thumb. Football players, for instance, have more muscle and greater muscle density than the average person. At the same time they carry very little fat. For this reason, the most accurate way to measure body fat is through hydrostatic (underwater) weighing. Fat is

1
6
9

IDEAL WEIGHTS FOR ADULTS BY BODY FRAME

Metropolitan Life Insurance Height/Weight Table (1959)+ (Weight in lbs.)*

MEN				WOMEN			
Height (No Shoes)	Small Frame	Medium Frame	Large Frame	Height (No Shoes)	Small Frame	Medium Frame	Large Frame
5'2"	115-123	121-133	129-144	4'10"	96-104	101-113	109-125
4"	121-129	127-139	135-152	5'0"	102-110	107-119	115-131
6"	128-137	134-147	142-161	2"	108-116	113-126	121-138
8"	136-145	142-156	151-170	4"	114-123	120-135	129-146
10"	144-154	150-165	159-179	6"	122-131	128-143	137-154
6'0"	152-162	158-175	168-189	8"	130-140	136-151	145-163
2"	160-171	167-185	178-199	10"	138-148	144-159	153-173
4"	168-179	177-195	187-209				

*Includes one pound for ordinary indoor clothing.
+Many established researchers consider the 1959 table of the Metropolitan Life Insurance Company more consistent with good health than revised tables with higher values.

Profile of an Overweight Person

- **Breakfast skimper**

- **Takes big bites; eats too fast**

- **Doesn't drink enough water**

- **Gets little, if any, exercise**

- **Uses salt freely**

- **Likes caffeinated drinks**

- **Is a nibbler—constantly eating**

- **Eats mostly refined foods—white breads, white rice, juices, candies, ice cream, etc.**

buoyant and weighs less under water. This difference allows for calculations of what percentage of a person's body is composed of fat.

One football player consistently weighed in over his maximum allowable weight. He just couldn't lose. Someone finally weighed him under water and found his body fat to be only 5 percent! (Ideally, a man should have 10 to 15 percent of body weight as fat. For women, 15 to 20 percent.)

Where can I get weighed under water?

Look for places that advertise health screening tests. Some of them have tanks of water for this purpose. Others use swimming pools. But it's an inconvenient and complicated process.

A simpler, more practical test is the pinch test. Trained health professionals use calipers to measure the thickness of skin folds at different places on the body. With the proper tables they can then calculate body fat percentages with fair accuracy.

You can do a simplified pinch test yourself. Reach over to your left side, just below the last rib, and pull the skin and fat away from the underlying muscle. Hold it between your thumb and index finger and squeeze. If the space between your thumb and finger is more than three fourths of an inch, you're in trouble!

Obesity can be dangerous. Disease, disability and premature death follow in its train. Next to lowering your cholesterol and quitting smoking, attaining and maintaining an ideal weight is the greatest favor you can do for yourself.

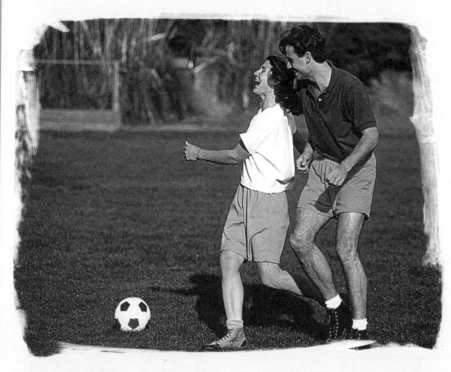

Whether we are obese or not still depends on the relationship between the amount of food we eat and the energy we use.

Application

Knowing your ideal weight is important. Studies show that people who remain near this target live longer, healthier lives. Find out how close (or far) you are from your ideal weight.

Tale of the Scale

The bathroom scale tells the story of our eating and exercise habits. It can also, for better or worse, predict our health in coming years.

Clinical Weight Definitions			
IDEAL	**WEIGHT**		
-10%	0	+10%	+20%
UNDERWEIGHT	NORMAL	OVER WEIGHT	OBESITY

How do you rate? Complete this easy exercise to find out. Before you begin, you will need to know your weight. Also have a calculator handy for calculating percentages.

Calculating Your Ideal Weight

For Men:

1. How many inches over five feet are you? _____

2. Multiply that number by six. _____

3. Add 100 to get your ideal weight. _____

For Women:

1. How many inches over five feet are you? _____

2. Multiply that number by five. _____

3. Add 106 to get your ideal weight. _____

For Women and Men:

Large-boned men and women should multiply their ideal weight by 1.05 to get an ideal weight adjusted for their build. Small-boned persons multiply by 0.95.

Normal Weight

Multiply your Ideal Weight by 1.09 = _____

If your weight is below this number, you are in the safe range. Regular exercise and a healthy diet will boost your energy and endurance while keeping your weight stable.

Overweight

Multiply your Ideal Weight by 1.20 = _____

If your weight is below this number but above normal weight, you are classified as overweight. Your weight has reached a level where it can affect your health and self-image. It is important to take action now to get your weight under control. Make the optimal diet and daily exercise a priority.

Obesity

If your weight takes you past overweight, then stop! You are in danger and need to take immediate action. Don't let anything stand between you and daily exercise. Learn to cook healthy meals and put the principles learned in the previous seven chapters into action. If you change your lifestyle now, you can feel years younger and enjoy a longer, healthier life.

Your Challenge:

A support network can keep you going when you feel like giving up. Find someone else interested in losing weight. Working together will make reaching your goals twice as easy —and twice as enjoyable. Also, graph your weight periodically and then post the record to keep you motivated.

It will boost your energy, increase your attention span, and help you lose weight—and it's legal! What is it? A good BREAKFAST

Jumpstart Your Day

Many people can't face food when they crawl out of bed. A quick cup of coffee is a standard adult breakfast. An increasing number of children arrive at school having eaten nothing at all.

Why bother with breakfast?

A group of scientists spent 10 years studying the effects of different kinds of breakfasts versus no breakfast at all on people of different ages.

A good breakfast, they concluded, can help both children and adults be less irritable, more efficient and more energetic. Breakfast helped children score higher on tests written before the noon recess. The steady influx of energy apparently stabilized glucose levels in the brain, improving mental function and attention span.

Other studies have even linked healthy breakfasts with less chronic disease, increased longevity and better health.

A good breakfast, by the way, is one that provides at least one third of the day's calories. Start your day with a whole-grain cereal, whole-grain bread, and a couple whole, fresh fruits, and you'll find that your energy level stays high throughout the morning.

What's wrong with orange juice and a Danish?

You need something with more fiber in it. Although fiber isn't digested by the body, it does absorb water as it moves through the stomach and intestines. The resulting spongy mass acts as a gen-

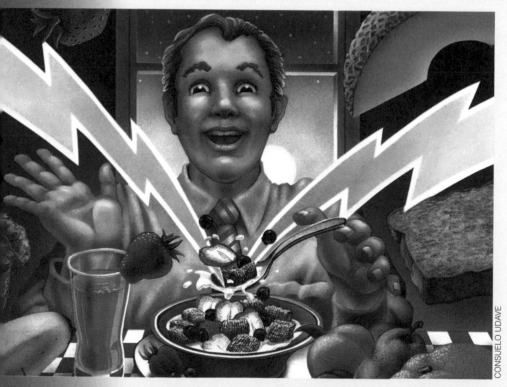

CONSUELO UDAVE

FOOD IS FUEL. *The brain cells have no stored blood sugar—no energy stores. A lot of people are needlessly fatigued because they're not eating early in the day. They skip breakfast.*

tle barrier to the food particles suspended in it so that they are not absorbed too quickly.

On the other hand, fiberless foods, especially sugared foods and drinks, quickly pass into the bloodstream, and cause blood sugar levels to rise and fall rapidly. No wonder energy and efficiency levels drop off in the later morning hours when little or no fiber-containing foods had been eaten at breakfast!

But I'm not hungry until midmorning!

Probably the biggest reason people feel that way is that they eat a large meal in the evening. (TV snacks don't help either!) When they go to bed, their stomachs are still busy digesting all that food. Since digestion goes into a "slower gear" during sleep, sometimes food is still in the stomach in the morning. But the stomach needs rest too. An exhausted stomach does not feel like taking on a big breakfast.

The solution?

- Eat a light supper at least four hours before bedtime, or even skip supper a few times.
- Eat or drink nothing but water or fruit between supper and bedtime.

If you do these two things, you'll be ready to break the fast of the long night.

Won't skipping breakfast help me lose weight?

Surprisingly, no. The Iowa Breakfast Studies demonstrated that the omission of breakfast does not have an advantage in weight reduction. It's actually a disadvantage because those who omit breakfast accentuate their hunger and eat more snacks and food the rest of the day to make up for the lack. They also suffer a significant loss of efficiency in the late-morning hours.

But I don't have time to eat breakfast.

Many people are in the habit of staying up late, then sleeping in as long as they can in the morning. Although a few people

Sugar in the morning?

You bet. Millions of us start the day with dessert, whether it's frosted Pop-Tarts, marshmallow-laden cereal, chocolate yogurt, or a muffin the size of a small TV. Then we spend the next 14 hours chugging more sweets, from a midmorning Danish to a vanilla shake at lunch to cookies after dinner. Meanwhile, soft drinks rise around us like flood-waters: we're swigging nearly 54 gallons a year per person!

work more efficiently at night, most don't fit that timetable.

Try going to bed early enough so you can wake up in the morning feeling refreshed and with time to spare. Begin the day by drinking a glass or two of water to rinse and freshen your stomach. Pull on your gym clothes and get some active exercise, like a brisk walk. Shower and dress for the day. Then fix and eat a hot breakfast.

This works with children, too. Put them to bed early enough so that they wake up in time to join the family around the breakfast table.

A good breakfast boosts your energy, increases your attention span, and heightens your sense of well-being. You'll be less apt to cheat on your diet by snacking. And you'll be in better control of your emotions.

What a great way to start your day!

BREAKFAST CHOICES				
	Calories	Fat (gm)	Salt (mg)	Chol. (mg)
STANDARD AMERICAN DIET				
Bacon (3 sl.)	129	12	574	60
Scrambled Eggs (3)	330	24	1230	675
Hash Browns (1 C)	355	18	3265	0
Danish Roll (1)	274	15	595	35
Hot Cocoa (1 C)	213	9	295	25
Orange Juice (1 C)	120	0	6	0
TOTAL	**1421**	**78**	**5965**	**795**
THE OPTIMAL DIET				
7 Grain Cereal (1 C)	159	1	400	0
Banana (1)	95	0	3	0
NF Milk (1 C)	88	0	318	0
Grapefruit (1/2)	66	0	5	0
Tofu (1 C)	118	7	1233	0
H. Browns, no oil (1 C)	101	0	22	0
W. W. Bread (1 sl.)	61	1	330	0
TOTAL	**688**	**9**	**2351**	**0**

How to Pick a Cereal

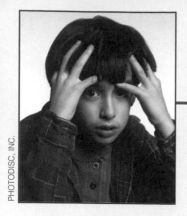

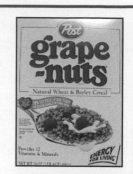

It's tough to pick a cereal these days. Do you go for fiber, or the least fat and sugar? Whole grains, or more vitamins? Or what the kids demand?

At $4.50 a pound, many cereals cost as much as or more than a pound of cheese, chicken breasts, or sirloin steak. That's because 55 percent of the price goes into marketing and profits—twice as much as the average for other foods.

- Be wary of names and claims. You can trust claims about nutrients, low-fat and high-fiber. But *Honey Nut Cheerios,* for example, has more sugar than honey and more salt than nuts. Check the ingredient list. If there is less fruit than sugar, skip it!

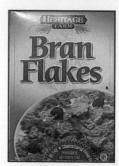

- Look for whole grains (to reduce cancer risk). Check ingredients to make sure the wheat and oats are "whole" or "rolled" and the rice is brown. Bran is also good.

- Check the fiber. Cancer experts advise up to 40 grams a day (most Americans get 10 to 15 grams). This means eat lots of whole grains, along with fruit, beans, and vegetables. Look for at least 10 grams of fiber per meal, and 15 grams if you are constipated.

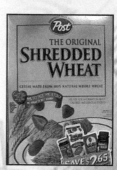

- Minimize sugar. It doesn't matter if it's honey, brown sugar, corn syrup, or fruit juice. They all have the same problems. Look for cereals with no more than five grams of added sugar per serving.

- Limit sodium. Look for the least amount of sodium.

- Watch out for fat traps. Most cereals are low in fat, but beware of granola and muesli. Stick to cereals with no more than three grams of fat per serving. Why not try a seven-grain cereal? You can find it in most supermarkets. Pour it into your Crockpot at night. Add enough water. Turn it on, and while you're sleeping your Crockpot is working. You wake up and a piping-hot delicious breakfast cereal is waiting for you. Just add some fresh fruit, a few raisins or dates, and some milk substitute, like rice milk, and you're purring. You started your day right. You're off and running!

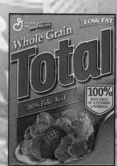

> "I've yet to meet an overweight person who doesn't skip breakfast and snack at night."
>
> –Pat Harper, R.D.
> American Dietetic Association

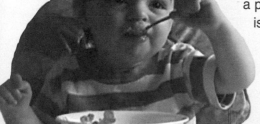

THE LUDINGTON GROUP

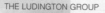

Application

A good breakfast boosts your energy, increases your attention span, and heightens your sense of well-being. Studies have now linked healthy breakfasts to less chronic disease, longer life, and better health.

Make the Most of Your Day

Many studies have emphasized the importance of breakfast. If you want to make the most of your day, fuel your body early with the right stuff. The following questions will help you examine your morning eating habits.

The Breakfast Quiz

1. Do you skip breakfast often? Mom was right: Breakfast really is the most important meal of the day. If you skip breakfast, you are starting the day at a disadvantage.

2. Do you get up in time to eat a good breakfast? If not, how could you change your routine to give yourself time for a nutritious morning meal? _____

_____

3. Are you hungry in the morning, or is your appetite a late riser? The preceding pages offer two solutions to this problem. What are they? _____

_____

4. Is your usual breakfast high in fiber from whole fruits and grains? The fiber and complex carbohydrates in whole foods provide a steady release of energy that most processed breakfast foods lack. It will keep you going strong all morning.

5. Is your breakfast high in fat and cholesterol? A traditional breakfast of eggs and sausage can be the most deadly meal of the day. Breakfast meats are loaded with fats, cholesterol, and salt. Egg yolks can send your cholesterol skyrocketing. The sausage-and-egg breakfast needs to go the way of the dinosaur if you want to avoid early extinction.

Based on what you have learned, how can you improve the quality of your breakfasts?

_____

_____

_____

Your Challenge:

Make eating a good breakfast a priority. Note any changes in your energy level and productivity. Here is a recipe to help get you started.

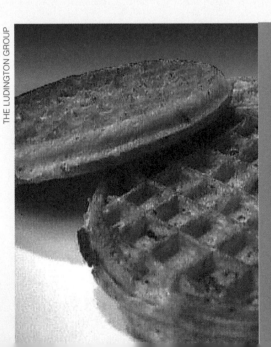

THE LUDINGTON GROUP

Cashew Oat Waffles

Blenderize the following ingredients until smooth. Bake in a preheated waffle iron for 10-12 minutes:

    1-1/2 c. regular rolled oats
    2 c. water
    1/3 c. raw cashews
    1/2 t. salt

Top with mashed bananas, fresh or frozen berries, applesauce, or crushed pineapple.

FAIL-SAFE FORMULA

Eat More, Weigh Less!

Every second adult in the United States is overweight. Despite 20 years of increasingly sophisticated diets, the average person is now nine pounds heavier.

That sounds pretty grim. Is there a brighter side?

Actually, there's a Mr. or Ms. Goodweight inside each one of us—it may just be stuck behind layers of discouragement, bulges of overindulgence, and mounds of misconceptions. We need to locate that special person inside and begin restoring the health, energy, and self-confidence that's been buried far too long.

How do you do that?

By finding a lifestyle that maintains health, increases energy, lowers the risk of disease, reduces food bills, and allows people to eat as much as they want and still lose weight without feeling hungry.

Surely that's an impossible dream!

Not really. Obesity occurs when calories eaten exceed the calories used by the body for physical activity and maintenance of its functions. These leftover calories are stored as fat. By the time 3,500 extra calories have accumulated, one pound of fat will have been deposited.

Adding an extra pat of butter (100 calories) to the daily diet will total up to 10 extra pounds of body fat in one year! On the other hand, omitting dessert (500 fewer

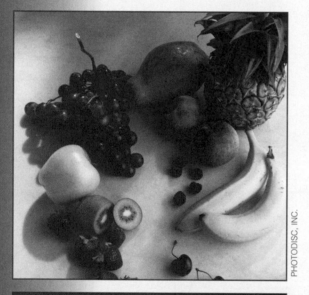

PHOTODISC, INC.

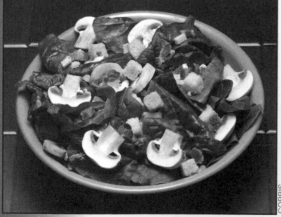

CORBIS

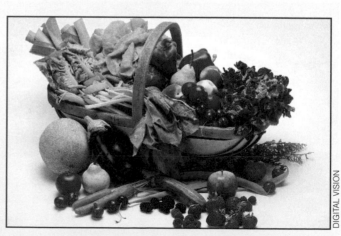

DIGITAL VISION

Each one of these salads has as many calories as you get from one tablespoon of most salad dressings.

Fast-food restaurants tempt from nearly every street corner with takeout service — but what they take out is nutrition!

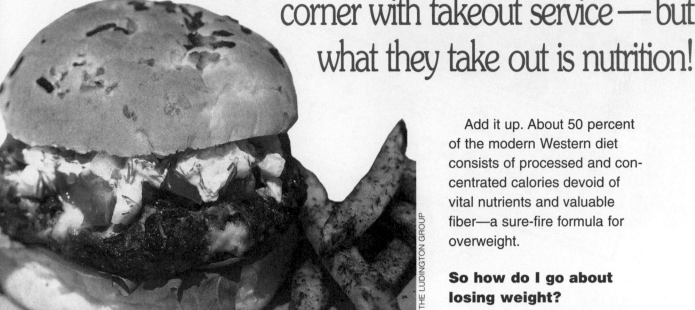

calories) for seven days will remove one pound of body fat.

The secret of success lies in finding a way to eat fewer calories instead of eating less food.

That sounds like a contradiction!

Today's world is full of contradictions. Popular magazines and TV screens brim with beautiful, slender people—and with full-color ads of rich, fattening foods. Supermarkets offer 25,000 slickly packaged, calorie-dense products, along with magazines touting the latest quickie diet. Fast-food restaurants tempt from nearly every street corner with takeout service—but nutrition is what they take out!

Modern food technology, has turned inexpensive, low calorie, high-volume foods into expensive, high-calorie, low-volume caloric bombs. It's now possible to eat a whole meal's worth of calories with only a few bites of food. No wonder people feel hungry and dissatisfied—and overeat!

How does it happen? *Processing* strips seven pounds of sugar beets of their bulk, fiber, and nutrients, producing one pound of pure sugar. Sugar and other refined sweeteners now account for more than 21 percent of daily calories eaten.

Technology takes 14 ears of corn and extracts one tablespoon of corn oil, which, along with its 110 calories, can be swallowed in one gulp! Extracted fats and oils account for another 20 percent of daily calories.

Grains, robbed of fiber and nutrients, can be turned into alcohol accounting for another 9 percent of empty calories many adults consume every day.

Add it up. About 50 percent of the modern Western diet consists of processed and concentrated calories devoid of vital nutrients and valuable fiber—a sure-fire formula for overweight.

So how do I go about losing weight?

If you love food but want to lose weight, then—

Eat more . . .

● Fresh and steamed vegetables, but go easy on sauces and salad dressings.

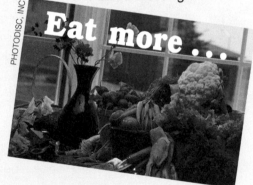

● Whole grains—cooked cereals, brown rice, whole-grain breads and pasta.

● Tubers and other vegetables—potatoes, yams, squash, and all kinds of beans, lentils, and peas.

● Fresh, whole fruits.

These *foods as grown* are filling, nutritious, inexpensive, and low in calories.

177

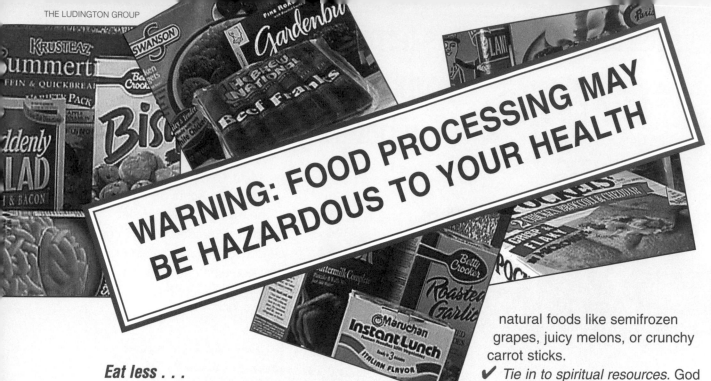

WARNING: FOOD PROCESSING MAY BE HAZARDOUS TO YOUR HEALTH

Eat less . . .

- Refined, processed, and concentrated foods. They are high in calories and price and low in nutrients and fiber.
- Nuts, meats, and rich dairy products. While these foods are nutritious they have little fiber and bulk and are very high in fat and calories. Meats and cheeses, for instance, are 60 to 80 percent fat.

CORBIS

Anything else?

✔ *Drink plenty of water*—six to eight glasses a day. Try herb teas, mineral water, or just plain water. Keep the sodas for special occasions.

✔ *Walk briskly every day.* Keep at it until you can walk at least 30 minutes without fatigue or shortness of breath.

✔ *Beware of weak moments:*

- If one cookie leads to a dozen, don't eat the first one.
- Don't buy problem foods. If they are not around, you won't be tempted.
- If you feel bored, frustrated or lonely, go for a walk, drink a glass of water, read a book, call a supportive friend. Or you can feast on

natural foods like semifrozen grapes, juicy melons, or crunchy carrot sticks.

✔ *Tie in to spiritual resources.* God didn't make nobodies. He created you for health and prosperity.

It's time to put an end to those unbalanced semi-starvation diets that leave you frustrated, dissatisfied and craving more to eat. Begin a lifestyle that will recondition your habits toward a lifetime of better health. By avoiding popular trends and choosing the right kinds of foods you can eat more and still lose one to two pounds a week.

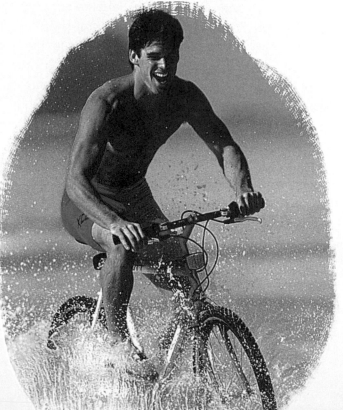

Application

It is possible to eat as much as you want and still lose weight. The secret is knowing which foods to eat and which to avoid. Whole plant foods that promote good health and prevent disease are also ideal for taking weight off and keeping it off—for good.

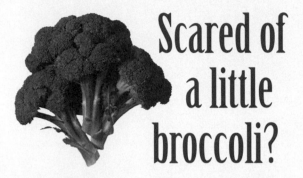

Scared of a little broccoli?

Food Selection

For most of us, getting permanent control of a ballooning waistline requires a radical shift in diet. The table below summarizes the food selection principles presented in this book.

Weight loss Tips: Attitude

Focus on the hundreds of foods that you *can* eat, not on those you shouldn't.

Be kind to yourself. It takes time to adapt to a new way of eating and living. Be patient and don't give up if you make a mistake or slip back into old habits. You are making a long-term investment in yourself. Keep going.

Eat freely from the following:

✔ **Fruit: All fresh fruit (avocado and olives sparingly)**

✔ **Vegetables: All vegetables, greens, herbs, squash**

✔ **Legumes: All beans, peas, lentils, garbanzos**

✔ **Tubers: Potatoes, yams, sweet potatoes**

✔ **Grains: All whole grains, breads, pastas**

✔ **Nuts: Eat sparingly**

Eight Steps to Permanent Weight Control

1. Build your diet around fruits, vegetables, grains, legumes, and other "as grown" foods.

2. Forget "quickie" diets. Make the Optimal Diet your diet. (See Coda, page 246.)

3. Reduce the oils, butters, dressings and other fats you add to foods.

4. Read labels carefully and choose foods very low in fat, sugar, and salt.

5. Make water your drink of choice. Avoid high-calorie beverages.

6. Kick the snack habit. Begin each day with a hearty breakfast that makes mid-morning snacking unnecessary.

7. Make exercise a part of your routine. Walk regularly.

8. Develop a support network with others who share your interest in making positive lifestyle changes.

Your Challenge:

Begin to integrate everything you have found helpful in the past 10 lessons. You can release the slender person inside of you and enjoy a happier, healthier life.

Unit Review:

This is the last of 10 units devoted to weight control. As you have worked through them, we have encouraged you to try many new behaviors. Now that you have had a chance to experiment, we hope you will make them a permanent part of your life. (See "Eight Steps" list above.)

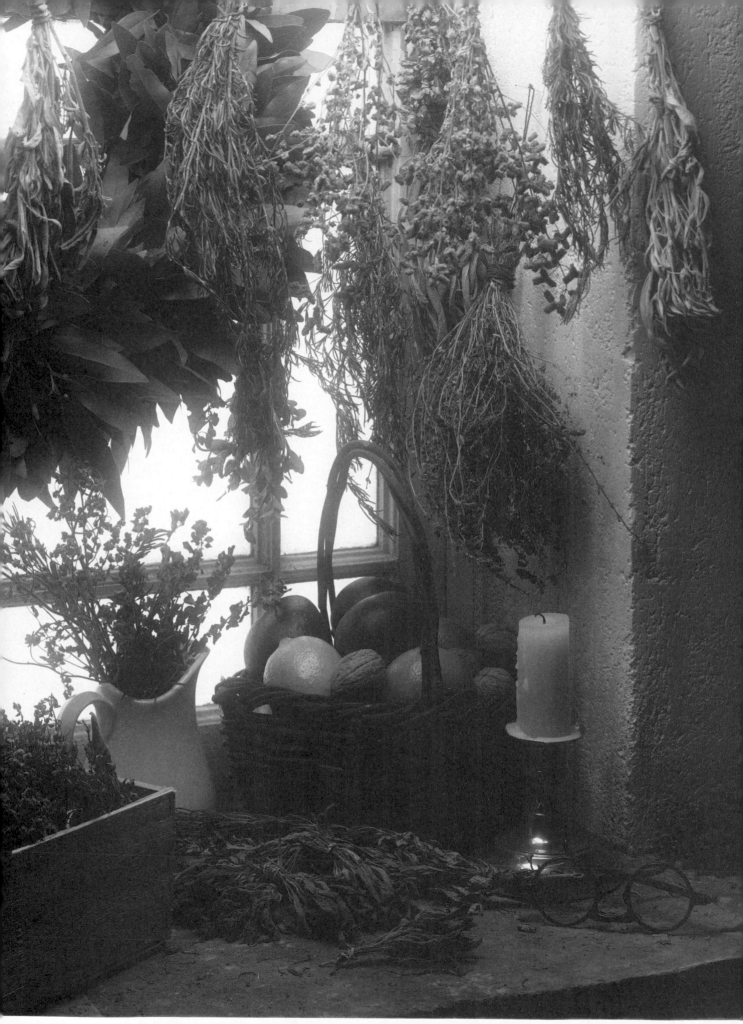

NATURAL REMEDIES

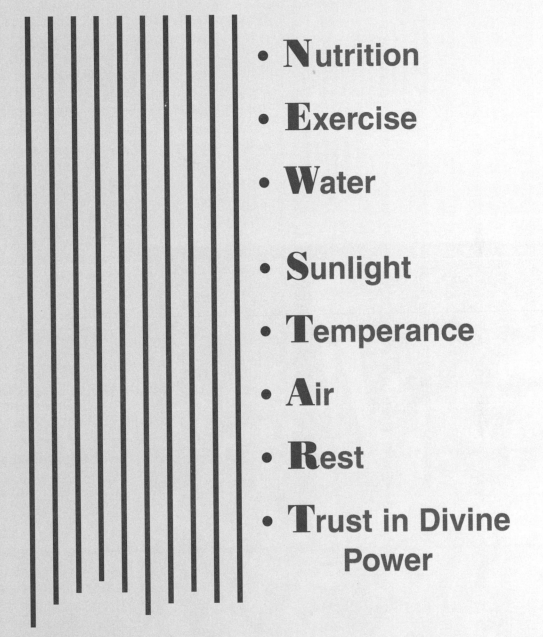

- **N**utrition
- **E**xercise
- **W**ater
- **S**unlight
- **T**emperance
- **A**ir
- **R**est
- **T**rust in Divine Power

"Now the Lord God had planted a garden in the east, in Eden; and there he put the [man and woman] he had formed. And the Lord God made all kinds of trees grow out of the ground—trees that were pleasing to the eye and good for food." Genesis 2:8, 9

NUTRITION

N E W S T A R T

The Ultimate Diet

Vegetarians are sprouting up all over—more than 16 million in the United States alone. Once stereotyped as food fanatics or leftover hippies, vegetarians are now widely respected. They are considered healthier and their diet more ecologically sound.

Why go to the trouble of being a vegetarian?

Seven out of 10 Americans suffer and die prematurely of three killer diseases: heart disease, cancer, and stroke. In his comprehensive report to the nation, titled *Nutrition and Health,* C. Everett Koop, M.D., stated unequivocally that the Western diet was the major contributor to these diseases. He confirmed that saturated fat and cholesterol, eaten in disproportionate amounts, were the main culprits. He reminded people that animal products are the largest source of saturated fat as well as the only source of cholesterol. To compound the problem, Dr. Koop pointed out, these foods are usually eaten at the expense of complex-carbohydrate-rich foods such as grains, legumes and vegetables.

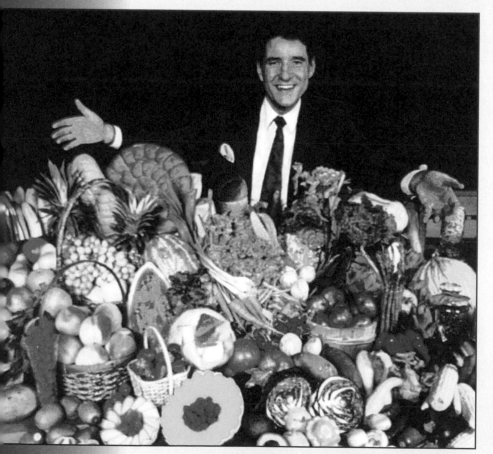

The average risk of heart disease for a man eating meat, eggs and dairy products is 45 percent. The risk for a man who leaves off meat is 15 percent. However, the coronary risk of a vegetarian who leaves off meat, eggs, and dairy products drops to only 4 percent.

An editorial in the *Journal of the American Medical Association* commented on these advantages. It said, "A total vegetarian diet can prevent up to 90 percent of our strokes and 97 percent of our heart attacks."

Going beyond prevention, Dr. Dean Ornish published studies proving, beyond a shadow of a doubt, that a very-low-fat vegetarian diet could reverse heart

"Then God said, 'I give you every seed-bearing plant on the face of the whole earth and every tree that has fruit with the seed in it. They will be yours for food.'" Genesis 1:29

BREADS and CEREALS

These foods have a high complex carbohydrate content and provide the body with energy. Sources: whole-grain bread, hot cereals, pasta, and brown rice.

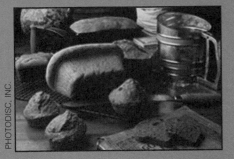

FRUITS and VEGGIES

This group is a primary source of phytochemicals and antioxidants, vitamins and minerals. Sources: for vitamin A, select dark-green, orange or yellow vegetables; for vitamin C, select citrus fruits, strawberries, tomatoes, and potatoes.

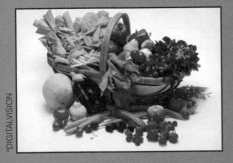

LEGUMES

Beans rate high in soluable fiber, protein, and energy, as well as phytochemicals and antioxidants. Because they contain a plant hormone called phytoestrogens, soybeans are hard to beat among the beans.

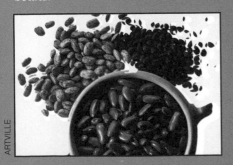

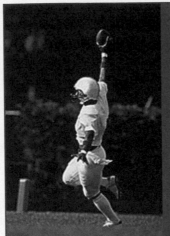

The Dallas...Vegeboys?

A few years ago the Super Bowl-winning Dallas Cowboys were rated the healthiest team in the NFL by the Professional Football Athletic Trainers Society. How did they do it? The players ate six daily servings of fruits and vegetables along with plenty of low-fat, grain-based foods such as bread and spaghetti.

Gone are the seasons during which beefy linebackers thought they had to eat a steady diet of red meat.

disease in patients scheduled for coronary-bypass surgery.

The risk for cancer of the prostate, breast, and colon is three to four times higher for people who consume meat, eggs, and dairy products on a daily basis when compared to those who eat them sparingly or not at all. In addition, vegetarian women have stronger bones and fewer fractures, and they lose less bone as they age.

Studies of long-lived vegetarian people like the Hunzas, who are healthy and active into advanced age, contrast sharply with the short life spans and increased disease rates of traditional Eskimos, who depend largely on what they catch from the sea.

Are there significant ecological effects?

Shifting toward a vegetarian lifestyle would greatly ease the environmental impact of our present meat-centered diet. Pollution from animal-based agriculture is greater than from all other

human and industrial activities combined. Overgrazing and intense cultivation of land for production of animal foods contributes substantially to the massive erosion and the irretrievable loss of 6 billion tons of valuable topsoil annually in America.

But the impact of a meat-centered diet goes beyond North America. In Central America, for example, irreparable damage with global implications continues on a daily basis. Americans eat more than 200 million pounds of Central American beef every year. Powerful landowners have destroyed nearly half the region's rain forests, turning them into grazing lands for the cattle needed to supply the ever-expanding hamburger chains. Some 55 square feet of land is needed to produce a single pound of hamburger.

Doesn't this impact the world's food supplies?

By moving away from a meat-centered diet, we could use our grains and beans to

1 8 3

Medicate yourself with food instead of pills.

feed the world's hungry people instead of the world's cattle and poultry. The amount of land needed to feed one person consuming a meat-based diet would feed 20 vegetarians. One acre of land yields only 183 pounds of beef, but 20,000 pounds of potatoes. To produce one pound of edible flesh from a feedlot steer requires 10 pounds of grain and soybeans. It's a poor conversion system that operates at a 10 percent efficiency level!

Are vegetarians able to meet their nutrient needs?

Easily. The recommended daily allowance (RDA) for protein is 45 to 60 grams for adults, which works out to about 10 to 15 percent of calories eaten. A beefsteak offers about 25 percent of its calories as usable protein. The protein content of grains usually exceeds 10 percent of total calories, and dried beans and peas carry close to 25 percent of their calories as usable protein. Even vegetables average about 20 percent of their calories as protein. So there is plenty of protein in plant foods, which are also low in fat, high in fiber, and cholesterol-free.

Studies show that complementary proteins and iron and calcium supplies are essentially nonproblems in humans eating a variety of plant foods, although pure vegetarians may require small supplements of vitamin B_{12}.

Will switching to a vegetarian diet affect my weight?

If you replace the meat in your diet with doughnuts, Twinkies, french fries, and other high-fat, high-sugar morsels, then, yes, you will probably gain weight.

If you choose, however, to eat more foods-as-grown, simply prepared, without those nutrition-depleted calories, you can shed excess weight and stabilize at a healthier level.

Any suggestions for making the transition?

Some people can switch to a vegetarian diet cold turkey, but others do it more gradually, eliminating red meat first, then poultry, fish, and finally dairy products.

Another idea is to begin with one or more meatless days a week. As you experiment with vegetarian dishes, you can gradually increase the number of meatless meals.

Switching to a less meat-centered diet is really not such a big deal. We already eat bean burritos, pasta, and other standard meatless fare. Stretch your imagination. Enjoy the varied tastes. Save on your food dollar. And savor a new level of health.

The evidence against meat continues to grow as it once did for cigarettes. The vegetarian diet is proving to be the ultimate diet—maximizing health, preventing disease, releasing food to the hungry, and preserving the planet. It's time for Americans to stop slaughtering 9 million creatures every day for food.

Take the first step toward a vegetarian diet—and begin to celebrate a healthier life!

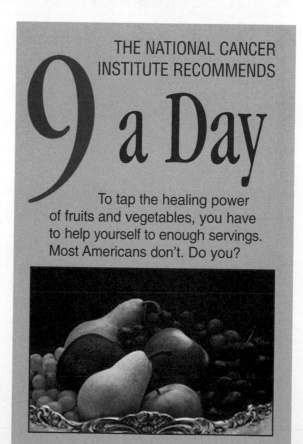

THE NATIONAL CANCER INSTITUTE RECOMMENDS

9 a Day

To tap the healing power of fruits and vegetables, you have to help yourself to enough servings. Most Americans don't. Do you?

Application

Vegetarians are no longer viewed as food fanatics and counterculture odd-balls. Studies confirm that most live longer, healthier lives, and they leave a softer footprint on the earth—they are ecologically tuned in. Making the transition to a meat-free diet can be a challenging adventure, leading to a new level of good health and well-being.

The Optimal Diet

By now you have been exposed to the optimal diet several times. Here are some questions to see how much you remember:

1. Are animal products necessary for good health and nutrition?
   __ Yes
   __ No

2. What is the average risk of heart disease for a man eating meat, eggs, and dairy products?
   __ 15%
   __ 35%
   __ 45%
   __ 75%

3. On average, vegetarians are:
   __ Heavier than meat eaters
   __ Thinner than meat eaters
   __ Weigh the same as meat eaters

4. Where do most of the calories in meat come from?
   __ Fat
   __ Protein
   __ Carbohydrates

5. Where is cholesterol found?
   __ All foods
   __ Peanut butter
   __ All animal products
   __ Plant foods

6. Meat-centered diets have been linked with:
   __ Heart disease
   __ Stroke
   __ Cancer
   __ All of the above

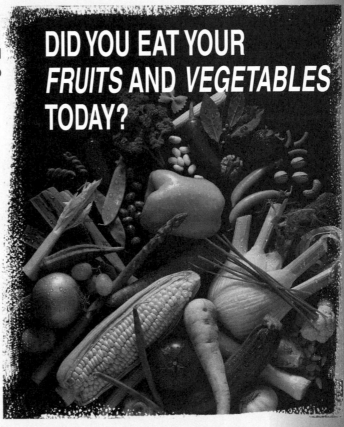

DID YOU EAT YOUR *FRUITS* AND *VEGETABLES* TODAY?

Lunch on the Go

For busy people, lunch is often a difficult meal. The temptation is to grab something quick. Fortunately, quick does not have to mean a burger from a fast-food restaurant. With some advance planning, you can take a healthful lunch wherever you go.

Your Challenge:

Meat can be hazardous to your health. Start eliminating it from your diet by making your own delicious lunches.

Answers
1. No 2. 45% 3. Thinner 4. Fat
5. All animal products 6. All of the above

EXERCISE

Modern Fountain of Youth

The fabled fountain of youth lured ancient adventurers into a lifetime of fruitless searching. In time it became a symbol for an impossible dream. That was yesterday. Today science seems able to put at least part of this dream within reach of nearly all of us.

In today's world, sweat is status and trimness is success. More and more modern executives are apt to be in prime condition.

What do you mean?

When the explorers were searching for a secret spring that would maintain perpetual youth, many people were dying in early adulthood of infectious diseases. Today improved sanitation and hygiene, along with antibiotics and vaccines, have almost eliminated those diseases. The battle has now shifted to lifestyle diseases. These are the maladies that are now robbing us of our energy, disabling us prematurely, and killing us s-l-o-w-l-y.

The good news is that greater vitality, better health and longer life can be ours through regular, brisk physical activity.

Do you mean EXERCISE? Can it really do all that?

Take a look at the facts. The adage "Use it or lose it" applies not only to muscles and bones but also to hearts, lungs, brains, blood vessels, joints and every other part of the body. A sedentary lifestyle is a direct route to an earlier grave. Inactivity kills us—literally.

A healthful lifestyle can hold back the aging processes as much as 30 years.

PHOTODISC, INC.

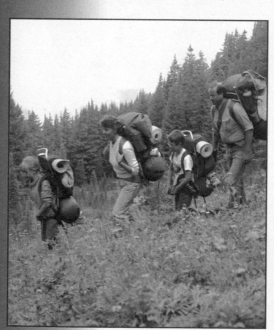

CORBIS

PHOTODISC, INC.

"The Lord God took the man and put him in the Garden of Eden to work it and take care of it." Genesis 2:15

Just being thin and "hip" isn't enough anymore. To be beautiful today, you have to be healthy and fit. And to be healthy and fit, you've got to exercise.

A strong genetic inheritance helps some people survive incredible odds. But just living longer isn't today's only concern. Along with their lengthened years people are looking for energy, good health, usefulness, and quality of life.

Just how does physical exercise help us live longer and better?

Here are some of the ways:

● Exercise helps us FEEL GOOD! Life becomes more fun, and the high that comes from exercise won't let you down later. Moreover, the hormones producing the exercise high are proving to be health promoting as well.

● Exercise strengthens the heart. This is important in a culture in which every sec-ond person dies of heart and vascular disease.

● Exercise lowers blood pressure and resting heart rate, protecting the heart and blood vessels.

● Exercise lowers LDL cholesterol levels in the blood and often raises HDL cholesterol, again decreasing heart and vascular risk. (LDL is the bad part of cholesterol; HDL the good part.)

● Exercise strengthens bones by helping retain calcium and other minerals.

● Exercise lifts depression. Outdoor exercise is one of the most valuable tools for fighting this common and disabling malady.

● Exercise relieves anxiety and stress. In our harried, pressured society, physical

activity is proving to be an effective antidote.

● Exercise increases overall energy and efficiency in all areas of our lives.

● Exercise helps maintain desirable weight levels. It builds muscles and burns fat. Moderate exercise blunts appetite by temporarily increasing blood sugar levels.

● Exercise improves circulation, and that makes for clearer minds, better sleep, and faster healing of damaged body areas.

What kind of exercise are you talking about? Not everyone can jog, or run marathons.

Every one of these listed benefits can come from plain, simple walking. Walking is the ideal

PUT MORE ZEST IN YOUR LIFE!

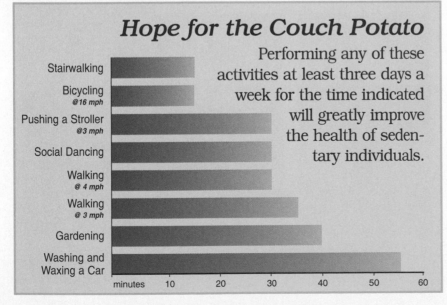

Hope for the Couch Potato

Performing any of these activities at least three days a week for the time indicated will greatly improve the health of sedentary individuals.

	minutes	10	20	30	40	50	60
Stairwalking							
Bicycling @16 mph							
Pushing a Stroller @3 mph							
Social Dancing							
Walking @ 4 mph							
Walking @ 3 mph							
Gardening							
Washing and Waxing a Car							

187

Easy Ways to Stay Fit for Life

exercise. It's inexpensive. It's safe. Nearly everyone can do it. And it's fun! You can select your own speed, and you can stop when you want. As your fitness improves, you can gradually add speed and time.

Other good exercises are swimming, bicycling, gardening, yard work, and golf—if you leave the carts behind. For hardier souls, jogging, stair climbing, rock climbing, jumping rope, and skiing provide challenging variations. In bad weather, try stationary bicycles, trampolines, rowing machines, or simply walking or jogging in place. To be effective, active (aerobic) exercise should be brisk and continuous for at least 15 to 20 minutes. Most people can work up to this goal. A daily program of 30 to 40 minutes of active exercise will give you maximum benefits. To lose weight, and for diabetics needing to control their blood sugar, increase the time to one hour. You can divide the hour into two or three sessions if you wish.

Is it true that reaching a certain pulse rate is necessary for exercise to be effective?

There are exercise regimes for specific purposes. The concept of training heart rate is particularly useful in strengthening the heart. Weight and flexibility training is also proving to be valuable. Remember: even moderate activities, such as brisk walking, will improve fitness. Every step counts.

But I hate to exercise. It's boring!

We all do many boring things every day: brushing our teeth, cleaning the house, washing the car, mowing the lawn, doing dishes, going to work. But we do these things because we like the rewards: beautiful teeth, an attractive home, a clean car, a regular paycheck. After a while these activities become routine, an accepted part of our daily living.

Let's look at exercise the same way. Its benefits are far greater than a clean house—they will last a lifetime.

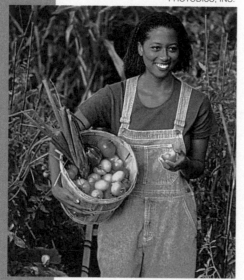

PHOTODISC, INC.

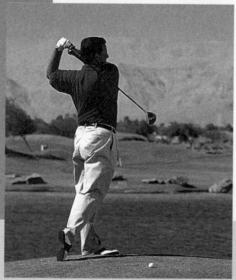

PHOTODISC, INC.

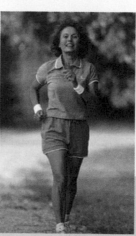

DIGITALVISION

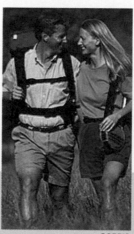

CORBIS

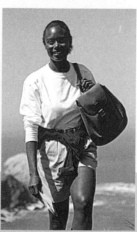

PHOTODISC, INC.

Application

Exercise slows down the aging process. It strengthens the heart, lowers blood pressure, relieves stress, preserves muscle function, and helps you maintain a desirable weight. You don't need expensive equipment or a health club membership to start. Walking can provide all these benefits and more.

The 10-Step Exercise Program

Have you tried exercise before and found that you just couldn't stick with it? If so, you should try the world's easiest exercise system. It's called the 10-Step Program.

All you do is make a commitment to the first 10 steps of a daily walk. That's it. You get out and take those steps every day. Once they're behind you, you can turn around and go home, if you wish.

The system works because it eases you past those difficult first steps. It gets you up and going. And if you are like most people, once you get going you will finish the entire walk.

The 10-Step Program also keeps you in the habit of exercising even when you can't manage your full routine. You might be sick, or traveling, yet in almost every situation you can manage 10 steps. In this way you maintain the exercise habit even when you can't exercise. That's important if you want to enjoy the benefits of fitness for the rest of your life.

Plan Ahead

A useful technique is to plan your exercise sessions in advance. If you are an early riser, try exercising before breakfast. If your morning is already too full, walk during your lunch hour or in the evening. The important thing is to find a time that is right for you.

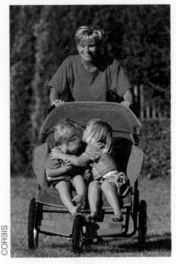

CORBIS

People Make Exercise Fun

Many people complain that exercise is boring. To liven up your sessions, include friends and family members in your exercise activities. If they won't join you, take the dog out for a stroll. Exercise can be enjoyable if you approach it with an attitude of fun and creativity.

Your Challenge:

Schedule your exercise sessions in advance and use the 10-Step Program to get you moving. Regular exercise is as necessary as air, water, and wholesome food. Don't let another day go by without it.

A newer concept for fitness recommends:

- Aerobic exercise for 30 minutes three times weekly.
- Alternate with 30 minutes of strength and flexibility training three times a week.

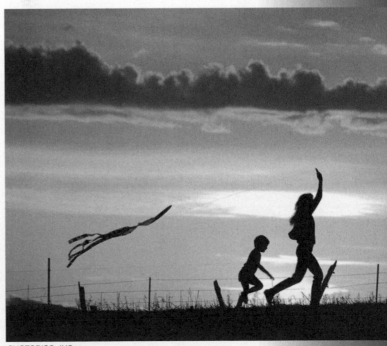

PHOTODISC, INC.

WATER

The No-calorie Wonder

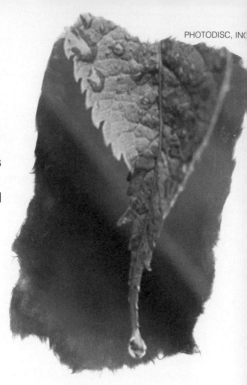

Forcing the body to work with limited amounts of fluid is like trying to wash the dinner dishes in a cupful of water. When you don't drink enough water, the body must excrete wastes in a much more concentrated form, causing body odor, bad breath, and unpleasant-smelling urine.

Don't most people get the water they need?

It's been said that the French don't drink water, only wine. We smile at this, but it's becoming a reality in America today. Our kids are drowning in soft drinks—soda pop has become their main beverage. The average teenager downs two to three cans a day, and some as many as six and seven. Many adults drink more beer than water. In addition, plenty of tea, coffee, and other beverages are consumed.

Notice what happens next time you go to a restaurant for a meal. You will usually be served a glass of ice water and then asked expectantly, "And what would you like to drink?"

How many glasses of just plain water does the average American drink? The truth for many is—hardly any.

"A river watering the garden flowed from Eden."
Genesis 2:10

HEARTBURN?

Drink some water every half hour. This will give you a regular stress break, and also wash the acid out of your esophagus and dilute it.

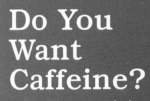
Does it matter what beverages I drink? They all contain water, don't they?

Our bodies are about 70 percent water, and our kidneys process more than 47 gallons of it in a day. Without it we'd look more wrinkled than California raisins!

But why is this colorless, tasteless, calorie-and-salt-free substance so absolutely necessary?

The answer lies in the physiological workings of the body. Water to the body is like oil to a car engine. It's the magic lubricant that makes everything else work. A drink of water is exactly what the body needs to carry out all

its life processes.

Beverages other than water, however, pose special problems. Many have calories that must be digested like food. Such calories may produce extra fat, blood sugar swings, and a slowed digestion. Many beverages increase the secretion of acid in the stomach. Some popular sodas contain phosphoric acid that can help deplete the body's calcium supplies, thus contributing to brittle bones.

Sugar in beverages requires extra water for metabolism. Recent studies have demonstrated that caffeine and alcohol dehydrate the body because they work as diuretics. This can contribute to fatigue, dry skin, indigestion, and headaches. The solution? For every alcoholic drink, for every cup of coffee, for every

cola, be sure you drink an extra glass of water.

Do the "no sugar" diet drinks solve these problems?

Diet beverages don't contain sugar, but they present other concerns. Nearly all beverages, sugared or not, contain chemicals that are added for color, flavor, preservation, and other reasons. Some of these may irritate delicate stomach linings, and some may also require the liver and kidneys to detoxify and dispose of them.

Drinking water eliminates all of these problems. It has no extra calories to slow down digestion or to add unwanted fat. It has no irritants to stress the sensitive linings of the digestive tract, fewer chemicals to threaten delicate body machinery, and no caffeine. It's readily available, and it's cheap!

How much water should I drink?

Drink enough to keep the urine pale. The body loses about 10 to 12 cups of water a day through the skin, lungs, urine, and feces. Food provides two to four cups of water, leaving us about eight glasses of water to drink.

Get into the habit of drinking water liberally. Drink on arising,

191

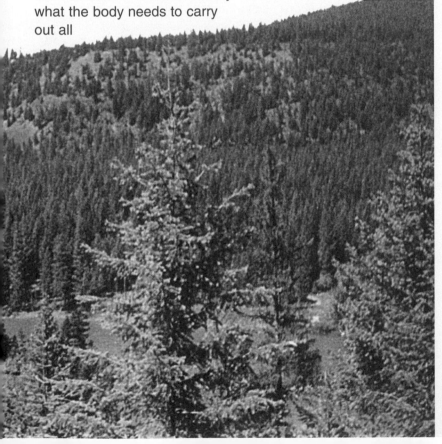

in midmorning and midafternoon. A drink of water is like an internal shower. It rinses the stomach and prepares it for its work.

So start the day right. Give that early-morning drink some zest by adding a twist of lemon. Then during morning and afternoon coffee breaks, reach for a glass of water and drink to your body's content. Tempted to snack? Replace it with a drink of water. It's magic!

Water is the perfect beverage, and one of life's greatest blessings. The next time you are asked, "Anything to drink?" you can say, "Yes, a glass of water is fine. In fact, it's perfect."

Bottled? or Tap?

With reports of contamination by heavy metals, nuclear wastes, fertilizers, pesticides, herbicides, and leaking fuels—some people are afraid to drink the water that comes out of their kitchen faucet.

With good reason, wouldn't you say?

Many Americans think so. Consumers spent $4 billion last year on bottled waters. But are they getting what they are paying for?

One problem is that the federal and state requirements are exactly the same for both bottled and tap water. Another concern is the absence of fluoride in bottled watter. Also, once opened, bottled water may be more vulnerable to bacteria due to the absence of chlorine.

Since most municipal systems are tested daily, if your water supply is up to standard, what comes out of your faucet may be just as safe as the bottled water you buy. And it's hundreds of times cheaper!

What can I do if my tap water is unsafe?

One way you can protect yourself is by installing your own filtering system: a good charcoal filter removes most contaminants and makes the water taste good.

If you depend on private wells, your local government may test your water for a nominal fee. National mail order testing services are also available.

But bottled waters taste so much better!

Sometimes they do, but not always. If you are willing to pay, there are many alternative choices (see sidebar on left).

The irony of it all is that most of us face more health hazards from not drinking enough water than we do from its possible contaminants.

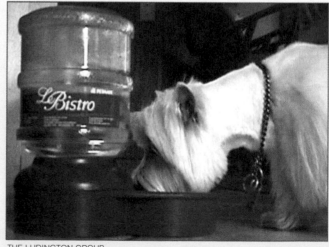

THE LUDINGTON GROUP

Application

Today North Americans drink more soft drinks and alcoholic beverages than water. These substitutes force the body to deal with calories and chemicals, and can disturb the process of digestion. The body needs water to function properly. When you want refreshment, choose the real thing—water.

Most People Should Drink More

Water really is the most healthful drink. We can only live a few days in its absence. Even though we all get enough to sustain us, most people don't drink enough for optimum functioning. We sip enough to survive, when we should be drinking enough to thrive. The result is unnecessary stress placed on the body's cleansing system and other functions.

Start Early

One way to make sure you get your daily quota is by drinking two glasses of water when you wake up in the morning. Do this before you get caught up in the activities of the day. With two glasses down, you only need to drink six more during the rest of the day. That is a feat everyone can manage. If you wait until you are thirsty, you probably won't get enough.

Worried About Contaminents?

In most cases, the health hazards we face from not drinking enough water are greater than those from possible contaminants in the water supply. If you are concerned, have your water tested, or install a good charcoal filter. A filter helps purify your water and makes it taste better.

NEED MORE ENERGY?
You could be dehydrated. Drink lots of water and find out.

Fighting Where the Battle Is

What makes more sense, eating fruits and vegetables needed for good health, or avoiding them on the off chance that they may contain pesticide residue?

Likewise, what makes more sense, drinking the eight glasses of water that your body needs to flush out toxins, or avoiding tap water for fear that it may contain something dangerous? Be good to yourself: start enjoying nature's super fluid today.

ART TODAY

5 to stay alive

8 to feel great

10 to rejuvenate

SUNLIGHT

Kiss of the Sun

Excessive exposure to sunlight can cause skin cancer as well as premature wrinkling and aging of the skin. In proper amounts, however, the sun's rays can be good for your health.

You say "proper amounts." Can sunlight be measured?

Yes. It's important to understand the power of sunlight. Most of us have observed how dim even the brightest electric light bulb appears in daylight. The intensity of light is measured in "lux," or "luxes." For example, outdoor light can reach 3,000 lux on a bright sunny day. A bright indoor environment may provide only 400 lux, less than 15 percent of daylight brightness.

In recent years melatonin, a natural body hormone, has been found to enhance sleep. Melatonin levels reach a peak in children, and fall slowly and steadily throughout adult life. This may explain why children sleep so much better than older people.

The body carefully regulates melatonin production. The process is largely controlled by the light-dark cycle. Optimal melatonin production occurs only at night, in a dark environment. The pineal gland, located in the center of the brain, is the "clock" that regulates this process at the right time.

Melatonin is not stored in the body. We need a liberal supply each evening to sleep well. Studies demonstrate that daily exposure to natural sunlight will boost melatonin output. Artificial light is a weak substitute, as are manufactured supplements.

Besides improving sleep, what else does sunlight have to offer?

Sunlight is an efficient germ killer. That's why it is important to sun and air out blankets, quilts, and other items that are not washed regularly and steril-ized in an automatic dryer.

"And God said, 'let there be light,' and there was light. God saw that the light was good, and he separated the light from the darkness." - Genesis 1:3, 4

Let there be light!

Proper amounts of sunshine also give the skin a healthy glow and help make it smooth and pliable. A moderately tanned skin is more resistant to infections and sunburns than untanned skin.

Also, sunlight elevates the mood for most people, producing a sense of well-being. (Just don't stay out too long and get sunburned!) Combined with active exercise, sunshine is an important adjunct in treating acute and chronic depressions. Remember, when depressed during winter's cold and gloomy months, try to catch any possible ray of sunshine.

What's more, the body is able to manufacture vitamin D by the action of sunlight on the skin. Vitamin D enables the body to pick up calcium from the intestines for use in building healthy bones. It prevents both childhood and adult rickets and aids in the prevention of osteoporosis.

Sunlight also helps to:

- enhance the immune system
- alleviate pain from swollen arthritic joints
- relieve certain symptoms of PMS
- lower blood cholesterol levels

Is there a flip side?

Sunlight is a major risk factor for skin cancer, especially in light-skinned people. Too much sunlight, for them, may be particularly damaging.

You should also know that burning the skin is extremely harmful for everyone. Every burn destroys healthy, living tissue. Repeated burns cause irreversible damage and can set up a person for skin cancer.

And if all that isn't bad enough, repeated sunburn and even repeated deep tanning of the skin gradually destroy its elasticity and its oil glands, producing wrinkling and premature aging.

Some studies suggest that a high-fat diet, when combined with exposure to sunlight, may also promote cancers of the skin.

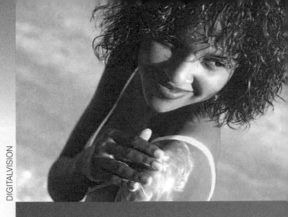

DIGITALVISION

Did You Know?

- *An extra hour of light a day may lift your spirits and affect your energy, sleep, fertility and even PMS.*

- *Seasonal variations in light levels can have a profound effect on mental health. This is clearest in people suffering from seasonal affective disorder (SAD)—a depressive illness that is successfully treated with light therapy.*

- *People getting more sunshine are less likely to get breast, colon or prostate cancer.*

195

What are some guidelines for safe, healthy exposure to sunlight?

- Modest tanning is protective, like putting sunglasses on your skin. But you must understand your own tolerance to sunlight. Fair-skinned people and redheads may have to begin with only five minutes of exposure to the sun per day. Darker-skinned people can

EARTH is a solar-powered world, 98 percent of its warmth coming from sunshine (the rest from geothermal heat). Solar energy lifts rain clouds, drives winds, and sparks the photosynthesis in plants, which feed all living things.

NASA uses bright light exposure to reset biological rhythms of the astronauts to decrease rocket lag (and jet lag).

Most of us no longer wake up with the dawn, spend the day outdoors, and sleep when it's dark.

begin with 10 to 15 minutes per day. Up to 30 minutes of sunshine, exposing as much of the body as possible, is a realistic goal for most people.

- Never, never burn! Malignant melanoma, the deadliest form of skin cancer, kills nearly 7,000 Americans a year; squamous cell carcinoma, more than 2,000. Sunburns raise the risk of both. A study in Israel found that Orthodox Jews, who wear coats and hats or shawls year-round, were much less prone to melanoma than were Israelis who regularly exposed their skin to the sun.

  Wear protective clothing, eyewear, and a protective sunscreen if needed. Be especially careful around snow or water and on cloudy days.

- If you have an outdoor trip or vacation coming up, prepare your skin by giving it progressive exposure in the days beforehand, to the point of pinking up.

- A few minutes of sunshine on your face and hands each day will produce all the vitamin D you need.

- Open up your house to the sunshine each morning. It will improve your health and lift your spirits.

- Just remember that artificial light is a very poor substitute for the real thing. Spend a little time each day soaking up some daylight.

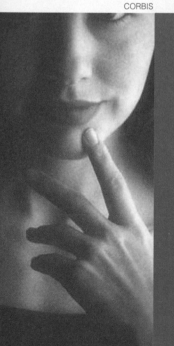

For thousands of years sunlight has been known as a mediator of life. But we know today that it can be healing or destructive; it can be the kiss of life or the kiss of death, depending on how we use it.

Application

Sunshine can be good for you. It kills germs, helps improve your mood, and allows the body to produce vitamin D. Yet while some exposure is good, too much can destroy the skin's elasticity and increase the risk of skin cancer. Enjoy sunlight and outside activities, but protect yourself from overexposure.

Friend or Foe?

Over the past few years, articles about the effects of the sun and the danger of skin cancer have driven many people into the dark. That's not all bad. Certainly you should use caution to avoid burning, but to avoid the sun altogether deprives you of one of nature's great healing remedies.

It's good to spend at least a few minutes in the sunshine every day. Studies have shown that, for some people, lack of exposure to light causes depression. Taking a sunshine break will give your body a dose of vitamin D, and will act as a disinfectant, killing bacteria on your clothes and skin.

During the summer do you:

__ Sizzle and sunburn?

__ Work on a deep, dark tan?

__ Tan lightly?

__ Stay out of the sun completely?

If you sizzle and burn or go for that deep tan, watch out! You are putting yourself at risk for skin cancer and damaging the elasticity of your skin.

On the other hand, lightly tanned skin is more resistant to sunburn and less prone to infection. Get outside in the fresh air. Soak up a little sunshine each day; just don't overdo it.

Ask Yourself

How often do you spend time in the sunshine?

__ Every day, weather permitting

__ Most days

__ A few times a week

__ Rarely

Sunlight Suggestions

1. Avoid going to sleep in the sun. It's a recipe for a severe sunburn.
2. Use sunscreen and sunglasses to protect yourself. A hat is also helpful to shade your face when you are working outdoors.
3. Be extra careful when you are around water or snow. The reflection from these surfaces can increase your exposure causing you to burn rapidly.
4. If you are swimming, remember to reapply your sunscreen when you are done. Better yet, use waterproof sunscreen.

197

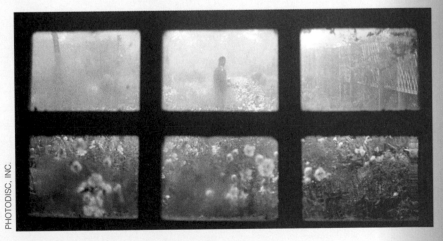

PHOTODISC, INC.

Open up your windows and let the sunshine in. It will kill germs, lift your spirits, and enhance your health.

TEMPERANCE

The Balanced Life

It was headline news: Carrots may prevent head and neck cancer. New research suggested that eating five or six of the crunchy tubers a day appeared to reverse leuko-plakia—a precancerous lesion occurring in the mouth and throat.

My friend Judith promptly purchased a machine that turned fresh carrots into juice.

"How much juice do you get from five carrots?" I asked her one day.

Her eyes flashed. "Oh, I don't stop there. With this machine I can drink five or six pounds of carrots every day!"

PHOTODISC, IN

Was that a good idea?

It's true that vegetables are an important part of a healthful diet. It's also true that they are increasingly being valued for their role in preventing disease.

But five pounds of one vegetable every day?

Judith's body eventually rebelled. Her skin took on a sickly yellowish color. Fearing hepatitis, she rushed to the doctor. He explained that carrots contain an orange-yellow dye known as beta-carotene. The body handles reasonable quantities of this substance, but excessive amounts are stashed away in the liver, skin, and muscous membranes, turning them the color of a carrot.

Did that experience straighten her out?

For the moment. But we humans are a curious lot. Sensationalized discoveries and quick solutions to complex health problems are almost irresistible. Before the carrot caper, Judith was swept into the excitement over oat bran. After months of mush and muffins,

"And the Lord God commanded the man, 'You are free to eat from any tree in the garden; but you must not eat from the tree of the knowledge of good and evil.'" Genesis 2:16, 17

however, she was ready for a change.

Do carrots actually protect us from cancer?

Carrots and other yellow fruits and vegetables are rich in beta-carotene, the substance that began to change Judith's skin color. Beta-carotene, which the body turns into vitamin A, is also a substance that appears to protect the body against certain cancers.

Vitamins can be divided into two basic types—

those that are water-soluble (dissolve in water) and those that are fat-soluble (dissolve in fat). Water-soluble vitamins (B-complex and C) are not a special concern, because excess amounts can usually be washed out through the kidneys.

But fat-soluble vitamins (A, D, E, and K) are another story. Any excess cannot be eliminated except as it is used. In excessive amounts, vitamin A begins to act like a toxin (poison) and may cause headaches, joint pains, damaged skin, and hair loss. Because of this potential toxicity, laws now limit the amount of vitamin A and other fat-soluble vitamins that can be put into supplements.

Beta-

carotene apparently doesn't have such limits. When the body receives beta-carotene it can make as much vitamin A as it needs and use the rest in other ways. That's why the trend these days is to substitute beta-carotene for vitamin A in vitamin capsules and tablets.

This distinction is important because it illustrates how the body uses food. Vitamins, minerals, and other nutrients in natural food occur in exactly the right forms for the body to use. It can pick and choose what it needs. But when we consume one food or

A balanced, healthful lifestyle may not grab headlines or create profitable markets, but it brings improved health that lasts.

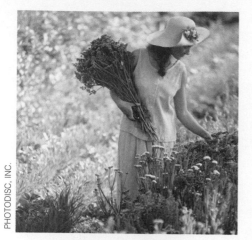

PHOTODISC, INC.

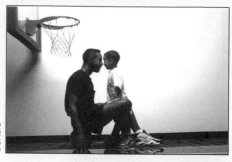

CORBIS

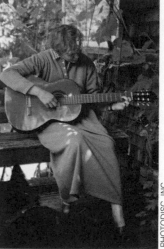

PHOTODISC, INC.

PHOTODISC, INC.

nutrient in excess, or tamper with the makeup of food, the whole balance can be upset.

So beta-carotene is good, but a whole lot of it isn't necessarily better.

This is a hard message for today's world. People do nearly everything to excess—they eat too much, drink too much, smoke too much, spend too much, party too much. *Moderation* is about as popular a concept as *wholesome.*

Then too, we live in an instant society with a quick-fix mentality, and it's difficult to accept that instant good health isn't also available. Each time a new fad splashes through the media there's no shortage of takers.

When I (Dr. Ludington) was a consultant for a popular health publication, I'd get a lot of phone calls from reporters. They'd try to get me to say such things as "Yes, eating a pound of alfalfa sprouts every day will strengthen the heart" or "Several capsules of rooted sea-weed will ensure a good night's sleep." No one wanted to hear my message about the good-sense, balanced diet the body really needs. I soon realized that even though I was giving them the right stuff, a health-ful, balanced lifestyle didn't grab headlines, sell magazines (even health magazines), or create profitable new markets for food products.

The human body is able to tolerate excesses of one kind or another for a long time—even six pounds of carrots a day! But the bottom line is that balance, not only in what we eat, but in our total lifestyle, is the key to enduring health and happiness.

The Key Is Balance

"I have never seen a person who died of old age. In fact, I do not think anyone has ever died of old age yet. To die of old age would mean that all the organs of the body had worn out proportionally, merely by having been used too long. This is never the case. We invariably die because one vital part has worn out too early in proportion to the rest of the body.

"There is always one part that wears out first and wrecks the whole human machinery, merely because the other parts cannot function without it.

"The lesson seems to be that as far as man can regulate his life by voluntary actions, he should seek to equalize stress throughout his being.

"The human body—like the tires on a car or the rug on a floor—wears longest when it wears evenly."

—Dr. Hans Selye

Application

Too much of a good thing is a bad thing when your health is involved. Common sense and moderation will do more for you than any health fad or miracle cure. Balance is the key to good health—learn to apply it in all areas of your life.

The Case of the Harried Sales Manager

Joe is a sales manager for a telecommunications company. At work he is always busy, talking with customers, motivating his sales team, or writing reports for a demanding boss. The pressure never lets up. For lunch he has a steak and salad if there are clients to entertain, or else he grabs a double cheeseburger and fries at a nearby fast-food restaurant. Sometimes there's no time for lunch at all. By the time Joe gets home at night, he's exhausted and cranky. "I feel like a wreck," he admits. "After work, all I want is to relax in front of the television. I know I should make some changes, but I'm not sure how to start."

Balance is "Common Sense in Action"

Imagine that Joe came to you for advice. What commonsense changes might you suggest to help him incorporate the principle of balance in his life?

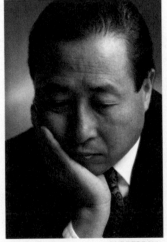

RUBBERBALL

_____

_____

_____

Joe's solution

Joe made a couple simple changes in his routine. First, he started bringing his lunch to work instead of eating out every day. Packing a lunch made it easy to eat more fruits, vegetables, and whole-grain foods, and helped him cut down on high-fat, high-calorie, restaurant fare. Second, Joe and his wife, Amy, now take a brisk walk in the evening when he gets home.

When asked if the changes have been worth it, Joe smiles. "I feel more relaxed and energetic. I've lost weight, and the walks Amy and I take together have become something we both look forward to. It's hard to believe the dramatic impact these changes have made in my life."

How about you?

What are some things you could do starting today to bring more balance to this part of your life? List your ideas:

_____

_____

_____

_____

_____

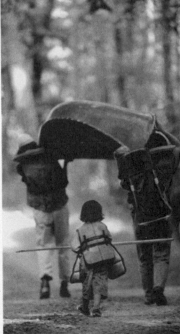

AIR

Don't Poison Your Home

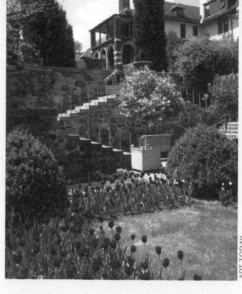

ART TODAY

House-plants do a lot more than enhance the appearance of our homes and offices. They enrich the air with oxygen and absorb carbon dioxide; some even remove toxic pollutants from the air we breathe.

Air is the breath of life. We are fully dependent on it for oxygen to operate the powerhouses in our cells. These powerhouses, called mitochondria, are the backbone of every activity carried on in our bodies.

You mean harmful pollutants can collect indoors?

Increasingly so. Many modern homes and office buildings are tightly sealed to save energy costs. But this advantage may be offset by poor ventilation and potential accumulation of indoor air pollutants.

Tobacco smoke, of course, is the most dangerous pollutant, but there are others.

Formaldehyde, for example, seeps from certain wood products, and other chemical fumes come from carpeting, copy machines, upholstery, cleaning products, and freshly dry-cleaned clothes. Carbon monoxide and nitrogen dioxide, two poisonous gases, may come from gas, oil, and coal furnaces, gas ranges, fireplaces, and kerosene heaters.

Other problems occur from dust, air mites, molds and fungi, ozone, lead, asbestos, pesticide residues, and, in some areas, radon gas.

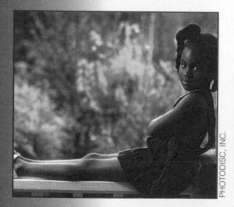

PHOTODISC, INC.

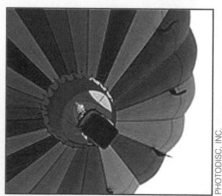

PHOTODISC, INC.

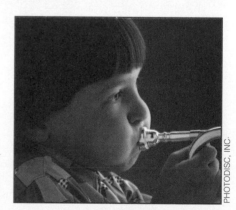

PHOTODISC, INC.

"So God made the expanse and separated the water under the expanse from the water above it. . . . God called the expanse 'sky.'" Genesis 1:7, 8

Air conveys life, vigor, and electrifying energy to every cell in the body.

How do these pollutants affect people?

Symptoms range from burning eyes, sore throats, coughing, and itching, to headaches, sluggishness, nausea, dizziness, feelings of exhaustion, and depression. This cluster of symptoms is sometimes referred to as "sick building syndrome."

What can people do to protect themselves?

There are two basic ways to protect ourselves, not 100 percent, but significantly.

First, we can control exposure. For example:

- Ban smoking indoors. Even secondhand smoke contains hundreds of harmful chemicals.
- Make sure all gas, oil, kerosene and coal-burning heaters and appliances are properly vented to the outdoors as well as coal- and wood-burning furnaces and fireplaces. And don't forget gas cooking ranges and clothes dryers.
- Keep heating and air-conditioning units well maintained. Clean air ducts and filters regularly.

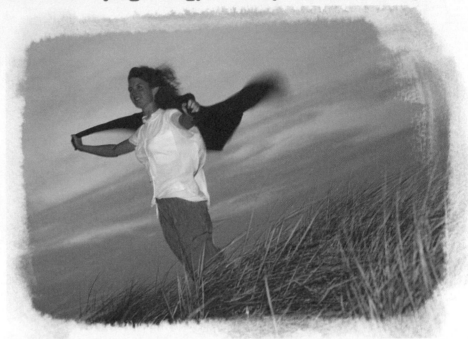

The heart sends blood streaming on its way, filled with red blood cells whose hemoglobin picks up fresh oxygen in the lungs and delivers it to every cell in the body.

- Keep chimneys open and in good repair.
- Use air fresheners, moth crystals, etc., sparingly.
- Avoid idling a vehicle in an attached garage or near an open window.

Second, we can improve ventilation.

The most obvious solution to indoor pollution problems is to open windows and set up good cross ventilation. Fresh air not only dilutes trapped fumes, thus decreasing their health threats, but enriches stale air as well. People often don't realize that in closed areas the same air can be breathed and rebreathed, over and over. The oxygen content decreases, and the carbon dioxide and other wastes increase, resulting in sleepiness, sluggishness, and headaches.

Here are some suggestions:

- Set air conditioners and heating systems to bring in 20 to 35 percent (or more) fresh air. Energy costs will be somewhat higher but health benefits will more than compensate for this.
- Air out your house at least once a day. On smoggy days, air out the house at night or in the early mornings. In most areas smog particulate matter drops considerably once the sun has set.
- Sleep with an open window. Set up cross ventilation in your bedroom if possible. You'll wake up feeling refreshed.

What about air-cleaning machines?

These machines can be expensive, complicated, and messy, and most have a limited range. However, people with allergies and certain lung ailments often find them helpful. And we recommend them for anyone exposed to air

Are you getting enough vitamin O₂?

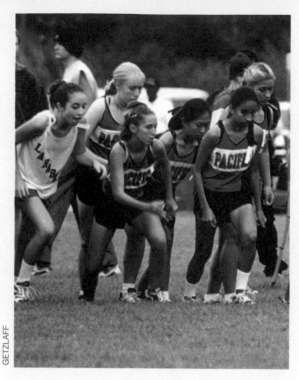

GETZLAFF

polluted with tobacco smoke at home or at work.

How does air relate to personal health?

Air is composed of about 20 percent oxygen, the rest being nitrogen along with a few other gases. Since the human body operates on oxygen, each one of its 100 trillion cells must receive steady, fresh supplies, or die. Oxygen is picked up in the lungs from the air we breathe, and delivered to our bodies via the red blood cells. Well-oxygenated cells are healthy and contribute to overall well-being. Anything that diminishes oxygen supplies to the lungs, or its delivery to body cells, is detrimental.

Air molecules can also be positively or negatively charged. Polluted air is usually full of positive ions. It's commonly found on freeways, at airports, and in closed, poorly ventilated areas.

Air containing an abundance of negative ions is plentiful around lakes, in forests, near rivers and waterfalls, at the seashore, and after a rainstorm. This kind of air is refreshing and gives people a lift.

Another "feel good" technique is to stop where you are and take a few slow, deep breaths several times a day. This gives your body an extra "shot of oxygen" and helps unload carbon dioxide.

Yet another way to flush your body with oxygen is to exercise. Activity opens up blood vessels and speeds those oxygen-laden red blood cells on their rounds.

And remember the houseplants. Placing at least one plant for every 100 square feet of indoor space is recommended. Live plants not only "eat" many toxic pollutants and freshen the air with oxygen; they probably slip in some extra negative ions as well!

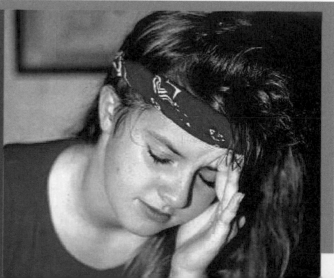

Oxygen is vital to each of the trillions of cells that make up your body. Poor breathing habits, or poor air to breathe, can rob the body of this vital element. Bad air and poor breathing habits promote negative emotions like depression and irritability. It can also cause headaches and chronic feelings of fatigue and exhaustion.

Application

The human body operates on oxygen. Make sure yours gets enough by exercising, keeping your house well ventilated, and pausing frequently to take slow, deep breaths.

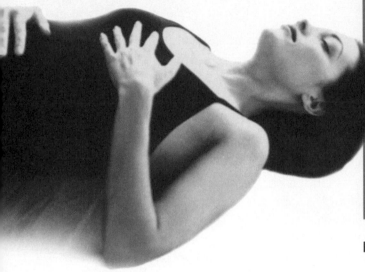

Place one hand on your chest and the other on your stomach. Breathe normally for a few moments, noting the movement of each hand as you inhale. Which hand rises more dramatically? If it's the one on your belly, take it off and pat yourself on the back. You have excellent respiratory technique. But if it's the hand on your chest, you'd better take a deep breath—though you probably can't. You're breathing wrong!

Air Inventory

Right now, without changing anything about the way you are sitting or breathing, answer the following questions:

1. How are you sitting right now? Is your spine straight, or are you slouching? Are your shoulders rolled forward?

2. Observe your breathing for a few moments. Is it shallow or deep?

3. Do the clothes you are wearing, or the chair you are sitting in, restrict your breathing?

4. Is the room you are in well ventilated with fresh air, or is it closed and stuffy?

5. Have you (or will you) exercise today?

6. Have you eaten a high-fat meal today? (A high-fat meal reduces your blood's ability to carry oxygen.)

7. When was the last time you got up and moved around? Have you taken a break or done some deep breathing during the past couple hours?

Breathe Deeply

Take a moment to try this simple breathing exercise. It will energize and refresh you.

Stand or sit with your back straight. Exhale deeply through your mouth. Now, draw the air back into your lungs. As you do, imagine it going right down into your belly, filling it. Feel your stomach expand as you inhale.

When your lungs are full, slowly begin to exhale. Tighten the muscles of your stomach as you gently push the last bit of air out.

Repeat the process, slowly, five or six times.

Do this exercise when you wake in the morning and several times during the day. If possible, step outdoors into the fresh air. Refresh body and mind by giving yourself a caffeine-free boost.

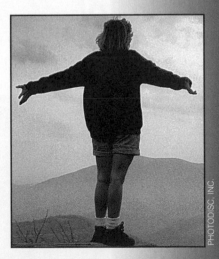

Your Challenge:

Practice frequent deep breathing and experiment with other tips in this chapter.

Healthy by choice, not chance!

REST

How Much Is Enough?

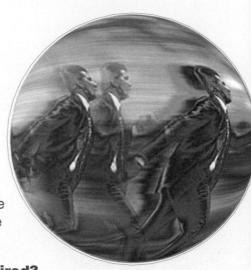

Life today is fast-paced, exciting—and exhausting. Insomnia is epidemic. People are gulping down millions of sedatives and tranquilizers, desperate for rest that will restore their energies.

Why am I always tired?

You may have an illness, such as a cold or the flu, that is sapping your energy. Or you may be depressed.

Many otherwise healthy people, however, work in confining sedentary jobs with deadline pressures and emotionally draining problems. These people are not likely to feel rested when they get out of bed in the morning.

In addition, few people get through a day anymore without a pick-me-up, usually coffee, tea or a cola. Caffeine is a central nervous system stimulant and a common cause of insomnia.

What about chronic fatigue?

Besides tiredness and a lack of energy, there is also an increase in irritability. Tempers get short, and patience goes out the window. Everything requires more effort, until finally the simplest tasks seem overwhelming.

Fatigue also sabotages creativity. Judgment suffers and efficiency goes. And if unrelieved, fatigue can culminate in exhaustion and full-scale depression.

Tired of being Tired?

"And God . . . rested from all the work of creating that he had done." Genesis 2:3

Average sleep time has declined 20 percent in the twentieth century.

How does rest relate to these problems?

- Rest allows your body to renew itself. Waste products are removed, repairs are effected, enzymes are replenished, energy is restored.
- Rest aids in the healing of injuries, infections and other assaults on your body, including stress and emotional traumas.
- Rest strengthens your body's immune system, helping protect you from disease.
- Proper rest can add length to your life. In a large population study of health habits a few years ago, it was found that people who regularly slept seven to eight hours each night had lower death rates than those who averaged either less than seven hours or who slept longer.

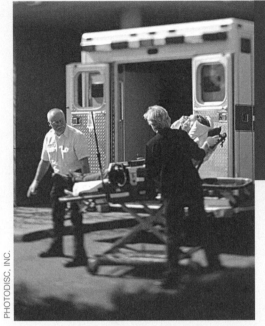

PHOTODISC, INC.

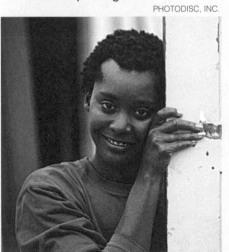

PHOTODISC, INC.

How much rest do I need?

People need different kinds of rest, and a relaxing night's sleep is a good start. Newborn babies sleep from 16 to 20 hours, while young children need 10 to 12 hours. Adults vary widely in their requirements, but most do best on seven to eight hours per night.

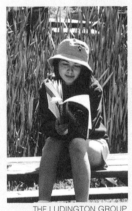

THE LUDINGTON GROUP

People also need a change of pace. During World War II Great Britain instituted a 74-hour work-week but soon found that people could not maintain the pace. After experimenting, they found that a 48-hour workweek, with regular breaks, plus one day of rest each week, resulted in maximum efficiency.

Society also recognizes the need for other breaks

The National Transportation and Safety Board estimates 100,000 car crashes causing 1,500 deaths and 71,000 injuries are caused each year by drowsy drivers.

from time to time. The long weekend is now an American institution and yearly vacations have proven their value.

What about sleep medications? Are they helpful?

During normal sleep the body passes back and forth between periods of light and deep sleep. During light sleep dreaming occurs; this apparently provides a natural outlet for the pressures and tensions that build up during the day.

Medicated sleep, however, while producing a welcome state of unconsciousness, suppresses that dream stage. And even though people believe they have slept soundly, they may not feel refreshed and energetic the next day as a result.

In emergencies sleep medications may be helpful, but will contribute to chronic fatigue if continued over time.

Others use alcohol to help them relax and go to sleep. But alcohol-induced sleep is not as restorative as natural sleep.

2 0 7

Did You Know...

• *It's not only how much you sleep, but when and how regularly that matters.*

• *Fatigue is one of the most common of the complaints that propel people to the doctor.*

• *Teenagers need an average of nine hours sleep, but most don't get it.*

• *Some 70 million people have too little or very disturbed sleep every night.*

• *In a recent survey, 51 percent of men and 42 percent of women said they would go to sleep earlier if they didn't have television or Internet access. Being wired might make you tired!*

Some people overfill their lives just as others overeat.

How can I sleep better?

✔ Take frequent breaks during the workday. Walk around, get a drink of water, take some deep breaths.

✔ Daily engage in 30 to 60 minutes of active exercise. Exercise relaxes, restores energy, helps banish depression, and combats nervous tension.

✔ Maintain as regular a schedule as possible for going to bed, getting up, eating, and exercising. The body flourishes on regular rhythms.

✔ Eat the evening meal at least four hours before bedtime. An empty, resting stomach is more conducive to quality rest.

✔ Try a lukewarm (not a hot) bath. It is a helpful relaxation technique.

✔ Count your blessings. Fill the mind with gratitude and thanksgiving.

✔ A clear conscience and a grateful mind are the pillows to sleep on.

Rest is an important part of life's rhythm. And like a dancer, if we go with our rhythms, we will be in tune with ourselves.

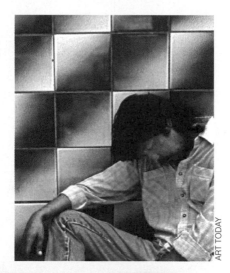

ART TODAY

THE PACE of modern society makes ever greater demands on us. But each week God gives an oasis in time that can help us find a new meaning in life for ourselves, our families, and others.

"Come ... to a quiet place and get some rest." Mark 6:31

Application

Rest is an important part of life's rhythm. Most adults do best with seven to eight hours of sleep each night. If you have trouble sleeping, don't reach for sleep medications. Take a warm, relaxing bath. Exercise daily. Maintain a regular schedule. Strive for a clear conscience and tranquil mind.

Sleep Quiz

Feeling tired? Have a hard time getting out of bed in the morning? The following questions are designed to get you thinking about your sleep habits.

1. I have trouble falling asleep at night.
   a. Usually
   b. Often
   c. Rarely
   d. Never

2. I usually get enough sleep and awake feeling rested.
   a. Usually
   b. Often
   c. Rarely
   d. Never

3. I use caffeinated drinks (such as coffee and soft drinks).
   a. More than 10 cups/day
   b. 5-9 cups/day
   c. 2-4 cups/day
   d. Less than 2 cups/day

4. I go to bed at night early enough to get a good night's sleep.
   a. Always
   b. Often
   c. Rarely
   d. Never

Trouble Falling Asleep

Many people occasionally have trouble falling asleep. Three common reasons for this are emotional stress, caffeine, and lack of exercise. Fortunately, all of these can be controlled.

Caffeine, found in coffee, tea, and many soft drinks, can be reduced or eliminated from the diet.

Emotional stress can also be reduced by handling disturbing problems earlier in the day, when you are rested. Don't wait till bedtime to bring up problems.

A regular exercise program may be the best medicine of all for ensuring a good night's rest. It reduces stress and provides a pleasant physical fatigue that helps you sleep more soundly.

Getting Enough Sleep

For many, getting to sleep isn't the problem—making time for it is. Busy schedules, bolstered by strong coffee, cut into the hours needed for sleep.

Your body is your most valuable possession. It may be tempting to skip sleep, but in the long run that is counterproductive. A parable by Stephen Covey from his book *The Seven Habits of Highly Effective People* illustrates this point:

"Imagine you are walking through the woods when you come upon a man feverishly trying to saw down a tree. The man looks exhausted. He says he has been sawing on the same tree for five hours.

"Why don't you take a break for a couple minutes and sharpen that saw?" you ask. "It will cut faster."

"No time for that," he gasps. "I'm too busy sawing."

Here are some tips for getting some good shut-eye tonight:

- *Go to bed and get up at the same time each day.*

- *Avoid caffeine.*

- *Don't use alcohol as a sedative. It makes the brain restless later in the night.*

- *Exercise early in the morning or late in the afternoon but no later than three hours before bedtime.*

TRUST IN DIVINE POWER

The Ultimate Life

"**I**s this all there is?" sighs the aging baby-boomer, surrounded by his very considerable possessions. Having bought into the *grab all you can get* philosophy of the 1980s, he has every material thing his heart desires. Yet he feels curiously empty and disappointed.

Isn't that a common human problem?

Yes, and it's getting worse. More and more Americans are living longer, healthier lives than ever before. Yet surveys show that they feel less and less satisfied.

Our hopes are continually being inflated by grandiose and unrealistic advertising, self-help gurus who promise the moon, and our childlike faith in medicine's ability to cure all of our ills. As disappointments pile up, we shuffle along looking for the missing pieces of our lives.

Are people ever really satisfied?

Early on we dream of wealth, fame and success, of having what we want and doing as we please. But can you think of a multimillionaire athlete who isn't itching for a bigger contract? Or a wealthy celebrity who hasn't felt drawn to do yet another commercial, endorse a bigger product or produce a new book? Where is the business executive who wouldn't jump at the next big deal

"There is a way that seems right to a man, but in the end it leads to death."

Proverbs 14:12

"You will keep in perfect peace him whose mind is steadfast, because he trusts in you." Isaiah 26:3

CORBIS

Trust in Divine Power

. . . means getting to know God well enough to trust Him for present and future well-being.

WHO CAN YOU TRUST?

Trust is like a bank account—if you build it up through daily deposits, it's there when you need it for an emergency.

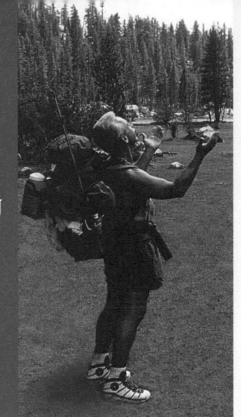

THE LUDINGTON GROUP

or lust after another merger?

On another level, do you know a teenager who is satisfied with his/her looks? clothes? friends? On the face of it, humans appear to be creatures of insatiable desires.

Is this why so many people turn to drugs?

In today's fast-paced life, people often feel so pressured and stressed, so full of pain and disappointment, and so hopeless that they become increasingly willing to gamble their health and even their lives on almost anything that promises relief, no matter how temporary. "Follow your feelings," they are urged. "If it feels good, do it." "Hurry, life is passing you by."

For every skid row bum there are scores of closet alcoholics. And for every street punk looking for a hit, there are many so-called respectable people numbing their pain with prescription pills.

But lasting joy doesn't come in snorts, and well-being doesn't come from bottles and pills. You can't shoot up peace of mind. Gratitude and compassion aren't sold in the drugstore or on the street.

So where can I get joy, peace—those good things?

The Bible says that following our "fleshly" or "natural-feelings" leads to negative results like immorality, debauchery, selfish ambition, drunken orgies, fits of rage.

The Bible also says that God wants better things for us, such as peace, joy, and healing (Galatians 5:19-21). These gifts, however, come through the cultivation of our spiritual nature.

Are such spiritual themes really relevant to life today?

You bet! Look at alcoholism, for instance. The medical miracles and the technological advances of the past half century have hardly touched this disease. Alcoholics Anonymous (AA) continues to offer the most consistently effective treatment with the best long-term results. AA uses a 12-step program that involves a recognition of human helplessness and the acceptance of a Higher Power. Similar 12-step programs, based on the philosophy of AA, are proliferating in almost every area of human need. They are bringing healing to thousands for whom medical care, drugs, counseling, and other human solutions have failed.

Today we are witnessing a renewed search for values, a resurgence of faith, and an increasing acceptance not only of a Higher Power but of a personal, caring God.

Humans find focus, purpose and meaning beyond creature comforts, needs and desires through a relationship with God and adherence to His commandments.
—Dr. Laura Schlessinger

211

Could this be just another fad?

This so-called fad has strong roots in reality. One of the most exciting breakthroughs in recent years has been the discovery of the strong and close relationship of the physical, mental, emotional, and spiritual components of human beings.

This is a radical departure from the past. For centuries it was believed that body, mind, and spirit were separate entities that functioned independent of each other.

Now we're discovering that things like anger, fear, resentment, and distrust can actually produce effects on the body that weaken its immune system and open the door to disease. Conversely, positive emotions like love, joy, faith, and trust produce protective substances that strengthen the immune system and protect the body from disease. Harboring bitterness and hatred, nurturing negative thoughts and feelings can make us sick; cherishing positive thoughts and feelings can make us well—literally.

What does cultivating my "spiritual nature" involve?

It could involve getting acquainted with your Bible, singing praise songs, and praying for the special "fruit of the Spirit" that God wants you to possess—*"love, joy, peace, patience, kindness, gentleness, self-control"* (Galatians 5:22, 23).

We are *"fearfully and wonderfully made"* (Psalm 139:14). We don't arrive in this world with only the minimal equipment needed for survival. We are each given a conscience to keep us on track; a full range of feelings and emotions to enrich our lives; and a brain that we can never use up or wear out.

Health and fitness are not enough. Neither are wealth, fame, good looks, or power. God has reserved a "special place" for Himself in every person's heart; as long as that space is vacant, everything this world has to offer will not fill it.

The ultimate lifestyle will be a life of spiritual growth that will supply the missing pieces and fill the empty spaces. The result will be a life of quality and fulfillment that will stretch into eternity.

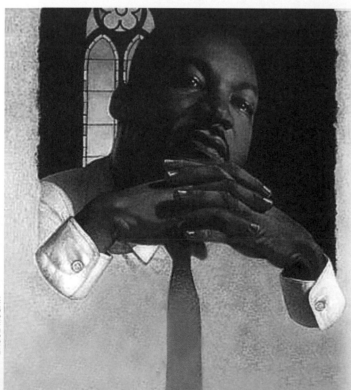

BRUCE McGAW

A for-real relationship with the true God, our Creator, is never optional—it is the very root of health.

Application

The ultimate lifestyle includes not just health and fitness; it also includes spiritual growth. Trust in God supplies a missing piece in our lives. It brings quality, fulfillment, and hope for the future.

Beyond Good Health

Good health is not the pinnacle of existence. Many who are otherwise healthy carry within themselves a deep longing for something more. At the root of our being is the need for greater purpose and meaning in life.

Poets and wise men have long affirmed this. Today even scientists are beginning to look into the spiritual dimensions of life.

Time

Like all things of value, cultivating the spiritual side of our nature takes an investment of time. Attention must be shifted from immediate concerns to deeper, more eternal issues. We need to take time for stillness, away from the commotion and noise of our everyday lives.

We need time to explore the deeper side of ourselves, to read inspiring words, or just to walk in the sunshine and fresh air.

When was the last time you allowed yourself to really enjoy the people closest to you? How long has it been since you joined with others who find faith and inspiration in a Higher Power?

We live today in a most exciting and yet para-

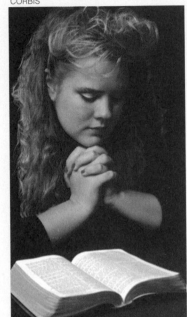
CORBIS

doxical age. We can tune our radios and TVs to sounds and pictures coming from outer space or across the ocean. And yet many persons fail to tune their souls to God and to hear His voice.

The Spiritual Dimension

Where do you turn for renewal? What is at your core, your center of being?

Your Challenge:

Take some time to step back and think about what is truly important to you. Look beyond the clamor of daily activity to the universal themes of life. Choose an inspiring book, listen to some uplifting music, give thanks for the marvelous gift of life and health. Every breath you take is a miracle. Every morning is a new start.

Religion, then, is not a piece of information for the mind. It is a way of life, which includes all that we are, all that we do, all our hopes and aspirations, all the moments of our lives. Mario Veloso

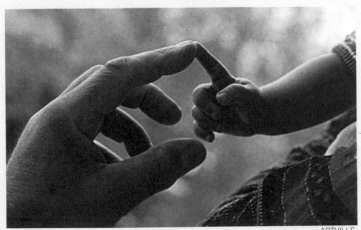
ARTVILLE

Body and Soul

People who have close ties to others, who share time and thoughts and worries and laughter with kindred souls, reap profound health benefits.

The relation that exists between the mind and the body is very intimate. When one is affected, the other sympathizes. The condition of the mind affects the health to a far greater degree than many realize....

"Courage, hope, faith, sympathy, love, promote health and prolong life. A contented mind, a cheerful spirit, is health to the body and strength to the soul." E. G. White, *Ministry of Healing*

MIND-BODY CONNECTION

- **Mind Power**

- **Depression**

- **Stress**

- **Endorphins**

- **Habit Formation**

- **Forgiveness**

- **Love**

OUR THOUGHTS AND FEELINGS are the nutrition of our minds. Just as we need a certain balance of vitamins, proteins, and other nutrients for our bodies to reach maximum health and energy levels, we also need a specific balance of mental "nutrients" for a happy, tranquil, and creative mind.

MIND POWER

You Are What You Think

We are constantly exposed to and attacked by chemicals, germs, and viruses—so why don't these bad things overwhelm us? When our immune system is healthy and well, the bad things that attack us are fought off, and our health is preserved.

Aristotle once said that a healthy body and a healthy mind were somehow intertwined, but the idea has travelled a rocky road ever since.

I thought that was pretty well accepted these days!

Yes and no.

Some scientists still question a direct link between emotion and disease, because they are not able to prove conclusively that a person's state of mind is able to cause or cure a specific disease.

What is emerging, however, is a better understanding of the body's immune system. While scientists can't take one particular emotion, such as anger, and relate it to a specific disease like a heart attack, they can now measure the body's immune response to specific stresses.

What is the immune system?

The human body is protected by millions of fighting units circulating in the bloodstream. These consist of different types of soldiers, each group having its own specific function. Central Control can order out new units when disease invades the body. During times of peace the numbers are reduced and the fighters become patrols. This is a simplified explanation of the immune system.

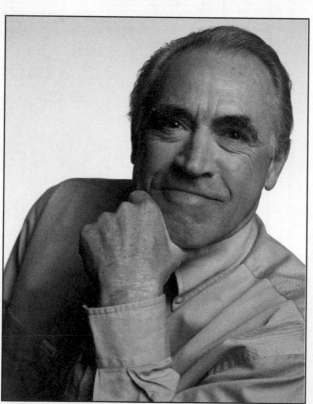

What affects the immune system?

A healthful diet, physical fitness, and positive emotional states can stimulate and strengthen the body's immune system. On the

"For as [a man] thinks in his heart, so is he." Proverbs 23:7, NKJV

Every day we encounter hundreds of germs that could make us sick or even kill us.

other hand, illness, drugs, and excessive stress can weaken it. AIDS occurs when the entire immune system has been decimated.

Emotions can affect it?

Definitely. Scientists report that people in depressed and negative emotional states may be especially vulnerable to diseases

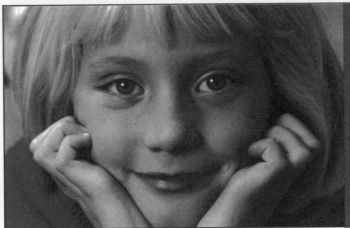

CORBIS

It may sound Polyannaish, but staying optimistic in difficult times may keep you well.

affecting the immune system, such as asthma, rheumatoid arthritis, and cancer.

How can feelings affect health?

Some scientists call it the placebo effect. Perhaps the best way to explain it would be to illustrate it with a story.

Working late one night,

I (Dr. Diehl) was nearly overcome by sleepiness.

Remembering that my secretary keeps a jar of instant coffee in her desk, I added several tablespoons of the powder to a cup of water, gulped it down, and waited.

Within 10 minutes I felt energized—yes, caffeine mobilizes blood sugar. Then came heightened alertness—yes, it also stimulates the nervous system. I rushed to the bathroom, confirming that caffeine is also a diuretic. The boost lasted the three hours I needed to finish the project.

THE BODY grieves too. Rates of illness and death tend to be higher among those who have recently lost a spouse.

Nursing home patients allowed some say in day-to-day decisions, such as what food they'll eat, often outlive those who accept more passive roles.

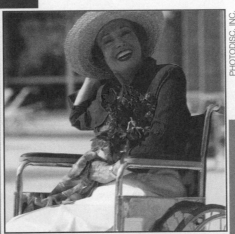

PHOTODISC, INC.

A factor called "JOY"—meaning mental resilience and vigor—was the second-strongest pre-dictor of survival time for a group of patients with recurring breast cancer.

The aggression, competitiveness, and materialism of modern living with its lack of ethical and spiritual values is as damaging to our health as it is to our environment.

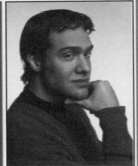

PHOTODISC, INC.

217

Placebo's healing power

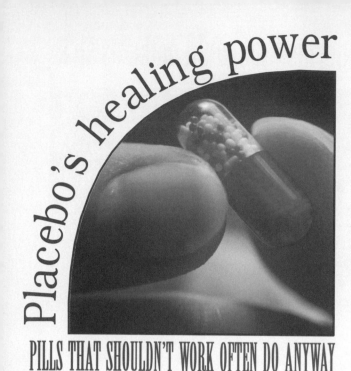

PILLS THAT SHOULDN'T WORK OFTEN DO ANYWAY

Next morning I confessed to my secretary. She listened and began to smile.

"I'm glad my coffee helped," she said. "But didn't you notice that it was decaffeinated?"

It worked because you thought it would work.

Yes. This placebo effect is commonly used to test new medicines. One group of test subjects is given the real thing, while another group receives the look-alike. Surprisingly, placebo subjects often report results as good as, and sometimes even better than, the results of those who receive the actual medication.

In short, thoughts and emotions directly influence the mind, which, in turn, powerfully affects the body. On record are reports of people who believed they were going to die on a certain day, and they did, even though no direct cause could be found.

Will positive emotions, then, strengthen the immune system?

Studies suggest that a stable emotional life is as important to good health as more traditional influences such as improved diet, regular exercise, and the avoidance of alcohol, tobacco, and other drugs.

Positive emotions and sensible health practices, it appears, can stimulate the production of endorphins. These mysterious substances are manufactured by the brain and can produce remarkable feelings of well-being. Apparently they pep up the immune system as well. Endorphins, in other words, help make you feel better while they also help make you well.

So I can cure myself by thinking nice thoughts?

You should never neglect whatever physical cures exist for a health problem. Giving up smoking, watching your weight, getting regular exercise, taking medication—all of these things are important.

But in addition, keep an eye on your attitude. As King Solomon said: *"A cheerful heart is good medicine, but a crushed spirit dries up the bones"* Proverbs 17:22.

And Paul adds: *"Whatever is true, whatever is noble, whatever is right, whatever is pure, whatever is lovely, whatever is admirable—if anything is excellent or praiseworthy—think about such things"* Philippians 4:8.

In a study of women, the happier their marriages were, the stronger their immune defenses.

The brain's first job is to keep us well and out of harm's way. The mind can accomplish this by deciding not to smoke cigarettes and by choosing to select healthful natural foods.

The immune system itself is an astonishing piece of work, rivaling the brain in its complexity and almost as difficult to track.

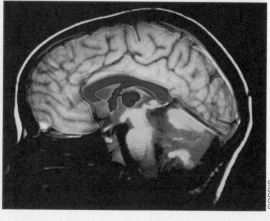

Application

Thoughts and emotions directly influence the mind, which in turn affect the body. Research suggests that a stable emotional life is as important to good health as more traditional factors, such as exercise and diet.

Questions Are the Answer

We've seen that the mind and emotions have a powerful influence in our physical lives. But how do we harness that power to work for us? One answer is through the power of questions.

Questions Have the Power to Focus

A question is like a lens, turning the focus of your attention toward a specific problem or situation. When you ask yourself a question, your mind automatically goes to work looking for an answer.

The right questions can affect all areas of your life—relationships, attitudes, creativity, and ability to solve problems.

Five Powerful Questions

Here are five questions only you can answer. If you back up your answers with action, each of them can have a tremendous effect on your life. Be specific, and ask yourself the following:

1. What is the one thing I could do that would have the greatest positive, long-term effect on my life?

_____
_____
_____

2. What is one thing I could do that would improve my relationship with someone I care about?

_____
_____
_____

3. Ask this one often: What is there in my life, right now, that is worth being happy about?

_____
_____
_____

4. What can I do today to develop a more healthful lifestyle?

_____
_____

5. Here's one to ask yourself when you are in a bind: If it were someone else in my situation, what would I tell them to do?

_____
_____

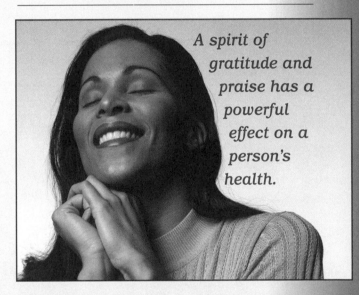

A spirit of gratitude and praise has a powerful effect on a person's health.

Don't Ask Yourself Negative Questions

Don't ask yourself such questions as, "Why am I so dumb?" or "Why can't I stick to an exercise program?" Those kinds of questions focus your mind in a negative direction. Instead, rephrase them in a positive, productive way: "What can I do in the future to avoid this mistake?" or "How can I adjust my schedule to make exercising easier?"

Your Challenge:

Use these five questions and try to come up with several more of your own. You will be surprised at the power of this simple technique.

DEPRESSION

The Hopeless Feeling

Depression can be a serious, life-threatening illness—a major cause of suicide. Depressive disorders affect an estimated 30 million Americans throughout the socioeconomic spectrum, people of every age, race, religion, or education. Billions of tranquilizers and antidepressants are gulped down each year in desperate efforts to cope. Yet the problem grows.

Aren't feelings of depression a natural part of life? Don't most of us get depressed from time to time?

Feelings of depression are some of the most common emotions that humans experience. Depression is a normal emotion, but it can also be a symptom of a wide variety of medical and psychological illnesses.

Feelings of hopelessness and discouragement are frequently produced or exaggerated by the advertising media. Products are presented that supposedly can magically transform people into capable, energetic, and happy new persons. When this does not take place at once, many people experience disappointment and further erosion of self-confidence.

How do people know whether it's serious or not?

First, people need to understand the difference between discouragement and depression. Everyone is occasionally discouraged. Discouragement is a small dip in mood that good thoughts, prayer, and positive thinking can often lift. Discouragement usually has a defined cause, and is usually temporary.

Depressions are characterized by feelings of sadness and dejection, often accom-

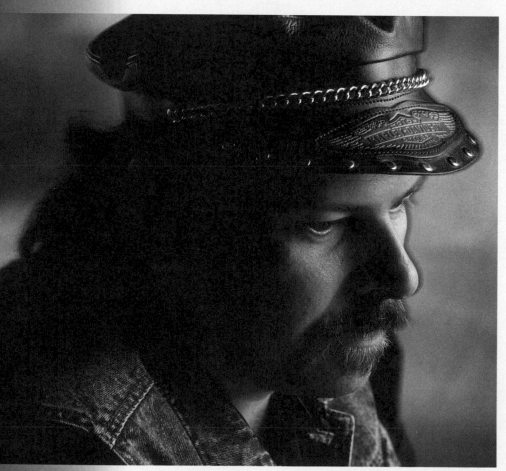

"Praise be to . . . the Father of compassion and the God of all comfort, who comforts us in all our troubles." 2 Corinthians 1:3, 4

panied by lessened physical activity. Feelings of unreasoning anxiety and a sense of hopelessness are often present. Let's look at some of the more common types:

- **The Blues**

  The most common type of depression is often referred to as "*the blues.*" A person may feel weepy, sad, discouraged, unable to cope, hopeless. These moods may be brought on by excessive fatigue, excitement, or stress, or sometimes for no apparent reason. Such depressions are short and self-limiting. They rarely require treatment. People commonly bounce back to their usual selves in a few days.

- **Reactive Depressions**

  These depressions typically result from intense life crises, such as losing a loved one or a job, going through a divorce, having children leave home, moving to a new location, or suffering a serious illness. At such times people are often unable to cope with their regular lives and responsibilities. A time of pulling back, of withdrawing, is needed to allow healing to take place. Supportive measures will usually take care of this, although more aggressive treatment may be needed if the depression is severe or prolonged.

- **Biological Depressions**

  In contrast, these depressions come and go, usually with no discernible cause. They are often inherited, passed down in a family from parent to child. These depressions usually

respond to treatment, although they may persist for several months despite treatment.

- **Somatic Depressions**

  These more serious depressions usually interfere with adequate physical functions. Symptoms include problems in almost every system of the body, but they most commonly involve the gastrointestinal tract and the sleep cycle. Some individuals will deny being depressed, but their bodily functions turn down, and their physical state has all the aspects of a depression. That's why psychiatrists call this a *somatic* depression—a depression expressed by altered body function: the body function is depressed even though the conscious mind may not be.

- **Psychotic Depressions**

  These are depressions in which individuals lose touch with reality; they require professional care.

What can be done for depressed persons?

Nearly all depressions respond to basic, common-sense measures. For example:

✔ *Purposeful Tasks.* All of us need to do some kind of productive work, whether heading a corporation, washing a car, or cooking a meal. A depressed person in particular needs the feeling of completion, accomplishment, and satisfaction found in doing something useful each day. These experiences build on

DEPRESSION can appear suddenly for no apparent reason, or it can be triggered by stressful life events.

themselves, especially if the person receives recognition and encouragement.

✔ *Structure.* Whether depressed or not, we all need structure in our lives to keep mentally sound. Without something to get out of bed for, something to do, even the most stable person can at times become depressed.

✔ *Simple Diet.* Eating a simple diet of fresh, natural foods at regular intervals gives increased energy and decreases the physical stress of body functions. Depressed people especially should avoid concentrated sweets and heavy, rich meals. Eating only fresh fruit for a day or two will do wonders in clearing the mind and banishing fatigue.

✔ *Adequate Rest.* Periods of quietness and calm are especially important in today's fast-paced pressured life. Chronic sleep deprivation can initiate or intensify depression. Most people do best when they get seven to eight hours of sleep a night. A few extraordinary individuals may need less, but even they must watch for signs of chronic fatigue. People who need more than nine hours of sleep are either unusual, ill, or convalescing. A person sleeping this much on a regular basis is likely to be depressed.

✔ *Daily Exercise.* One of the most exciting findings of recent years has been the profound effects of exercise on emotional well-being. Regular active physical exercise elevates mood, improves sleep, relieves stress, promotes health, helps to prevent disease, and increases the overall sense of well-being. The good news for depressed people is that the improvement in mood and attitude occurs through the release of endorphins in the brain. These "feel-good" hormones are activated by physical exercise. A brisk one-hour walk each day will do more good for many depressed people than medication.

Is There More?

Even severely depressed people can make simple everyday choices, such as deciding whether to get up in the morning or stay in bed; whether to watch television all day or look for more strengthening activities; whether to dress and groom themselves or stay in a bathrobe. Such simple, everyday choices matter a great deal because they mold our capabilities for making choices tomorrow. It is by making good choices that people grow and become stronger.

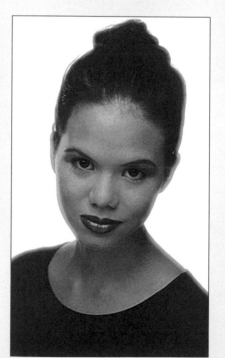

Even people with serious mental problems can improve their ability to deal more favorably with their life situations.

Encourage the depressed person to develop a list of goals. Write down positive and interesting activities. Then work on one item at a time.

Checking each one off as it is done enhances the feeling of accomplishment.

People's attitudes and belief systems are at the root of all effective treatment. A person must understand that feeling bad or worthless is not the same as being bad or worthless. Feelings are temporary and they change, much like the weather.

To be worth living, life must have meaning and value. Otherwise a chronic emptiness and a fluctuating sense of despair may creep in and spread. We must, therefore, search to find reasons for living and codes to live by. This quest may lead to a progressive awareness of the reality of a God who cares about us. As spiritual growth takes place, it can bring answers to anxiety, fear, guilt, and resentment. And it can restore energy and release a new zest for living.

What about medical treatment?

Medications are frequently needed for psychotic depressions under professional care. Medications may also be indicated for certain biological depressions, such as bipolar affective disorders (manic-depressive mood swings).

Ideally, one should not need to take medication for emotional and psychological problems. At times when medications are needed, their use should be for a specific reason and for a limited time. Chronic use, especially of sedatives and tranquilizers, can lead to dependency and may actually deepen the depression.

Depressions that are unusually severe or last a long time need professional treatment. This treatment may include counseling, anti-depressant drugs, or both. But even with professional help there are limits as to how much can be accomplished without the full participation of the patient. When people partner with their physicians, taking increasing responsibility for their lives, recovery can be greatly hastened.

Depression is no longer the dead-end, discouraging affliction it once was. By improving physical health, developing positive mental attitudes, making good choices, pursuing worthwhile activities, and developing spiritual goals and values, most people will be able to deal with their feelings of depression and live rewarding, productive lives.

"God has said, 'Never will I leave you; never will I forsake you.'"

Hebrews 13:5

Application

Our health, happiness, and longevity, as well as our relationships with family, friends, and associates, and our spiritual life—are interrelated and interdependent. Improving our health, pursuing worthwhile goals, developing positive mental attitudes and nurturing spiritual values can help us deal more effectively with our feelings of depression and hopelessness.

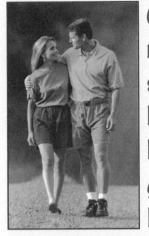

Close relation-ships go hand-in-hand with good health.

The Power to Choose

One of the things that sets us apart from other creatures is our ability to make choices. We can think about our actions, and we can choose between alternatives.

Family and Social Relationships

We are social creatures, and most of us do best when we experience a sense of community and belonging that comes from our relationship to others. When we feel isolated or in conflict, it is much easier to slip into depression.

A Higher Power

Through the ages millions have found comfort in time of need by turning to a Higher Power for strength and wisdom. Stories of people overcoming problems that seemed unsolvable are abundant.

It is easy for the hustle and bustle of life to crowd out time for spiritual nourishment. Yet those who have endured trying times can vouch for these values. Is your spiritual life the source of inspiration, strength, and renewal that it could be?

Here are some suggestions for boosting self-esteem and beating the blues. Write "OK" beside the ones that apply to you, and put a "?" beside those you would like to adopt.

_____ Look your best. Wear clothes that enhance your confidence.

_____ Play upbeat music.

_____ Speak well of yourself and others.

_____ Remember that you are unique. There is no one else like you.

_____ Make a list of your good qualities and focus on them.

_____ Realize it's OK to make mistakes.

_____ Consider a part-time job, a college course, an exercise class—a study group.

_____ Read self-help books. Take an "assertiveness" class.

_____ Go to a place of worship (even if you are not religious). Absorb the peacefulness.

_____ Play with a pet. Play with children.

_____ Take a long relaxing soak in your tub.

_____ Buy a surprise gift for someone.

_____ Clear up misunderstandings; don't let them fester.

_____ Relive happy times and remember pleasant memories.

_____ Help someone else.

_____ Nurture your spiritual life.

223

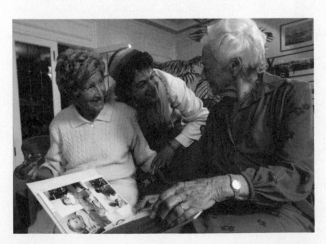

STRESS

Beating Burnout

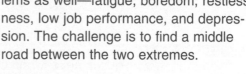

B urned out." "Overloaded." "Exhausted." "Overwhelmed." These are some of the words we use to describe the impact of stress on our lives. In our time-pressured society, few escape without feeling—at least some of the time—that they are battling stress.

Stress has been linked with almost every medical problem we have—heart attacks, strokes, hypertension, ulcers, colitis, asthma, arthritis, even cancer. Yet too little stress can invite problems as well—fatigue, boredom, restlessness, low job performance, and depression. The challenge is to find a middle road between the two extremes.

What is stress?

Stress occurs in any situation that requires making a change. Most people define stress by problems that confront them and concerns they have to deal with.

Some stress, often defined as "eustress," can improve our awareness, promote alertness, and result in superior performances. Some examples might be sports competition, theatrical performances, skiing down a smooth slope, winning a race, receiving a job promotion. The stress involved in these situations can produce feelings of extreme pleasure.

Other stresses may not be quite so exciting yet cause strong feelings of satisfaction: a romantic evening, praise from a coworker, a child's good report card. Still other stresses may make us weary although they are good in themselves: a wedding, or a family reunion. Then there are stresses that exhaust and depress:

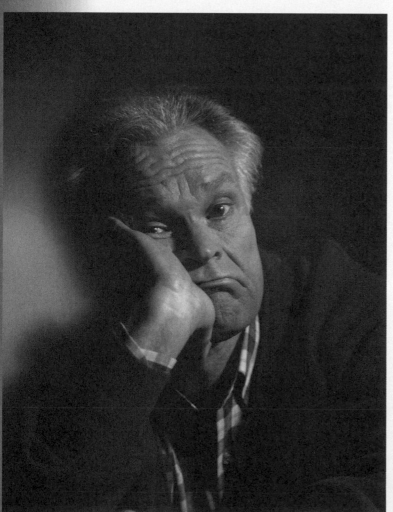

PHOTODISC, INC.

a job loss, legal problems, rebellious children, divorce, the death of a loved one.

Health has been called the ability to adapt to life's stresses. If so, healthy people must find ways to pace themselves by keeping their stress in a positive balance.

Are stress problems getting worse?

The pace of modern life has thrown us into a kind of time warp. We are constantly urged to go now, see now, buy now, enjoy now. After all, as the ads tell us, we have only one chance in life, and we'd better grab all we can.

But after a few years of grabbing, getting, going, seeing, buying, we begin to feel battered and disappointed. The inevitable *pay later* comes along: burnout, debts, poor health, depression, and loss of interest in life. It's a vicious cycle that has trapped many well-meaning men and women.

What can we do about it?

To understand stress, we must recognize a critical distinction: the difference between "stressors" and "stress." "Stressors" refer to outside forces that we must deal with. "Stress" refers to the response of the individual to these stressors. We now know that it is not *what* we have to deal with (stressors)

but rather *how* we deal with it (response) that dictates the severity of stress in our lives.

For example, picture a very cranky man walking to work in the pouring rain, cursing all the way. What is going on inside this man? Now picture three delighted children playing in the same rain. What is going on inside these children? Who has more stress? The difference is not in the circumstances but in the attitude toward those circumstances.

To cope with the "distress" in your life, your first step is to recognize and identify the significant stressors you are dealing with. The awareness that the stressor and the stress response are not identical is critically important. So take time

right now to list the 10 leading stressors in your life (on the Application page). Identifying these stressors opens the way for you to begin planning a process to cope with them.

Could you explain some of these coping processes?

There are many techniques that work, but here are some of the more important ones.

● *Healthy Adaptation* means that you recognize the stressor and do something positive about it. Ignoring or denying the problem is an unhealthy response as is escapism.

● *Proper Planning and Organization.* These steps are required to determine what it will take to accomplish a task before you begin.

● *Positive Mental Attitude.* Don't be anxious about the future; take one day at a time. Worry tends to incapacitate, but seeing the problem as a challenge tends to motivate.

● *Commit to a cause that helps others and is approved by God.* Isaiah

225

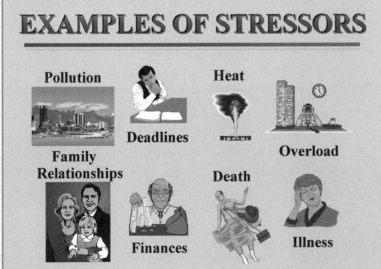

EXAMPLES OF STRESSORS

Pollution

Deadlines

Heat

Overload

Family Relationships

Death

Finances

Illness

NEIL NEDLEY, *PROOF POSITIVE*

If you removed the rocks, the brook would lose its song.

58 is one of the Bible's most sublime prescriptions for health.

● *A Healthy Lifestyle.* It's difficult to seriously damage a healthy body with stress. You can help protect your body against the harmful effects of stress with these simple stress inoculations:

✔ *Regular active exercise* for at least 30 minutes a day. Exercise produces endorphins, the feel-good hormones that protect the body against stress. Sunshine and fresh air also produce endorphins, so outdoor exercise is doubly beneficial.

✔ *A simple, vegetarian-centered diet.* The body easily handles such a diet. The result is increased energy, efficiency, and endurance.

✔ *No cigarettes, alcohol, caffeine, or other harmful drugs.* These substances all chalk up substantial *pay later* debts, often beginning the next day.

✔ *Adequate rest.* This includes a good night's sleep and regular times for relaxation and recreation.

✔ *Liberal use of water inside and out.* Drink enough water to keep the urine pale (six to eight glasses a day). A hot and cold shower each morning starts your day off right.

✔ *Stable life anchors.* A religious faith, a loving home, a job that makes you feel worthwhile, inspiring friends, a purpose for living—these are all vaccines against stress.

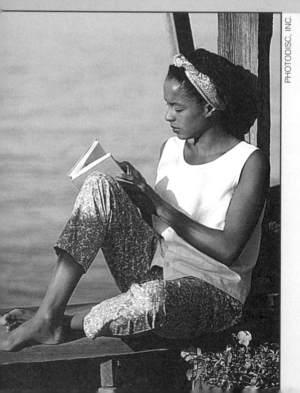

PHOTODISC, INC.

● *Think on Elevated Themes (see Philippians 4:8).* What we see and hear is under our control—movies, radio, TV, magazines, newspapers. Madison Avenue is successful because they use these mediums to focus attention on what we do not have, making us discontent. Remember: "The man who has little and wants less is richer than he who has much and wants more."

● *Trust in God* will provide a buffer against stress and a hedge against anxiety. Trusting God involves complete confidence in our heavenly Father to act on our behalf in the way and at the time that is best for us, according to His will.

As you can see, much of life does give us a choice. Don't procrastinate! Choose to enjoy life as it goes by. Praise the sunshine and the rain. Smell the flowers, return the smiles, play with children. This approach to life costs little and avoids hangovers. It exacts no pay later debt. Instead, it pays generous dividends.

Application

There are many things you can do to prevent stress from taking its toll. Regular exercise, a healthful diet, and stable life anchors all play a part in combating the effects of physical and emotional pressure.

Overcoming Stress

Too much stress is a very real problem in our society. Learning to deal with it has become an important health issue since studies began linking stress to a host of physical ailments. In most cases, running away is not the answer. We must develop more positive methods of coping.

Handling Overload

Sometimes it is possible to feel emotionally stressed without knowing why. When that happens, it is helpful to make a list of the things that are bothering you. Getting the sources of your stress onto paper allows you to focus and take action. Instead of overeating, overdrinking, or escaping into some time-wasting activity, you can identify the source of the problem and work towards a solution.

List Your Top Stressors:

_____
_____
_____
_____
_____
_____
_____
_____
_____

What Can You Do?

Read these symptoms of stress, and check the ones that apply to you.

Do you suffer from:

❑ Increased irritability or impatience?
❑ Changes in sleep patterns?
❑ Changes in appetite?
❑ An increase in health problems?
❑ Difficulty in concentrating?
❑ Lack of energy?
❑ Lack of interest in things you used to enjoy?
❑ A sense of being "cut off" or isolated?
❑ A feeling of being "out of control"?
❑ Thoughts of suicide?

List three suggestions for managing stress that seem most valuable to you:

1. _____
2. _____
3. _____

227

STRESS in the short term is vital, but over time it turns destructive. Research is now showing how chronic stress breaks down the body and makes way for disease.

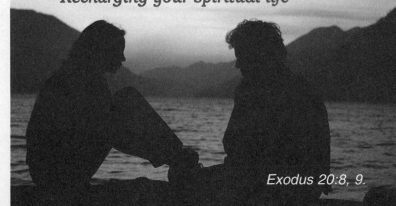

God gave one day each week for:

• *A weekly break from stressful living*
• *Time for family and friends*
• *Recharging your spiritual life*

Exodus 20:8, 9.

ENDORPHINS

The Happy Hormones

FEEL-GOOD drugs are almost irresistible. From cocaine to caffeine, people are reaching more and more for something that can help ease the numbing stress and paralyzing pressures that make up so much of modern life. But as evidence mounts that these drugs are destructive, scientists are discovering that a healthy body can make its own feel-good substances that are both protective and health-promoting.

You mean a person's body actually makes "drugs"?

Yes. If drugs are defined as chemical substances, then the body makes thousands each day. If drugs are defined as substances used as medicine to treat disease, the answer is still yes. The human body is engaged in constant efforts to heal itself.

What kinds of "good drugs" does the body make?

The most potent human-made feel-good drugs are the narcotics. Narcotics block pain and produce feelings of extreme well-being. They are valuable in controlling severe, unavoidable pain. Over time, however, they can become destructive and addictive.

Scientists have found that the body produces narcotic-like substances of its own. These can be lumped together under the general term *endorphin*.

Want to see these hormones in action? The next time you stub your toe or smash your finger, notice how quickly the intense pain fades and a comforting numbness sets in. People injured in accidents and soldiers wounded in battle seldom realize at first how badly they are hurt. Athletes can even fracture bones in the heat of competition and not feel the pain—until the game is over. These are examples of the body's endorphins at work.

HOPE

An experiment was done with two rats. One was placed in a pail of water. He swam vigorously for 20 minutes, finally got tired, and drowned.

Another rat was treated the same way, except that just as he gave up, he was rescued. A few days later he was put back in the pail, and this time he swam an hour and a half before giving up.

Why? He had HOPE. He'd escaped once—maybe it would happen again!

Hope is a powerful motivator!

He who has little, and wants less, is richer than he who has much, and wants more.

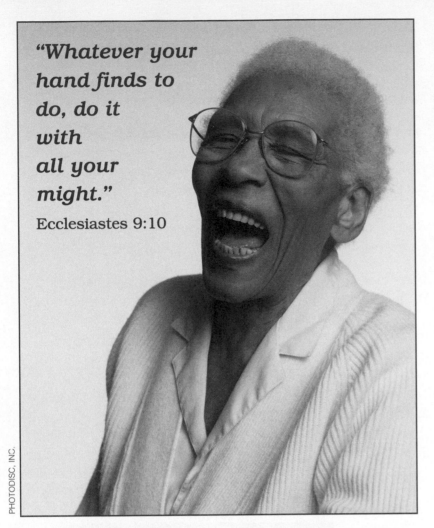

"Whatever your hand finds to do, do it with all your might."

Ecclesiastes 9:10

Norman Cousins opened the door to a new field of research when he helped heal himself of a fatal, hopeless disease by using positive emotions such as joy, laughter, love, gratitude and faith, along with sensible health practices. Since then, scientists in the field of psychoneuroimmunology have isolated many of the substances these emotions produce in the brain. They are the endorphins. They not only block pain, but can also promote healing, strengthen the immune system, and produce wonderful feelings of well-being.

Are you saying that the way we think and feel can either damage or help heal our bodies?

Emotions are a very special part of our humanity. Clinging to persistent, negative emotions can promote disease, while nurturing positive emotions benefits every part of the body. For instance, physicians are learning that they must not shut the door of hope on

Years ago Dr. Hans Selye found that fear or anger could trigger a blast of adrenaline in the body. The extra adrenaline produced a surge of energy that enabled the person either to fight or flee the source of danger.

Research later demonstrated that feelings of fear and anger can harm the body if they are experienced over long periods of time. Other negative emotions such as grief, hatred, bitterness, and resentment, if prolonged, can also exhaust emergency mechanisms and weaken the body's defenses against disease.

If negative emotions can be destructive, what about positive ones?

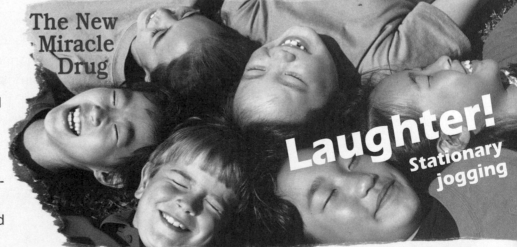

The New Miracle Drug

Laughter!

Stationary jogging

Your whole body can benefit from a good laugh.

terminally ill patients. The caring physician who, with confidence and optimism, tells a patient, "I have a feeling you are going to be that one person in ten who conquers this disease," will often be surprised by a fulfillment of his prophecy. This is quite different from his saying, "You have only a 10 percent chance of surviving."

How else can we encourage the production of these special hormones?

We have known for a long time that physical exercise is beneficial to health. But scientists began noticing that the good feelings that came from exercise could not be explained by their fitness effect alone. Something more was happening, and that something more proved to be an increase in endorphins.

Could this feeling just be a result of positive thinking?

The action of both narcotics and endorphins can be reversed by a particular chemical. A person whose pain is relieved with morphine will almost immediately lose that effect if this chemical is given. A person who is feeling a heightened sense of well-being from the body's production of endorphins will also lose that effect if the chemical is given. It's that specific.

But, yes, endorphin production is a result of positive thinking. Solving conflicts, banishing hatred and resentment, cultivating a loving, generous, thankful disposition, finding a strong faith—all these will boost the production of endorphins in our brains and strengthen the ability of the body to resist disease. And the physical benefit of a daily walk is the frosting on the cake.

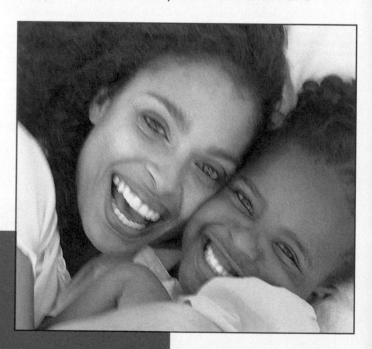

How to Raise Endorphins

- Daily active exercise
- Seek some solitude each day
- Be loving and kind to others
- Learn to say "no"
- Get enough sleep
- Don't procrastinate, plan your days
- Give away "stuff"
- Laugh a lot

Happiness is an inside job.

Application

The body makes its own feel-good substances—endorphins—that are both protective and health-promoting. Physical exercise and a positive mental attitude boost the production of these endorphins in the brain and increase the body's ability to fight disease.

The Happiness Quiz

Part 1

It's easier to be happy when you feel healthy. Which of the following are you doing to boost your state of mind physically?

❑ *Exercise daily* (preferably in the fresh air): Studies show that exercise is one of the most effective cures for the blues. Certainly it is the least expensive.

❑ *Avoid caffeine:* Too much caffeine shortens your fuse and decreases your tolerance to life's stresses. It can also cause insomnia, robbing your body of much-needed rest.

❑ *Avoid Alcohol:* Alcohol is a depressant, yet many people turn to it during periods when they are experiencing negative emotions. That's like pouring gasoline on a fire. You don't need a depressant when you are feeling down.

❑ *Eat a low-fat, cholesterol-free diet:* Build it around whole grains, vegetables, legumes, and fruits. On this diet you will feel better, look better, and have more energy. All of these benefits create an environment in which positive emotions can flourish.

❑ *Get enough fresh air:* A well-ventilated house and frequent deep breathing helps keep your blood oxygenated. This is essential for being mentally and emotionally in top form. Fresh supplies of oxygen help keep you awake and alert.

Part 2

The mind and body are linked. Just as it is difficult to be happy when you are feeling the effects of physical illness, it's also hard to feel healthy when you are in conflict with yourself or others.

The following habits cultivate a happy, thankful attitude. How many of them are you developing?

❑ *Count your blessings:* Every one of us has much to be thankful for. Paying attention to what is good in your life rather than being overwhelmed by troubles is one key to a joyful existence.

❑ *Work toward harmony in relationships:* If you nurture the negative emotions of bitterness, envy, and jealousy toward others, you rob yourself of much joy. On the other hand, developing a forgiving, caring attitude brings happiness and friendship into your life.

❑ *Work for the good of others:* Reaching out beyond yourself to touch others helps you as much as it does those whose lives you brighten. Your emotional focus moves away from your own problems, and you feel good about yourself.

❑ *Take time for spiritual renewal:* The great men and women of all time have drawn strength and inspiration from their faith in something greater than themselves. This faith has helped them overcome obstacles and achieve greatness. Pausing from the rush of everyday life to contemplate the deeper things, reaching out to a power beyond one's self, may be the most effective means of bringing happiness back into your life.

231

Your Challenge:

Look back over the Happiness Quiz. Are there things that you aren't doing that might give your emotional life a boost? Choose one item; focus on it a few days—then make it a habit.

HABIT FORMATION

How to Change

Hard to get up in the morning? Hate to exercise? Can't shed those extra pounds? Most of us long to be different—to live healthier, more disciplined lives. Yet our most determined efforts to change too often come to nothing.

✔ **YOU DETERMINE YOUR DESTINY BY THE CHOICES YOU MAKE EACH DAY.**

✔ **HOW YOU THINK AND FEEL SHAPES YOUR CHARACTER.**

✔ **YOUR CHOICES ACTUALLY MAKE PHYSICAL AND CHEMICAL CHANGES IN YOUR BRAIN AND NERVOUS SYSTEM.**

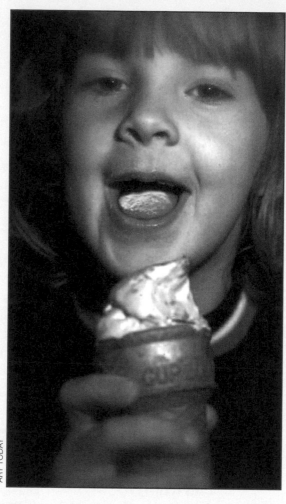

ART TODAY

Why is it so hard to change?

Habits are what tie us down—and our lifestyles are often little more than the sum total of our habits. True, they can oil the machinery of our lives, helping us glide through our days, saving time and energy. (Who would want to have to stop and *think* how to tie a pair of shoelaces, after all?)

But habits can make our lives more difficult as well—and if you doubt that, try changing sides of the bed with your spouse tonight!

How are habits formed?

As you're probably aware, your brain sends messages to the rest of your body through nerve cells. Each nerve cell has a central processing headquarters and a

"The wrong desires that come into your life aren't anything new and different.... And no temptation is irresistible. You can trust God to keep the temptation from becoming so strong that you can't stand up against it.... He will show you how to escape temptation's power."

1 Corinthians 10:13, TLB

People are walking bundles of habits. *William James*

long sending fiber (or *axon*) over which it relays messages. Nerve cells also have lots of tiny receiving fibers (or *dendrites*) for incoming messages.

Frequently used axons form tiny bumps; scientists call these bumps boutons, from the French word for buttons. And the more boutons a nerve cell has, the more easily and quickly it's able to transmit messages.

This helps us understand how habits are formed in the nervous system. Any thought or action repeated over and over builds little boutons on the ends of the affected axons, making it easier to repeat the same thought or action. It's almost as though the repetition wears a groove in the brain, much as repeatedly walking over the same place in a lawn will wear a path in the sod.

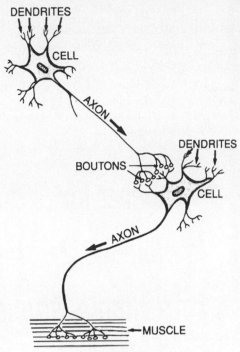

Once these pathways are formed, can they be changed?

Boutons, unfortunately, do not go away when they are no longer used. And because the old pathways are still there, the chance of falling back into a bad habit is always present, as when an alcoholic "falls off the wagon."

But people can change, can't they?

Yes, but only by building new habits that are stronger than the old. The new choice must be made repeatedly, over and over.

That sounds tough!

It can be at first. But in time more boutons will appear on

the new pathway than on the old one, and the "path" will wear deeper. As it becomes easier to take the new route, the new habit is being established.

How long does this take?

Most people find it takes about three weeks to form one new habit. A few years ago, for instance, a woman named Anya Bateman decided to start flossing her teeth. What had been a tiresome chore, she learned, evolved into a bedtime ritual in less than a month. Encouraged, she applied her three-week plan to breaking her habit of eating too many sweets. Next she broke her habit of criticizing her husband, then formed a new habit of praising her kids. The results were so astounding that they were published in *Reader's Digest.*

Likewise, just as some people become accomplished musicians by so many hours of daily practice, we can become a better person by consis-

The repetition of anything —good or bad—causes the habit to become confirmed in our lives: and fixed habits determine our character.

By choosing our habits, we determine the grooves into which time will wear us. Frank Gilberth

233

EVERYTHING CHANGES!

I have a coin in my hand, and I give it to you. Now the coin is not the same! It is older, smaller (lost a few molecules), has a different temperature, there are different cells on it (from your hand), and its magnetic and gravitational lines have changed.

Living or not, everything in the world is undergoing change. You are constantly changing.

How you change is up to you.

tently making good moral choices. And even if we lose a battle now and then, we won't lose the war—not as long as we get right back onto that new "path" we're trying to form.

So if you've always wanted to get some more exercise, try starting tomorrow. Get up a half hour earlier and hit the pavement with a brisk walk or jog. Sure, it may be tough at first—but in three weeks you'll have shed a few extra pounds, and you'll be on your way to a healthier lifestyle.

_____
* Anya Bateman, "Three Weeks to a Better Me," *Reader's Digest*, September 1983.

"Whoever loves discipline loves knowledge, but he who hates correction is stupid." Proverbs 12:1

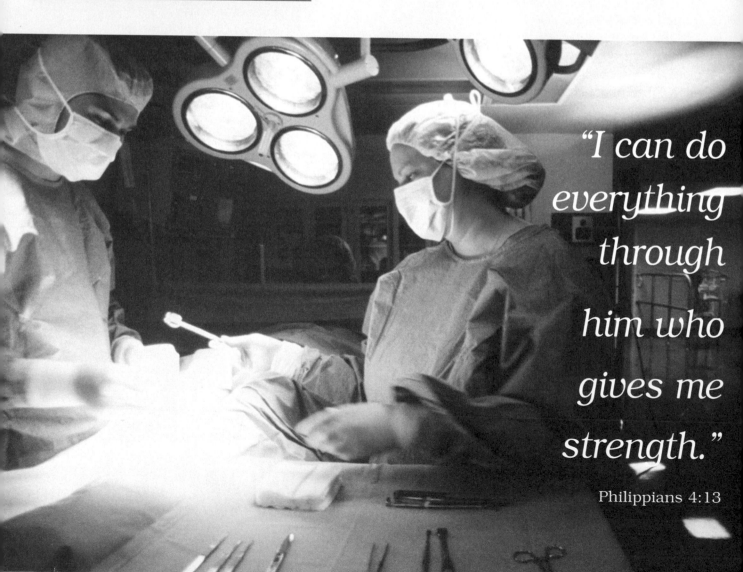

"I can do everything through him who gives me strength."

Philippians 4:13

Application

Why do good, strong, sensible people hang on to their bad habits when they know better? These people just grew into their habits while they were young, and now find it impossible to slip out of them. They are like a cucumber allowed to grow in a bottle until it is too big to take out.

Seven Lifestyle Factors

In the well-known Alameda County study, researchers followed 7,000 people for nine years. They were able to identify seven lifestyle factors that influenced how long people lived. They found a striking relationship between death rates and seven common health practices:

1. Don't smoke

2. Exercise regularly

3. Either don't drink alcohol, or drink only moderate amounts

4. Get seven to eight hours sleep nightly

5. Maintain proper weight

6. Eat breakfast daily

7. Don't eat between meals

Findings:

- The fewer of the above health practices followed, the greater the likelihood of death.

- Only 5 percent of those who followed all seven practices died during the nine-year period.

- From 12 to 20 percent of those who followed three or less were dead in nine years.

- Those who followed the greatest number of these health habits experienced only half the risk of disability as those with the poorest habits.

- Of men in the 60- to 94-year-old range, those who ate breakfast regularly and did not snack had half the risk of death of men who skipped breakfast and snacked.

Your Challenge:

How many of these health practices do you follow regularly?

Which ones are you going to adopt today?

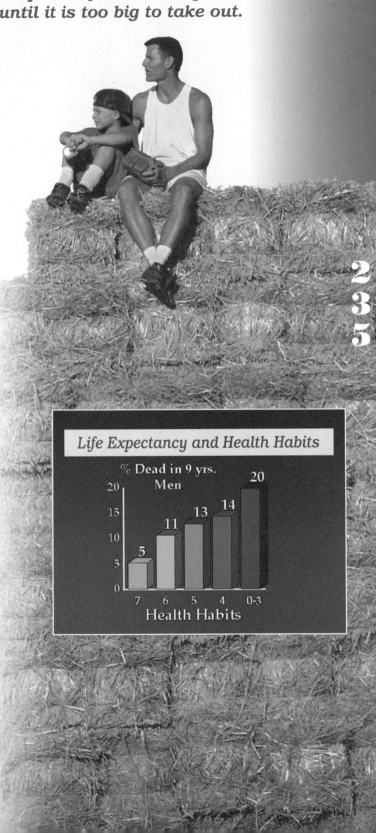

Life Expectancy and Health Habits

% Dead in 9 yrs.
Men

Health Habits	7	6	5	4	0-3
% Dead	5	11	13	14	20

FORGIVENESS

The Key to Peace

A touching story by Ernest Hemingway tells of a great quarrel between a father and his teenage son. Their relationship shatters, and the son leaves home. The father soon regrets the episode and goes in search of his son. But the city of Madrid is so large, so confusing—the father hasn't a clue where to look. He decides to put an ad in the paper. "Dear Paco, meet me at 10:00 a.m. tomorrow in front of the newspaper office. All is forgiven. I love you. Dad."

The next morning the father finds hundreds of Pacos in front of the newspaper office, searching, hoping . . .

That many young men longing for a father's forgiveness? That's heartbreaking!

Our world is full of hurting, heartbroken people—people who've been mistreated, neglected, alienated, victimized; people who are angry, resentful, bitter, lonely, depressed, fearful, and guilt-ridden; people consumed by hatred and self-pity.

But our world is also full of people longing for love, acceptance, compassion, and forgiveness, for someone to care, for spiritual comfort and peace of mind.

The spiritual hunger of people in this country is reflected in the skyrocketing sales of books on religion, spirituality, and inspiration. One of the largest book distributors reported a cumulative growth in religion titles of nearly 500 percent from June, 1994 to the third quarter of 1996, an additional 40 percent increase in 1997, and a 58 percent rise in the first quarter of 1998. "This kind of growth for any category of books is unprecedented," he said.

Still, why are the answers so hard to find? Why do so many of us continue to live lives of quiet desperation?

New medicines come and go— but love has passed the test of time.

"Bear with each other and forgive whatever grievances you may have against one another. Forgive as the Lord forgave you."

Colossians 3:13

Studies indicate that people shown affection are less likely to see a doctor or feel sick. They also report a zest for life, love for work, and a sense that their existence is meaningful.

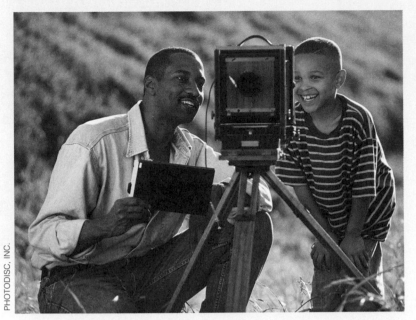

One reason is that too many of us fail to realize that the cause, the root, of most of our problems lies within ourselves. For example, a wealthy, well-educated but deeply depressed woman sought counsel. She suffered from recurrent headaches, ulcers, and obesity. "I'm bloated with fat," as she put it.

"He did it to me," she sobbed. Her husband, a respected politician, had had an affair. "I hate him for it, and I hate the woman even more.

See what she's done to me? She's ruined my life."

The affair had occurred 13 years before, yet the woman remained obsessed with her bitterness and anger.

What then can we do for people who can't forget; when past pains refuse to be healed?

We could also ask What does their hatred do for them? To what worthwhile place does it take them? Why do they allow the hurts of the past to make a mockery of their lives today?

They need to know about the healing option. A painful memory is a mental wound, and they must let it heal. They must stop picking at the scab. They can't afford to keep an emotional scrapbook of their painful memories, because this is what imprisons them.

As the woman began to understand these principles, she realized how wrong it was to mortgage her present by clinging to her past. She needed to let the dead past bury its dead. She found comfort in the apostle Paul's testimony in Philippians 3:13, 14: *"But one thing I do: Forgetting what is behind and straining toward what is ahead, I press on toward the goal to win the prize for which God has called me heavenward."* Paul knew that the present was what mattered, and he lived the present with zeal.

It's been said that our attitude toward the past is far more important than the past itself. Attitude involves choice. What do we let life do to us—with its unfairness and its hurts? Make us bitter? Or will we choose to let the difficulties in life make us better?

237

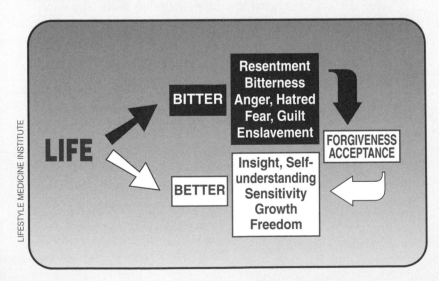

Bitter or Better? Are those the only options?

It pretty much boils down to that. Once a scientist watched a moth struggling to get out of its cocoon. It seemed that it just could not force its way through such a small opening. After watching awhile, he "helped" the moth by enlarging the hole. The moth emerged with a swollen body and shriveled wings. It never flew. It needed that struggle through the small opening to force the fluid into its still-developing wings.

You're saying that we actually need hardships?

This world is a university of hard knocks. We owe it to life not to get bitter. Bitterness shrivels the spirit, causing spiritual atherosclerosis. Just as too much of the wrong kind of food hardens our arteries, nurturing the wrong kinds of emotions can harden our attitudes. Troubles, difficulties, and disappointments *can* push us to grow—in insight, in understanding, and in finding new directions for our lives.

Our depressed woman began to realize that she had to move away from her "poor me—pity me" attitude and begin to tackle her problems and learn to solve them.

"The moment I started to hate that woman," she reflected, "I began to be her slave. For 13 years she has had a tyrannical grasp on my mind and my body. NO MORE! I know now that I can learn something positive from the most desperate situation. That woman will not steal my joy for even *one more day* of my life."

> *We cannot change our past . . . we cannot change the fact that people will act in a certain way. We cannot change the inevitable. The only thing we can do is play on the one string we have, and that is our attitude. . . . I am convinced that life is 10 percent of what happens to us and 90 percent how we react to it.*
>
> —Charles Swindoll

Your Beliefs Can Affect Your Health

People who regularly attend religious services have been found to have lower blood pressure, less heart disease, lower rates of depression, and generally better health than those who don't.

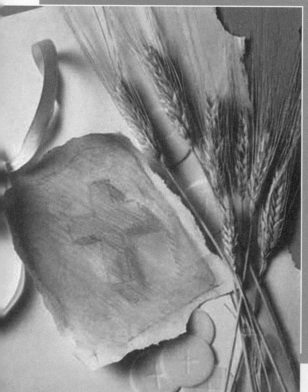

Also—

- *People who go to church have strong networks of friends who look out for them.*
- *Religious people are less likely to smoke, drink, and have other unhealthy habits.*
- *Taking part in prayer may lower harmful stress hormones.*

Basically, then, it was a change in her attitude that made the difference.

And a big difference it was! Here is another "attitude" story:

A high-society woman periodically checked into a luxurious suite of a New York hotel. She sought quiet time—to rest, to think, and to regain perspective. One time she heard a piano playing next door. Furious, she expressed her feelings in no uncertain terms.

The manager apologized profusely for putting Anton Rubenstein in the suite next door.

Rubenstein? The great one? The woman's attitude totally changed. She listened, she *loved* the music, and she treasured every day the renowned pianist was there. What had been noise before was now heavenly music!

It's what we value, not what we have, that makes us rich.

A little understanding goes a long way!

Most of the time. One place many of us still stumble is over racial problems. Recently a popular Black columnist* for the Washington *Post* put the question in perspective by painting the larger picture. Here is a part of her editorial:

"I've felt hatred rage through me, washing away every barrier of reason and compassion. Hatred seeped through the crevices of my good sense, exploited the strains of my everyday life, and chilled my compassion. Once hatred takes hold, it is hard to contain. When I'm in its grip, hatred can look sane and necessary. At such times I've screamed my loudest, cursed my rawest, and flailed away at my supposed enemy, until I'm exhausted; until I find my way back to love.

"Focusing too closely on hatred distracts me from a power more lasting and formidable—'the one power I can't afford to forget.'"

Beautiful! But aren't there some who do such horrible things that we shouldn't forgive them, much less try to love them?

The Bible reminds us that it is easy to love the lovely people—what's hard is to love the unlovely. Mrs. Hannah's only child was raped and murdered by a man who was subsequently put in prison for life.

Mrs. Hannah hated this man intensely, and prayed that every day of his life would be even more miserable than hers.

One day "Gideon" (a man who supplies hotels, motels, and other public places with Gideon Bibles) came to her home and asked if she would care to inscribe a Bible for this murderer. She angrily refused.

Mrs. Hannah struggled on for weeks—for months. She finally realized she was trapped in her own prison of misery. There was no focus in her life, no joy, no triumph.

Finally Mrs. Hannah knelt down and pleaded with God to forgive her feelings of bitterness and hatred. Then the burden lifted, and she experienced peace.

She called "Gideon" and asked him to bring back the Bible—she was ready.

She opened the Bible and wrote—"Mrs. Hannah loves you." When the prisoner read this message, tears dribbled down his cheeks. He'd grown up an orphan. Never had he been told that anyone loved him. That one sentence changed his life. He trained to become a prison chaplain, and spent the rest of his life ministering to other prisoners.

And on that very day the old, bitter, hateful Mrs. Hannah died, and a new Mrs. Hannah took her place. She too realized she'd been imprisoned. It took forgiveness to set her free.**

At best we have a limited number of days in our lives. Isn't each day too precious to be marred by unforgiving thoughts?

Right on! Besides, do we really want to inflict the pain and misery on ourselves that we feel when we're not willing to forgive?

We need to ask ourselves—
- Are there people I need to forgive?
- Do I need to forgive myself?

People who learn to forgive suffer less anxiety and depression and have higher self-esteem. And they enjoy better health. A wise man said, "If you cannot forgive, you will live lonely, and the wine of life will be soured for you forever."

Love is more important than being right. Forgiveness opens the heart.

While being crucified by His tormentors, one Man prayed—*"Father, forgive them, for they do not know what they are doing"* (Luke 23:34).

To err is human, to forgive divine.

239

We cannot grow mentally, spiritually, or socially without practicing the grace of forgiveness.

*Donna Britt, *Washington Post*
**Source of story unknown

The Ultimate Gift

"Love the Lord your God with all your heart and with all your soul and with all your mind.' This is the first and greatest commandment.

"And the second is like it: 'love your neighbor as yourself.'"

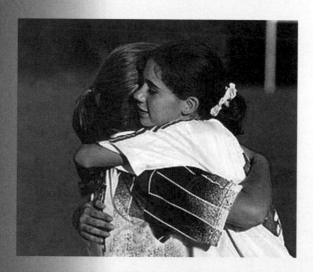

LOVE

Mirror, mirror, on the wall,
Am I skinny? Am I tall?
Am I really who I see?
Do my friends know the REAL me?*

Perhaps you know yourself very well—know who you are and where you're going.
Maybe so.
Maybe not.
Probably not.

Why do you say that?

Because, deep down, most of us harbor feelings of low self-esteem. Although Americans now live longer, more prosperous lives, surveys show they feel less and less satisfied. We are increasingly a nation of whiners and hypochondriacs.

"If I could write a prescription for the women of this world," says Dr. James Dobson, "I would provide each one of them with a healthy dose of self-esteem and personal worth. I have no doubt that this is their greatest need."

Is it just women? Don't men have the problem as well?

Feelings of worthlessness and low self-esteem are certainly no respecter of persons. They cross lines of gender, race, age, color, and ethnic origin. People today are bombarded with overinflated expectations, grandiose hopes, and unrealistic representations of life. When their dreams fade and their hopes crash, when disappointments pile up, many become disillusioned and discouraged. Other people always seem to be doing better than they're doing.

They've missed out somehow. Life is passing them by.

How about children?

Most problems with self-esteem have their roots in childhood. What happens during the first five years pretty much sets children's attitudes for the rest of their lives.

Many children grow up feeling unloved, neglected, and unwanted. They are yelled at and otherwise abused. Surrounded with too many negative messages and rules, they often become sullen, rebellious, hostile, and difficult to handle.

Savor the things that bring you untarnished pleasure and satisfaction — food, friends, music, and the outdoors.

Someone's opinion of you does not have to become your reality.

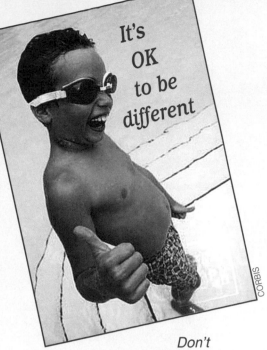

It's OK to be different

When they become teenagers their feelings of worthlessness intensify. They long to be attractive, to be popular, or even just noticed. Their low level of self-confidence suppresses their talents and their personalities. The result is loneliness, isolation, perhaps bad relationship choices, and often drugs and prostitution.

That's a lot of bad news. Are there any good answers?

"When all else fails, try God."

The phrase may sound trite, but the answers are there. God certainly didn't intend for any of us to suffer from low self-esteem. *"I have loved you with an everlasting love,"* He tells us; *"I have drawn you with loving-kindness"* (Jeremiah 31:3). And the Master Teacher

Himself, when summing up the great commandments, said that you shall *"love your neighbor as yourself"* (Mark 12:31).

Ultimate self-esteem comes from knowing who we are, why we are here, and where we are going. The Bible answers these questions in a beautiful and meaningful way.

● *Who are we?*

We are God's unique creation (Genesis 1:27). Among all the billions of people who have been born on our globe, there are no duplicates—not even among identical twins.

And that isn't all. We're told that God *"knit [us] together in [our] mother's womb."* He knows when we sit down and get up. He understands our thoughts. Read for yourself Psalm 139, which spells out God's care from our earliest conception.

And the same God continues to love us unconditionally. *"Are not five sparrows sold for two pennies? Yet not one of them is forgotten by God.*

Indeed, the very hairs of your head are all numbered.

Don't be afraid; you are worth more than many sparrows" (Luke 12:6, 7).

● *Why are we here?*

To take care of the earth and its people, and to spread the good news of a God who is present and who cares about us (Genesis 1:26; Mark 12:31; 16:15).

● *Where are we going?*

God has told us that His house has *"many rooms"* and that He is preparing a place for us to live with Him! (John 14:1-3).

And that's not all. He also promises that if we believe, we will *"have eternal life"* (John 3:16).

I'm impressed! God's plans and purposes for us completely upstage even the most spectacular of our human achievements!

Yes, and we need to help people understand what value each of us represents to our Creator. It's only

2
4
1

Most of us honestly admit that we seek a renewing purpose in life, a sense that life matters and that we can contribute something to the world.

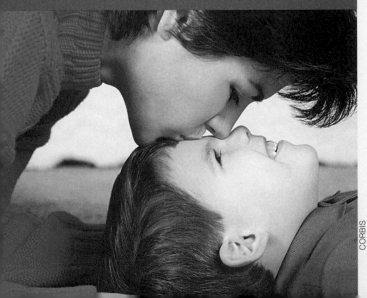

CORBIS

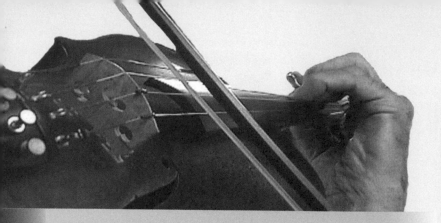

TOUCH OF THE MASTER'S HAND

'Twas battered and scarred, and the auctioneer
Thought it scarcely worth his while
To waste much time on the old violin,
But held it up with a smile.
"What am I bid, good folks?" he cried.
"Who'll start the bidding for me?
A dollar, a dollar—now two, only two—
Two dollars, and who'll make it three?"
"Three dollars, once, three dollars, twice,
Going for three." BUT NO,
From the room far back a gray-haired man
Came forward and picked up the bow;
Then wiping the dust from the old violin,
And tightening up all the strings,
He played a melody pure and sweet,
As sweet as an angel sings.

The music ceased, and the auctioneer,
With a voice that was quiet and low,
Said: "What am I bid for the old violin?"
And he held it up with the bow.
"A thousand dollars—and who'll make it two?
Two thousand—and who'll make it three?
Three thousand once and three thousand twice—
And going and gone!" said he.
The people cheered, but some of them cried,
"We do not quite understand.
What changed its worth." The man replied:
"The touch of a master's hand."

And many a man with life out of tune,
And battered and torn with sin,
Is auctioned cheap to a thoughtless crowd,
Much like the old violin.
A "mess of pottage," a glass of wine;
A game—and he travels on.
He's going once, and going twice,
He's going—and almost gone!
But the Master comes, and the foolish crowd
Never can quite understand
The worth of a soul and the change that's wrought
By the touch of the Master's Hand.

—*Myrna Brooks Welch*

when we realize this value that we gain true self-esteem.

The Master Teacher knew this. When we love ourselves, when we learn to fully appreciate this life God has given us, we can reach out to others—and learn to love them too.

Dr. Laura Schlessinger sums up this concept in one of her books: "People find focus, purpose, and meaning beyond creature comforts, needs and desires through a relationship with God and adherence to His commandments." She continues, "For me it has meant a better and richer life, and a new significance in my work."

Do these concepts belong in a health book?

Obviously it takes a lot more than healthy food and regular exercise to make life worthwhile. People need dignity and respect. The need to love and be loved is as essential to health and well-being as are fresh air and clean water.

Too many people base their self-esteem on what other people think of them. But people's opinions are fickle, unstable, and certainly undependable.

Then there are people who are really in the gutter. They've been so betrayed, so rejected, so battered by life, that they cease to see any value in continuing the struggle of living.

But the Master Healer never passed by a human being as worthless, and we can't either. With a restored sense of self-worth, we become willing to take risks. And taking risks in loving others is what life is all about.

"Dear friends,

✔ let us love one another, for love comes from God... *1 John 4:7*

✔ since God so loved us, we also ought to love one another... *1 John 4:11*

✔ let us not love with words or tongue but with actions." *1 John 3:18*

---

* Kay Rizzo

Loved people become loving people.

Application

This is not a radical or new idea! Our health, happiness, longevity, and self-esteem—as well as our relationships with family, friends, and associates, and our spiritual life—are interrelated and interdependent.

How much are you worth?

The story is told of a speaker who started off his seminar by holding up a $20 bill. In the room of 200 people he asked, "Who would like this $20 bill?" Hands started going up.

"I'm going to give this $20 bill to one of you, but first let me do this." He proceeded to crumple the bill into a small wad.

"Now who wants it?" The hands went up again.

"Well," he replied, "what if I do this?" He unfolded the crumpled bill and dropped it on the ground and started to grind it into the floor with his shoe. He picked it up, now all crumpled and dirty.

"Anybody want it now?" All the hands still went up.

"My friends," he said, "you have all learned a valuable lesson. No matter what I did to the money, you still want it, because it has not decreased in value. It is still worth $20.

Many times in our lives we are dropped, crumpled, and ground into the dirt by the decisions we make and the circumstances that come our way. We feel as though we are worthless. But no matter what has happened or what will happen, we never lose our value in God's eyes. Dirty or clean, crumpled or creased, we are still priceless to Him.

243

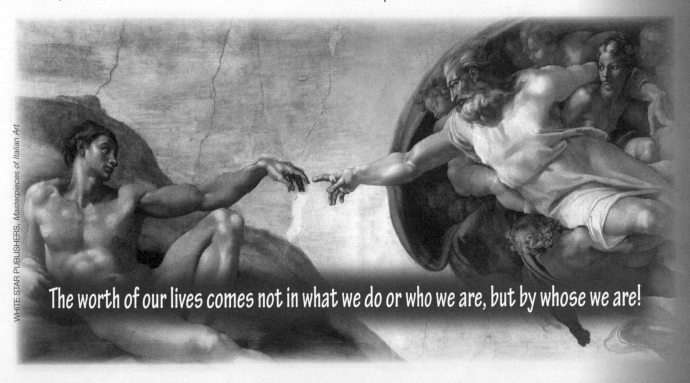

WHITE STAR PUBLISHERS, *Masterpieces of Italian Art*

The worth of our lives comes not in what we do or who we are, but by whose we are!

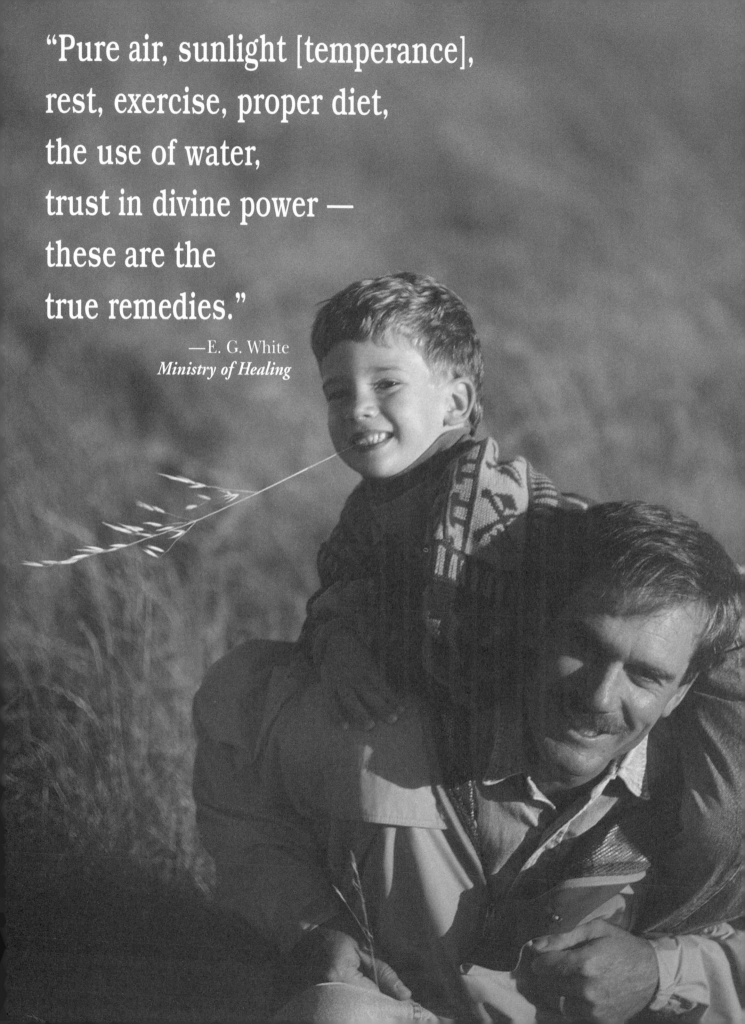

"Pure air, sunlight [temperance], rest, exercise, proper diet, the use of water, trust in divine power — these are the true remedies."

—E. G. White
Ministry of Healing

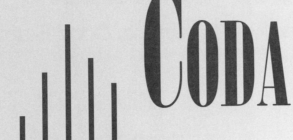

CODA

"The use of natural remedies requires an amount of care and effort that many are not willing to give. . . . [But] those who persevere in obedience to [nature's] laws will reap the reward in health of body and . . . mind." —E. G. White, *Ministry of Healing*

Eat for Health!

Basic Guidelines for a Lifetime of Good Eating

EAT LESS:

Visible fats and oils

Avoid fatty meats, cooking and salad oils, sauces, margarines, butter, dressings, and shortening. Use spreads and nuts sparingly. Avoid frying; sauté instead with a little water in nonstick pans.

Sugars

Limit sugar, honey, molasses, syrups, pies, cakes, pastries, candy, cookies, soft drinks, and sugar-rich desserts, like pudding and ice cream. Save these foods for special occasions.

Foods containing cholesterol

Avoid meat, sausages, egg yolks, and liver. Limit dairy products, if used, to low-fat cheeses and nonfat milk products. If you eat fish and poultry, use them sparingly.

Salt

Use minimal salt during cooking. Banish the saltshaker. Strictly limit highly salted products like pickles, crackers, soy sauce, salted popcorn, nuts, chips, pretzels, and garlic salt.

Alcohol

Avoid alcohol and caffeinated beverages such as coffee, colas, and black tea.

> "We cannot safely be guided by the customs of society. The disease and suffering that everywhere prevail are largely due to popular errors in regard to health." —E. G. White, *Ministry of Healing*

EAT MORE:

Whole grains

Freely use brown rice, millet, barley, corn, wheat, and rye. Also eat freely of whole-grain products, such as breads, pastas, shredded wheat, and tortillas.

Tubers and legumes

Freely use all kinds of white potatoes, sweet potatoes, and yams (without high-fat toppings). Enjoy peas, lentils, chickpeas, and beans of every kind.

Fruits and vegetables

Eat several fresh, whole fruits every day. Limit fruits canned in syrup and fiber-poor fruit juices. Eat a variety of vegetables daily. Enjoy fresh salads with low-calorie, low-salt dressings.

Water

Drink at least eight glasses of water a day. Vary the routine with a twist of lemon and occasional herb teas.

Hearty breakfasts

Enjoy hot multigrain cereals, fresh fruit and whole-wheat toast. Jumpstart your day.

COMPARISON		
	U.S. Diet/day	The Optimal Diet/day
Fats and Oils	35-40%*	10-20%*
Sugar	35 tsp	under 10 tsp.
Cholesterol	400 mg	under 50 mg
Salt	10-15 gm	under 4 gm
Fiber	10 gm	40 gm
Water (fluids)	minimal	8 glasses

*of total calories

Live for Health!

Basic Guidelines for a Lifetime of Healthful Living

A checklist for making your new start:

Nutrition
- ✔ Nourish your body with healthful, full-fiber, nutrient-rich foods.
- ✔ Increasingly move toward a totally vegetarian lifestyle.
- ✔ Enhance digestion by breaking the snack habit.
- ✔ Schedule regular mealtimes, four to five hours apart.
- ✔ Eat larger breakfasts and smaller evening meals.

Exercise
- ✔ Strengthen your body and increase your enjoyment of life with daily active exercise, outdoors if possible.
- ✔ Aim for at least 30 minutes of exercise a day. Walking is the safest exercise and one of the best.
- ✔ Physical exercise reduces stress, combats depression, restores energy, improves sleep, and strengthens bones.

Water
- ✔ Rinse out and refresh your insides by drinking a glass or two of water on arising.
- ✔ Come alive with an alternating hot and cold shower in the morning.
- ✔ Lighten your body's metabolic load and increase circulation by drinking plenty of water—at least eight glasses per day.

"Through the agencies of nature, God is working, day by day, hour by hour, moment by moment, to keep us alive, to build up and restore us." —E. G. White, *Ministry of Healing*

Sunshine
- ✔ Pull back the drapes! Fill your home with sunshine! It will lift your spirits, brighten your day, and improve your health!
- ✔ Spend at least a few minutes outdoors every day.

Temperance
- ✔ Live a balanced life. Make time for work, play, rest, exercise, and hobbies.
- ✔ Nurture relationships and spiritual growth.
- ✔ Protect your body from harmful substances, such as tobacco, alcohol, caffeine, and most drugs.

Air
- ✔ Air out your house daily. Sleep in a room with good ventilation.
- ✔ Keep your lungs healthy by taking frequent deep breaths. Walk outdoors when possible.
- ✔ Fill your house with green plants that absorb carbon dioxide and increase oxygen.

Rest
- ✔ Reserve seven to eight hours a night for rest and sleep. The body needs this time to repair and restore the damage of daily wear and tear.
- ✔ Go to bed early enough to wake up feeling refreshed.
- ✔ Devote time to a change of pace. Attend church, go on a picnic, plant a garden, pursue a hobby, take relaxing, enjoyable vacations.

Trust
- ✔ A life of quality and fulfillment includes spiritual growth and development.
- ✔ Love, faith, trust, and hope are health-enhancing. And they bring rewards that endure.
- ✔ Trust in God augments all healing—physical, mental, emotional, and spiritual.

Summary

"Let Nutrition Be Your Medicine."

—*Hippocrates*

To win the battle against the epidemic of Western lifestyle diseases we must break with the lethal excesses of today's Western diet. We need a simpler, more natural way to eat, and live.

As incredible as it might seem, there is *one* diet that not only prevents most of these killer diseases but also helps reverse them. Such a diet consists of a wide variety of foods eaten *as grown,* simply prepared with sparing use of fats, oils, sugars, and salt. It contains very few refined, engineered products. Animal foods, if used, are strictly limited.

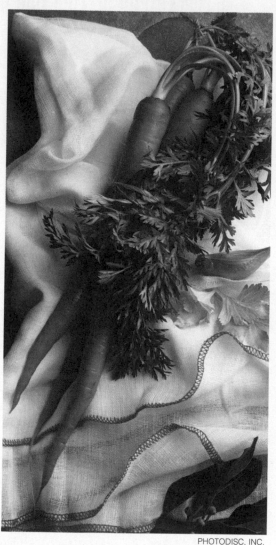

PHOTODISC, INC.

Adopting this simpler, more natural dietary lifestyle brings improved health and increased energy. We can eat larger quantities of food without gaining weight, and still cut our grocery bills in half. Where, indeed, can we find a better bargain than that?

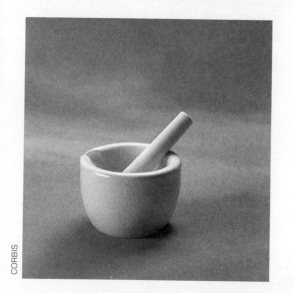

CORBIS

"Many transgress the laws of health through ignorance, and they need instruction. But [most of us] know better than [we] do. [We] need to be impressed with the importance of making [the] knowledge [we have] a guide for [our lives]." —E. G. White, *Ministry of Healing*

Index

249

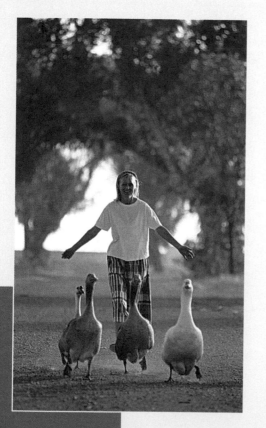

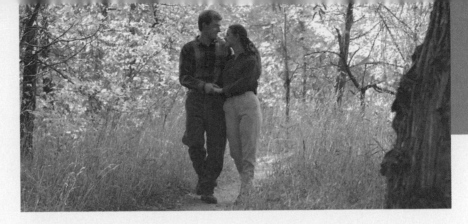

References

Barnard, Neal. *Eat Right, Live Longer.* New York: Harmony Books, 1995.

McDougall, John. *A Challenging Second Opinion.* New York: Penguin Books.

Messina, Virginia. *The Vegetarian Way.* New York: Crown, 1996.

Nedley, Neil. *Proof Positive.* Ardmore, OK: 1998.

Nelson, Ethel. *Burkitt—Cancer, Fiber—How a Humble Surgeon Changed the World.* Brushton, NY: TEACH Services, 1998.

Ornish, Dean. *Dr. Dean Ornish's Program for Reversing Heart Disease.* New York: Random House, 1990.

Robbins, John. *Reclaiming Our Health.* Tiburon, Calif.: H. J. Kramer, 1996.

Temple, N; Burkitt, Denis (editors), *Western Diseases—Their Dietary Prevention and Reversibility.* Totowa, N.J.: Humana Press, 1994.

White, E. G., *The Ministry of Healing.* Pacific Press, Nampa, Idaho: 1909.

Photos and Illustration Credits

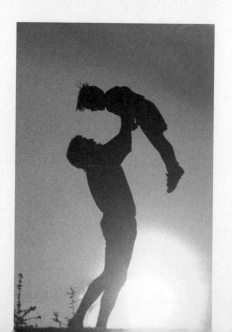

Educational Resources

BY CHERYL THOMAS PETERS, RD
JAMES A. PETERS, MD, DRPH, RD

More Choices

Simple solutions to eating well. Enjoy healthy, great-tasting meals in minutes! 150 savory, slimming, professionally developed recipes that promise to promote your health with patient proven plan to achieve your ideal weight and optimal health. Spiral, 160 pages US$14.99. Can$19.99.

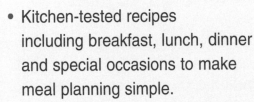

More Choices Cookbook also features:

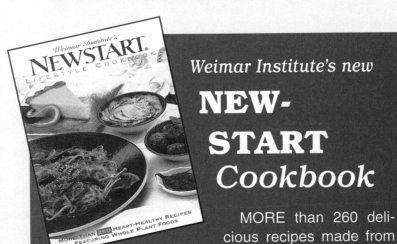

Weimar Institute's new NEW-START Cookbook

MORE than 260 delicious recipes made from whole plant foods—easy to prepare, economical, and nutritious. People everywhere today are convinced they should be eating better but few find it easy to make the shift. This book can make the difference for you. Highly recommended. From the famous Weimar Institute. Price US$19.95.

Better Health Productions
(909) 825-1888

- Kitchen-tested recipes including breakfast, lunch, dinner and special occasions to make meal planning simple.
- Incredible color-photography
- Menu planning tips
- Nutrition analysis
- Shopping guide
- Diabetic exchange
- Spiral bound book
  . . . and much more!

Call to order your copy now:

1-909-825-1888

Better Health Productions
P.O. Box 1761
Loma Linda, CA 92354
www.betterhealthproductions.com

Are you ready to take the next step?

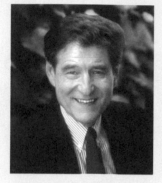

Then look for the CHIP program nearest you and enroll! Take 30 days—and change your life and health forever!

What's CHIP?

CHIP is an educationally intensive 30-day lifestyle intervention program with more than 40,000 graduates. Founded by Dr. Hans Diehl, the clinical results have been written up in major medical journals. Endorsed by the Physicians' Committee for Responsible Medicine and the Center for Science in the Public Interest, the Coronary Health Improvement Project (CHIP) focuses on markedly reducing coronary risk factors through the adoption of better health habits and wiser lifestyle choices.

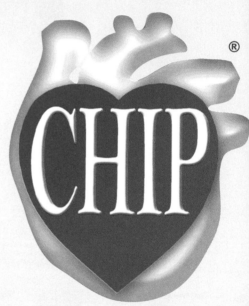

What will it do for me?

Overweight? It will show you how to eat more and still lose all the weight you want. *Hypertension?* It will lower your blood pressure. *Diabetes (type 2)?* It will help you to lower your blood sugar and your medication requirements. *Cholesterol?* CHIP will bring your cholesterol down on average 10-20% without medication. *Heart Disease?* It will show you how to slow down, halt and reverse coronary artery disease. *Depression?* It will give you the lift and energy you've been looking for.

Where can I find CHIP?

CHIP programs are conducted in more than 250 locations in North America—in cities, corporations, and churches. For more information, please call the Lifestyle Medicine Institute at: **909-796-7676**, or online at: www.CHIPglobal.org. We'll be looking forward to helping you with your new journey.

Dedicated to the remarkable women
of St. Matthews Baptist Church . . .

my encouragers, mentors,
and friends.

TABLE OF CONTENTS

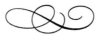

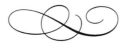

INTRODUCTION

The writing of this Bible study has been a mind and heart opening journey. Where I thought I was going is not even remotely close to where I ended, and the path has been serpentine at best. Funny how that happens, isn't it?

Shortly after resigning my fourteen year staff position at the church where my husband and I were, and still are members, I decided it would be helpful for me, and possibly others, to chronicle the discernment process that led me to that decision.

Although I had not seen handwriting mysteriously appear on the walls of my home or heard ethereal voices in the night, I knew God was leading me into a new area of purposefulness and some major life changes. A novel I had recently read about Zipporah, the wife of Moses, caught my interest and compelled me on a four month study through the books of Exodus, Leviticus, Numbers and Deuteronomy. I found countless lessons and parallels, which impacted me deeply and helped me better understand the path I had traveled to get to that particular place of transition in my life. I was amazed to discover a middle-aged, twenty-first century woman could have anything in common with a man who lived approximately 3400 years ago. My initial intrigue with Moses and four month study ultimately guided me through a career change, but it also extended to a two year in-depth writing adventure culminating in this study.

There has never been any argument Moses was one interesting fellow. As a man, he felt the joys of fatherhood, sorrow at the death of loved ones, and macho pride after rescuing damsels in distress. Yet, there is much more to set him apart in history: born a Hebrew yet raised an Egyptian; born in secret and hidden by a loving mother; died in secret and buried by a loving Father. He is mentioned in no less than thirty-one books of the Bible. In Judaism, he is remembered as the greatest prophet, leader and teacher the world has ever known; yet based on natural ability and personal confidence, he was certainly an unlikely leader.

Although I have no delusions of being remembered as the "greatest" at anything, the writing of this study has been akin to Leadership 101 as I have taken the days and events of Moses' life and juxtaposed my own circumstances along side his. Situations lived by Moses lend clarity to the path I walked; times of questioning, strange encounters, significant markers, evidence of provision and protection. I discovered it was more than the fourteen years I spent in one particular area of ministry that brought me to my own exodus, wilderness place, and mountaintop experience; it was a lifelong adventure of epic proportions.

Walking With Moses—Talking With God is written in a format that will encourage you to read not only the text and focus Scripture for each day, but to dig deeper for additional text which might bring broader understanding to each lesson. I hope you will take advantage of each question and inquiry throughout, allowing the interactive nature of the study to enhance your learning experience.

Just as the Israelites wove their way through the wilderness, we will follow a winding path as we make our way through the books of Exodus, Leviticus, Numbers and Deuteronomy. Volumes have, and will continue, to be written about the events in these four books, but we will stay focused on Moses and his leadership role in each scenario. Be prepared for a thematic/topical approach as opposed to one chronological in nature.

Whether you are flying solo or enjoying this study with a group, the style for each day and week will be the same. The introduction page of each week's study will outline the theme, daily topics, and a challenge for your heart and mind.

Unless otherwise noted, all Biblical passages are taken from the *New King James Version*. Consequently, access to this particular translation will be extremely helpful, although not essential, as you complete each day's written work. In addition to various translations of the Scripture, countless resources were used in the preparation of this study and are acknowledged within the text or in footnote form at the end of each day's study, and are included in the bibliography.

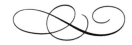

Week 1

PRAYING THE HARD QUESTIONS

Moses was a man of many questions, as we will see in our first week of study. We will jump right into our journey with Moses as he encounters God for the first time in an audible and visual way and gets his marching orders for the next forty years. I warned you in the introduction to our study we will not always move through the Scripture in chronological order, so be prepared for a bit of backtracking next week. But for now, let's look at the questions that defined Moses' commission, which will ultimately define ours as well.

This week, as you walk with Moses and talk with God, rest secure knowing God will call you, equip you and answer all your questions.

Day 1
Who Am I?

Text: Exodus 1-3:1, 3:7-12

Focus: *But Moses said to God, "Who am I that I should go to Pharaoh, and that I should bring the children of Israel out of Egypt?"* Exodus 3:11

My father is one of the most humble people I have ever known. He will step back to allow another to step forward, and quietly hold his opinion as others verbosely share theirs. Because of his meek demeanor, I have seen him be taken advantage of by those interested in their own personal gain. Do not misunderstand; he is not a weak man—quite the contrary. He is strong in his beliefs and unflappable in his faith. He simply does not force his ideas or intentions on anyone else. Quietly, he goes about his days, never seeking the regard of others.

For several years, Daddy was a Sunday School teacher for young married couples, and though he invested many hours in study, he never felt adequately prepared or qualified to teach. Occasionally, members of that class from long ago will remind him of a lesson learned under his tutelage or a truth he helped them embrace. He became a quiet mentor to the young men who worked as farmhands, treating each with fairness and compassion. As a respected member of the farming community, he was often called upon to bring his expertise and insight to a rural planning meeting or to give advice to a young farmer just starting out. In his typical selfless manner, he quietly and succinctly shared his time-tested knowledge, quickly adding that he was "no expert." I am certain many of those he has advised through the years would beg to differ and agree that he is an expert on many things: expertise gained by hard work, trial and error, a keen awareness of the workings of nature, and a sharp and inquiry mind.

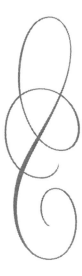

That was how I was raised, never to seek the limelight or draw undue attention to myself. I became the quintessential behind-the-scenes worker, not comfortable speaking in public or being acknowledged as a leader. I would gladly volunteer to cook for the church dinner; play the piano for the ensemble; run the sound board for the guest speaker; and type up the session notes afterwards; but I would never agree to be on the front line.

What about you? Are you an "up-front" person or do you prefer working behind the scenes allowing others to gain the applause? There is no wrong or right, better or best answer.

_____

_____

_____

In 1996, a new ministry was budding within the congregation of my church. I was already on staff and it was a relatively simple transition for me to be involved in the startup of the program—the proverbial at the right place at the right (or wrong, depending on your perspective) time scenario. I can think of countless circumstances that could have led to a much different outcome, but God was orchestrating, a point person was needed, and I soon found myself in the coordinator's role.

Have you found yourself in a leadership position that you did not seek or envision for yourself? If yes, briefly explain.

_____

_____

_____

_____

Has the position shown you strengths, talents, and abilities you did not know you possessed?

_____

_____

_____

_____

In Exodus 3:1 Moses was learning a new profession—tending the sheep of his father-in-law, Jethro. Each day it was his responsibility to find fresh water and green grass for the herd, protect them from predators, and lead them back to the compound before nightfall. On this particular day, Moses moved beyond the familiar grazing lands of Midian and found himself at the foot of the "mountain of God." I wonder if he ended at this spot simply by accident, as his mind was preoccupied with other things and veered off the regular path; maybe he had seen this particular mountain from afar and his curiosity finally got the best of him; or perhaps he simply was trying to find new pasture land for his wooly charges. Regardless of how it came to be, this day would be the start of an entirely new direction for Moses.

Have you had such an encounter? One day going about your daily routine, then suddenly confronted with a new plan or direction for your life? If so, explain where and how this came about.

_____

_____

_____

Moses did not see himself as a leader. As he looked back over his life prior to the encounter at the burning bush, he saw a history of contradiction, confusion and uncertainty. As God laid out the plan for the Israelites, and the leadership role Moses would play, we should not be surprised to hear him ask, "Who am I?"

Glance back through Exodus 1 & 2. List the circumstances that might have caused Moses to think he was unqualified to lead the Israelites.

_____

_____

Do you think Moses had a sense of his destiny even as a child? If so, explain why.

_____

_____

_____

_____

Now the man Moses was very humble, more than all men who were on the face of the earth.

Numbers 12:3

Moses was a slave by birth, the adopted son of Pharaoh's daughter, a murderer, a runaway and traitor to his adopted family, an alien in a foreign land, and a shepherd in his father-in-law's household. Consider for a moment how each of these situations might have prepared Moses for God's plan for the Israelites. He was a humble and unqualified man in his own eyes, yet a leader in the eyes of God (Numbers 12:3).

Proverbs 3:34: Surely *He scorns the scornful, but gives grace to the* _____ .

Proverbs 16:19: *Better to be of a* _____ *spirit with the lowly, than to divide the spoil with the proud.*

Does God see you differently than you see yourself? If so, briefly explain:

_____

_____

_____

_____

Moses received a divine assurance from God that all would be well. Fill in the blanks from Exodus 3:11-12: *But Moses said to God, "Who am I that I should go to Pharaoh, and that I should bring the children of Israel out of Egypt?" So He said, "_____ _____ _____ _____ _____ _____ . And this shall be a sign to you that _____ _____ _____ _____: when you have brought the people out of Egypt, you _____ _____ _____ _____ _____ _____."*

We will see later in our study how Moses does indeed return to this same place after he has successfully freed the Israelites. This first encounter simply sets the stage for each and every encounter yet to come on the mountain of God.

Have you returned to the place where you first felt God's call on your life? If so, give a brief description.

_____

_____

_____

Do you consider that place holy ground? If yes, give a brief explanation why.

_____

_____

◯ **Walking With Moses** ◯

God can and will take the circumstances of your past and use them to prepare you for His ultimate design for your life. Feelings of inadequacy have no place before a totally adequate God. You may ask "Who am I?" and rest assured God will answer you decisively.

◯ **Talking With God** ◯

God, thank You for calling me into Your service. Help me to see all the ways You have prepared me.

_____

_____

Day 2
Who are You?

Text: Exodus 3:13-22

Focus: *Then Moses said to God, "Indeed, when I come to the children of Israel and say to them, 'The God of your fathers has sent me to you,' and they say to me, 'What is His name?' what shall I say to them?"* Exodus 3:13

Names . . . we all have one or two and sometimes even three picked out for us at birth. Surnames come without choice, passed down through generations. Brides generally take their new husband's last name, although occasionally these days, it is the other way around; and sometimes, the new couple will keep both names and just throw in a hyphen. In addition to the legal names, there are pet names, nicknames (some flattering/some not) and variations of given names. Attached to those names are titles, distinctions made by occupation or association, and of course, plain, old adjectives.

Allow me to use myself as an example. My given name is Cinda, although my family calls me Cindy. My niece and nephews call me Cissy. My nickname when I was little was Skeezicks. When I went to first grade, there were two other six year olds named Cindy, so one got to keep Cindy, one became Cynthia, and I went back to Cinda. In high school, I went back to Cindy. When I started to drive, my nickname became A.J. (in honor of race car driver, A.J. Foyt), and in college, I decided Cinda sounded more grown-up. Through all those changes, my family resolutely called me Cindy.

When I married, I assumed my husband's last name. As my children came along, their names for me evolved from Momma, to Mom, to Mother, to "you are without a doubt the most annoying person in my life" (that's a story for another day). To the children at church, I am Ms. Cinda; to friends of my children, I am Mrs. King; and frequently, I am introduced as Greg's wife.

List the different names you are known by to family, friends, & colleagues.

_____ _____ _____

_____ _____ _____

_____ _____ _____

I have assumed the vocational names of director, coordinator, assistant, minister, writer, speaker, and teacher. Daily, I am called friend, companion, listener, caregiver, daughter, daughter-in-law, and a myriad of other descriptors.

What about your vocational names and other descriptors? List as many as you can think of: _____

_____

You get the picture, I'm sure. We each have various names, titles and descriptions that help us know who we are. Most of us know the origin/meaning of our given names and it is usually something that fits our individual personality rather well. Bottom line, I think most people like to be called by their "given" name.

Do you know what your given name means? If not, take the time to look on-line or check it out next time you are in the library or bookstore. It can be an enriching experience to know how your name corresponds with your personality and God-given traits.

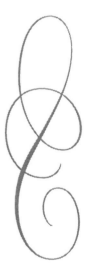

The Israelites were familiar with many names for God; each giving clarity to the distinctive characteristics of God.

El Elyon – Genesis 14:20: *And blessed be God* _____ _____.

El Roi – Genesis 16:13: *Then she called the name of the* LORD *who spoke to her, You are the God* _____ _____.

El Shaddai – Genesis 17:1: *When Abram was ninety-nine years old, the* LORD *appeared to Abram and said to him I am* _____ *God.*

El Olam – Genesis 21:33: *Then Abraham planted a tamarisk tree in Beersheba, and there called on the name of the* LORD, *the* _____ *God.*

In today's Scripture passage, Moses is not only wanting a specific name for God, he also wants credentials; a resumé of sorts, so the Israelites will know from whom Moses is taking orders.

What "name" does God give Himself in Exodus 3:14a? *And God said to Moses, "*
_____ _____ _____ _____ _____ _____
_____*."*

And just in case there is any question, Moses reminds the Israelites this is the same *"Lord God of your* _____*, the God of* _____*, the God of* _____*, and the God* _____*.* (Ex. 3:15)

How long will God be known as *I AM THAT I AM* (Ex.4:15b)? _____

How is the name God gave Himself in Exodus different from those given earlier in Genesis?

_____

_____

_____

_____

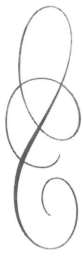

The name Moses was to use when he spoke with the Israelites and to Pharaoh had no limitations or specific characteristics.

A few years ago, I was compelled to learn and begin using the many names of God in my daily prayers. I gathered resources that explained the origin, as well as the scriptural and historical context of each. In addition to those already listed, I learned the Hebrew names:

- *Ab* – God the Father
- *Elohim* – God the Creator
- *Shapat* – God the Judge
- *Adonai* – God the Lord
- *Qedosh Yisra'el* – God the Holy One of Israel
- *YHWH (Yahweh)* – Lord (at the most intimate level)

And the Aramaic names:

- *Abba* – Daddy
- *Attiq Yomin* – God the Ancient of Days

Plus several additional Hebrew variations attached to Yahweh or Jehovah:

- *Jehovah Nissi* – the Lord is my Banner
- *Jehovah Sabaoth* – the Lord of Hosts
- *Jehovah Shalom* – the Lord is Peace
- *Jehovah Jireh* – the Lord will Provide
- *Jehovah Tsidkenu* – the Lord our Righteousness
- *Jehovah Rohi* – the Lord is my Shepherd
- *Jehovah Shammah* – the Lord is There
- *Jehovah M'Kaddesh* – the Lord who Sanctifies
- *Jehovah Rophe* – the Lord who Heals

It was an interesting study and gave me a deeper understanding of God—one God with so many names and attributes.

Since doing that particular bit of research, and as the design of each day is different, so too are my salutations. On some days, I specifically pray to *El-Roi,* "the one who sees me" and on other days I rest with *Jehovah-Shalom,* "the Lord is peace." With each name, I feel a renewed sense of relationship and an awe-filled familiarity. God knows when I call on *Jehovah-Jireh,* I need to know "the Lord will provide"; when I call out to *El-Shaddai,* I am recognizing Him as "God Almighty"; and, on those rare occasions when I wonder if He is really hearing me at all, I can rest in the name He gave Himself in Exodus 3:14—I AM.

When you call out to God, what name do you use? Is it different on different days?

_____

_____

_____

Does calling God by name boost your confidence? If so, explain how.

_____

_____

_____

_____

The Hebrew text of Exodus 3:14a, 'ehyeh 'asher 'ahyeh is translated "I am who I am." or "I will be who I will be."

God was definitive of His own identity and the nature of His power. His instructions to Moses were clear and decisive: Tell the elders of Israel deliverance is at hand, and then ask Pharaoh to allow the Israelites to journey three days outside of Egypt to offer sacrifices to God. Moses must have wondered why he was to only ask for three days when total freedom was the ultimate plan, but God continued giving details so Moses would understand the following days were going to be very eventful and were designed and destined to prove the awesome power of God.

Exodus 3:19-20: *But I am sure that the king of Egypt will not let you go, no, not even by a mighty hand. So I will stretch out My hand and strike Egypt with all My wonders which I will do in its midst; and after that he will let you go.*

Exodus 7:4-5: *But Pharaoh will not heed you, so that I may lay My hand on Egypt and bring My armies and My people, the children of Israel, out of the land of Egypt by great judgments. And the Egyptians shall know that I am the LORD, when I stretch out My hand on Egypt and bring out the children of Israel from among them.*

⌒◌ Walking With Moses ◌⌒

If you ask, God will reveal Himself to you. He has enough names and titles to fit every situation, every question, and every dilemma. God is the great I AM, forever and for all generations, and He is the One who has called you. He will guide you with His mighty hand.

⌒◌ Talking With God ◌⌒

God, help me to know You and call You by name. Lead and guide me by Your authority.

_____

_____

_____

_____

Day 3
What is in Your Hand?

Text: Exodus 4:1-9

Focus: *So the Lord said to him, "What is that in your hand?" He said, "A rod."*
Exodus 4:2

Prove it! If I have heard my children say it once, I have heard it a million times. I live in a house full of natural debaters and curious minds—always in search of facts to give credence to their particular opinions or philosophies. We have been known to stop in the middle of dinner to check a fact in the encyclopedia or a definition in the dictionary. In my husband's profession as an attorney, he is duty bound to prove the innocence or particular position of his clients. In one way or another, we are all out to prove something, either to ourselves or to someone else.

Moses was beginning to understand God was serious about using him to lead the Israelites out of Egypt, but he was unsure how he would convince anyone else of his commission. After all, other than a bunch of sheep, there was no one else to witness the conversation at the burning bush.

Exodus 4:1: *Then Moses answered and said, "But suppose they will not _____ me or listen to my voice; suppose they say, 'The LORD has not appeared to you.'"*

What three specific signs did God give Moses to prove he was called by God?

Exodus 4:2-5 _____

Exodus 4:6-8 _____

Exodus 4:9 _____

The Israelites did indeed ask for proof from Moses. *Then he did the signs in the sight of the people. So the people believed; and when they heard that the LORD had visited the children of Israel and that He had looked on their affliction, then they bowed their heads and worshiped.* (Ex. 4:30b-31)

Describe a time when you have been required to prove a particular calling or mission.

_____

_____

_____

_____

Were you able to list specific "signs" to prove you were called by God? If so, what were they? _____

_____

_____

Two of the three signs would be used before Pharaoh, although with less convincing results. Later in our study we will devote more time to the discussion of the rod turning into a snake and the water turning to blood, but for today, our focus will remain on the significance and the power of the rod or staff as a tool of deliverance.

We all have talents. And most of us have tools to go along with those talents. Some are literal tools we hold in our hands and others are natural abilities that help us do our jobs more effectively. When I cook for a crowd, I appreciate my sharp knives and oversized pots and pans. When I play the piano, I need the music, of course, and my reading glasses. And I can't imagine trying to write a book or anything else without my computer and spell check.

The tools that come with our natural abilities are a bit harder to nail down and tend to evolve over time. When I joined the church staff in 1992, my innate tools were the ability to cook for a crowd and not panic when an extra thirty people showed up unannounced for Wednesday dinner. As time went by, the ability to organize large events and rally volunteers became more prevalent. Later, God placed a calling in my heart and began cultivating the tools needed to be an effective leader. I'll admit, I was surprised and hesitant to believe I actually had the capabilities to do all God was nudging me to do, especially since most of it was far outside my comfort zone.

What is that in your hand? What are the literal tools that help you do your job better?

_____

_____

_____

What are the tools that come with your natural abilities?

_____

_____

_____

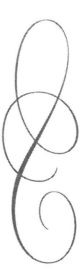

Moses must have thought God was asking a trick question when He posed the question in today's focus Scripture. God knew this was simply a rod, the shepherd's staff Moses used every day as he tended Jethro's sheep. It was the basic tool of every shepherd. How surprised Moses must have been when he threw it down and it turned into a snake! Naturally, he drew back from it (vs. 3). On this, Moses and I are definitely in agreement. I can tell you unequivocally, I don't like snakes and would not only have drawn back from it, but I would have been on down the road or scrambling atop the nearest boulder. Never, in my right mind, would I grab a snake by the tail, but that is precisely what God told Moses to do. *"Reach out your hand and take it by the tail"* (vs4). I have to wonder how much self-talk Moses was doing as he reached out his hand. "I know it's not really a snake. It only looks like a snake. It's my rod, the same staff I use everyday tending sheep." Yet, there it was, slithering across the ground, a living, hissing and potentially dangerous snake. Of course, Moses did as he was told and the snake became a rod again. From that moment on, Moses knew he held a tool in his hand which would be used to carry out the job God was laying out before him.

Do you question whether you have the tools needed to be an effective leader?
_____ yes _____ no

Describe a time when you were surprised by the way God used your natural ability or "tool" for His purpose.

_____

_____

Who are the Bible figures and what tools (literal or natural abilities) did they use to effectuate God's will in each of the following passages?

Genesis 6-9 _____

_____

Genesis 40-41 _____

_____

1 Samuel 17 _____

_____

Daniel 2 _____

_____

Matthew 3 _____

_____

Acts 9:10-19 _____

_____

Acts 16:11-15 _____

_____

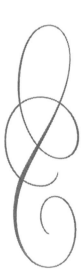

Often I have hesitated when God has nudged me to do the scary or unpleasant—to grab the snake by the tail. I want proof that what I'm about to do is really God's plan; after all, Satan disguised himself as a snake from time to time. It's only by faith that I am able to reach out my hand with the confidence God has a plan for my life.

Matteh is the Hebrew word translated as rod or staff. It is also the word used most often in the Old Testament meaning tribe. Allow your mind to wonder for a moment and consider our present text and scenario replacing the word "rod" with "tribe". The question would become "Moses, what is that you have in your hand—what or who are you feeling responsible for?" Moses said, "A tribe." The conversation continues as God tells Moses to let go of the *tribe* (throw it down); Moses sees the danger and complexity of trying to control or lead the tribe (Moses fled from it); and then God tells Moses to take the tribe in hand *"that they may believe that the LORD God of their fathers, the God Abraham, the God of Isaac, and the God of Jacob, has appeared to you."* (Ex. 4:5) Of course, I took a good bit of artistic license with that word exchange, but it certainly gives additional significance to the power and complexity of the future for which God was equipping Moses.

◦⁄◦ Walking With Moses ◦⁄◦

Moses stood before the great I AM at the burning bush with nothing in his hand but his shepherd's rod or staff—a common tool he used as he went about his daily routine. That same tool would be used countless times throughout the journey to the Promised Land. God will use whatever you hold in your hand if you are willing to throw it down and grab it by the tail under God's leadership.

◦⁄◦ Talking With God ◦⁄◦

God, help me to see and use the tools You have given me.

_____

_____

_____

_____

Day 4
Is there Someone Else? – Part I

Text: Exodus 4:10-17

Focus: *But he said, "O my Lord, please send by the hand of whomever else you shall say."* Exodus 4:13

I have never been comfortable speaking in public. It may not be a phobia, but it is certainly outside my comfort zone. As a young child I hid behind my parents and certainly never spoke to an adult unless absolutely necessary. At that age, it was okay to be shy.

In high school, I was ridiculed for having a pronounced lisp and was mortified each week as I was called to the office for speech therapy. The therapist did not keep a regular schedule so I was at the mercy of the school secretary, who seemingly took pleasure in embarrassing students, her raspy voice crackling through the intercom for the entire class to hear "Please send Cinda to the office for speech therapy." I would gather my things and dart from the room as quickly as possible in an effort to escape the stares and laughter of my classmates.

As a senior, with fear and trembling, I stood at the front of Mr. McCullough's Communications class and struggled through my required speeches—demonstration, personal narrative, fiction, and so forth. Although I usually received an acceptable grade for concept, composition and organization, the teacher's comments always reflected my lack of confidence. He stopped me in the middle of one speech and laughingly said, "Smile, you're among friends." I wasn't so sure since some of the "friends" were the same ones who snickered as I was notified the speech therapist had arrived.

Describe a situation when your confidence was shaken by the outward responses and words of those around you.

_____

_____

_____

_____

I overcame or outgrew most of my lisp, but my fear of public speaking was rock solid. My knees shook all the way through college and I developed some very effective ways to avoid being called on—never make eye contact with the teacher, hide behind the person seated in front of you, keep a confused expression on your face, and never, never volunteer. Had I known when I registered at Georgetown College oral examinations were a requisite for graduation, I probably would have reconsidered. I did not sleep or eat for days prior to standing before the department representatives to deliver my final speech and answer questions proving mastery of my declared major and minors. Relief does not adequately describe the feeling after that torturous event. In 1983, I married into an entire family of public speakers and a husband who could not understand my trepidation. For natural born speakers, organizing thoughts and putting them to words is a very easy task. I can get the thoughts together, but somewhere between my brain and my mouth, everything turns to mush.

Fortunately, my first few jobs kept me safely behind a desk and not a podium, until I accepted a position at a beautiful historic home. Daily I found myself in front of a group of children or senior citizens as I welcomed them and provided a brief overview of the tour they were about to take. I was always nervous, but the site director insisted I was not only competent, but an effective communicator. I never really believed her, but I always will be thankful for her confidence and patience.

Describe a time when your confidence was buoyed and strengthened by the outward responses and words of those around you.

_____

_____

_____

_____

Has someone noticed gifts or abilities in you that you were not aware of yourself? If so, describe how these revelations were presented to you and by whom.

_____

_____

_____

_____

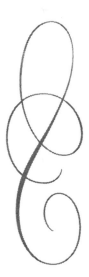

After joining the staff of my church in a very "behind the scenes" role, I again allowed others to do the talking. As my areas of ministry evolved, it became increasingly more difficult, but thankfully, just as God provided Aaron to speak when Moses could not, He provided those who would speak for me. For the first few years as I coordinated the ministries for women of the church, I would count on someone else to lead prayers, make announcements, and welcome guests.

Are you quick to find others to do the work God has called you to do? If so, describe a situation when this occurred.

_____

_____

_____

_____

Reread Exodus 4:13. The NIV says, But Moses said, *"O Lord, please send someone else to do it."* Have you tried to convince God someone else could do a better job than you? _____ yes _____ no

What was God's response to Moses? _____

_____

_____

_____

So the LORD said to him, "Who has made man's mouth? Or who makes the mute, the deaf, the seeing, or the blind? Have not I the LORD? Now, therefore, go, and I will be with your mouth and teach you what you shall say." (Ex. 4:11)

What was God's response to you? _____

_____

_____

_____

I stayed in the background planning and orchestrating details and logistics while others took the podium. It was a good plan, until God evidently wearied of my hesitancy. I remember the moment vividly. I was in Lexington, Kentucky with approximately 100 ladies from my church attending our fourth annual spring women's retreat. As the soloist sang "My Life Is In Your Hands," so beautifully penned by contemporary gospel artist Kathy Troccoli, I was overcome with the truth of the words. As the song came to a close, I wiped tears from my eyes, and with a quivering voice, took the microphone to officially welcome the ladies to the1999 Women's Retreat. It was a turning point, the start of a healing, and another step of the journey.

Describe a time when you took a bold step in the direction God was calling you.

_____

_____

_____

_____

Read Exodus 4:10 and Exodus 6:12. What do these verses tell you about Moses?

_____

_____

There has been great speculation throughout history as to why Moses described himself as "slow of speech and slow of tongue." Jewish Midrash recounts Pharaoh's ministers testing the loyalty of Moses as a toddler. In this story, Moses touched a brazier or metal bowl of hot coals to his mouth, causing a serious burn and a resultant speech impediment. Perhaps as a young child, he was frequently hushed so as not to draw attention to himself. After all, the other Hebrew boys his age had died at the edict of the cruel Pharaoh. As a teen, maybe he endured the ridicule of others in Pharaoh's courts as he lisped his way through his studies. As an adult in the house of Jethro, his strange dialect surely evoked comments from the other Midian shepherds.

Whether a physical or emotional impediment, God was, none the less, preparing Moses for a huge "behind the podium" job. As Moses stood before the burning bush arguing and attempting to convince God putting him in charge was a huge mistake, God had other ideas. Mercifully, He arranged for Moses to be reacquainted with his brother Aaron who obviously had no qualms about speaking in public (vs. 14 - 16). The brothers became a dynamic duo as God spoke to Moses, Moses spoke to Aaron, and Aaron spoke to the people. Moses orchestrated the details and logistics while Aaron's voice boomed the traveling instructions to the Israelites preparing to leave Egypt.

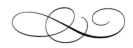

Midrash — story, inquiry, investigation

… refers to a method of exegisis of a Biblical text. The term "midrash" also can refer to a compilation of Midrashic teachings, in the form of legal, exegetical, homiletical commentaries on the Tanakh (Jewish Bible).²

… interprets and expands stories from the Bible. Midrash derives from the Oral Law of Judaism that dates back more than 3,000 years and is considered the mirror image of the Written Law. In layman's terms, Midrash fills the gaps or holes within the biblical narrative.

Can you relate to this story? Has there been a time when you empowered someone else to convey the message God had given you? If so, give a brief account.

_____

_____

_____

_____

I wonder who was more surprised, Aaron or Moses, when somewhere along the way, Moses found his voice. And what a voice it was! Jump ahead in the story and read Exodus 14:13 - 25. The Israelites were at the edge of the Red Sea, the chariots could be seen in the distance, a wave of panic moved through the masses as they realized there was no escape. Unlike the previous chapters, Exodus 14 does not mention Aaron or his participation in the big event recounted here. It was Moses' voice that rallied the spirits of the people as he raised his staff over the sea saying, *"Do not be afraid, stand still, and see the salvation of the Lord, which he will accomplish for you today"* (Exodus 14:13a). His knees might have been knocking under his desert robes, but he obviously applied those words to himself as well, and it was the beginning of a new era of leadership for Moses. He did his own talking for the next forty years and could truly say, *"The Lord is my strength and song, and He has become my salvation"* (Exodus 15:2a), even if he inwardly remained skeptical of his own abilities and qualifications.

Walking With Moses

God could certainly use someone else to do a task, but He has called you specifically and given you all the skills and gifts you need to accomplish His will. Do not miss what God has planned for you based on doubts about your own abilities.

Talking With God

God, please give me the confidence to do all You have called me to do.

_____

_____

_____

28

Day 5
Why Me?

Text: Exodus 5:1 - 6:30

Focus: *So Moses returned to the* L<small>ORD</small> *and said, "Lord, why have you brought trouble on this people? Why is it You have sent me?"* Exodus 5:22

As a child, I remember making a silent, yet solemn, promise to myself that if I ever became a parent, I would never say the words I often heard from my mother. In her frustration, after enduring moments of questioning, arguing, and complaining, she would breathe an exasperated, "Because I said so!" During my tumultuous teenage years, that particular phrase set in motion a verbal challenge that I was not quick to step away from. Alas, my poor mother.

Now, as a parent, I will admit, time and again I have broken that vow made so many years ago. I am convinced strong-willed children cause such definitive phrases to come into existence. And, although I will usually attempt to counter with every reasonable remark I can conjure, sometimes there is nothing left to be said, except "Because I said so!"

Briefly describe a time when you reluctantly heard and heeded the words "Because I said so!"

_____

_____

Listening to the voice of authority, whether a parent, employer, or spiritual leader, can be a challenge; willingly obeying that voice can seem impossible. In our creative intellects, we have our own plan or strategy to effectuate a particular outcome. Our minds whirl with possibilities and solutions. Consequently, when a superior states an absolute, it is human nature to question. Even if we eventually acquiesce, when things do not go well, we want to challenge the plan and institute our new and improved way of doing things.

Have you experienced a time when you were required to trust in another's plan, even when it was not going well? If so, give a brief description.

_____

_____

_____

_____

As much as I might hate to admit it, due to experience, education, or a combination of the two, the speaker of this time worn phrase is usually correct in their directive. I recall several times, while on the church staff, when my supervisor (who also happened to be the pastor), gave an instruction I did not agree with or think would produce the desired outcome. He would ask me to trust his discernment. Occasionally, things would not appear to progress as either of us had hoped, yet before I could speak a terse "I told you so," he would remind me of my agreement to trust him. Much to my dismay, in the end, many times he was right.

Moses found himself in a similar situation. After much questioning and side-stepping, he agreed to return to Egypt; with the stipulation Aaron would be on hand to do the talking. The two brothers stood before Pharaoh and requested the Israelites be allowed to go into the wilderness for a three-day religious festival and to offer a sacrifice to God. Pharaoh not only said a vehement no, but he instructed the slave taskmasters no longer to provide straw for the bricks the Israelites were forced to make.

Re-read Exodus 5:9. What was Pharaoh's plan to keep the Israelites from listening to Moses and Aaron?

_____

_____

_____

With no straw and the same number of bricks expected each day, the situation quickly became unbearable. The Israelite supervisors were beaten as the Egyptian taskmasters questioned, _"Why have you not fulfilled your task in making brick both yesterday and today, as before?"_ (Exodus 5:14b) In desperation, the supervisors went before Pharaoh asking for relief. His response was without feeling as he said _"You are idle! Idle!_

Therefore you say, 'Let us go and sacrifice to the LORD.' Therefore go now, and work."
(Exodus 5:17-18a)

The Israelites looked to Moses with anger as they accused him of bringing Pharaoh's ill-temper upon them. How confused they must have been. Moses had promised their deliverance yet now they were expected to work harder with less resources and harsher punishment. What kind of deliverance was this?

Once again Moses questioned God's divine plan and uttered those oft-said words, "why me?" *"Why is it You have sent me?"* (Ex.5:22b) He repeated the complaints of the people and bemoaned their ever worsening situation. Obviously, Moses still was not convinced God would or could do all He had promised when first they met at the burning bush.

Have you found yourself in a similar situation—you believe you are doing God's will and following a divine directive, yet every effort you make seems to backfire? Give a brief description.

_____

_____

_____

_____

Exodus 6 begins with a strong response to Moses' question in the previous chapter. If you will allow me to paraphrase, God answered Moses' cries of "why" with a resounding "Because I said so!"

Complete the following "I" statements God spoke to Moses in Exodus 6:

Verse 2b: *I am the _____.*

Verse 3a: *I _____ to Abraham, Isaac, and Jacob as _____ _____.*

Verse 4a: *I have also _____ my _____ with them.*

Verse 5a: *I have also _____ the groaning of the Israelites.*

Verse 5c: *I have _____ my covenant.*

Verse 6b: *I am the _____.*

Verse 6c: *I will_____ _____ _____ from under the burdens of the Egyptians, I will _____ you from their bondage.*

Verse 6d: *I will* _____ _____ *with an outstretched arm and with*
great judgments.

Verse 7a: *I will* _____ _____ *as my people,*

Verse 7b: *I will be* _____ _____ .

Verse 7c *I am the* _____ _____ _____ , *who brings you*
out from under the burdens of the Egyptians.

Verse 8a: *I will* _____ _____ *into the land which I swore to give to*
Abraham, Isaac, and Jacob;

Verse 8b: *I will* _____ _____ _____ _____ *as*
a heritage,

Verse 8c: *I am the* _____ .

Expanding my previous paraphrase, just a bit, God listened to Moses asking why and answered by saying "because I AM said so!"

ᴄ⁄ᴏ Walking With Moses ᴄ⁄ᴏ

Moses questioned God's plan and wisdom as he witnessed the increased hardship placed upon the Israelites, yet he did not turn his back on God's sovereign call upon his life. God sees the big picture for your life and the plans He has for you. Trust Him to be in control, even when you have questions.

ᴄ⁄ᴏ Talking With God ᴄ⁄ᴏ

God, help me to trust and not to ask why You have chosen me.

_____

_____

_____

_____

[1] Troccoli, Kathy. *My Life Is In Your Hand.* Careers-BMG Music Publishing, Inc. and Floating Note Music, 1994.

[2] Lazareth, William H., ed., *Reading the Bible in Faith: Theological Voices from the Pastorate* (Wm. B. Eerdmans Publishing Co., 2001, Grand Rabids, MI)

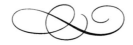

Week 2
STRANGE ENCOUNTERS OF THE GOD-KIND

Moses' life was filled with colorful individuals who not only set the stage for his upbringing in Pharaoh's courts, but helped shape his character and leadership qualities. This week we will take a look at some of the people who influenced Moses and the events leading up to the Exodus of the Israelites from Egypt. His experiences were anything but ordinary and could only be described as strange encounters of the God-kind.

This week, as you walk with Moses and talk with God, rest secure knowing God will use people of influence and defining moments to speak His will into your life.

Day 1
People of Influence

Text: Exodus 2:1-23

Focus: *And his sister stood afar off, to know what would be done to him.*
Exodus 2:4

My husband and I are the proud parents of two remarkable children. They are bright and beautiful, as different as night and day, and both adopted. We brought our daughter, Abby, home when she was just a few days old. Our son, Samuel, on the other hand, stayed in his native country of El Salvador for the first eighteen months of his life, as we waded through red tape and the infamous bureaucracy of international adoption.

In light of their varied genetic heritage, we have frequent conversations regarding what plays a larger role in the development of personality and temperament—genetics or environment. In many ways, they could not be more like my husband and me. Abby and her dad are articulate, opinionated (in a positive way, usually) and goal oriented. She and I are organized, creative, and enjoy solitude. Samuel and his dad are extremely talkative and always on the move. He and I share a love of animals and a curiosity for what makes things work.

Just as we are alike, there are also traits of each of the children we must attribute to genetics. For example, Abby is a gifted artist. Fully aware of our limitations, any artistic requirement beyond stick figures is assigned to her. Samuel has a keen intellect for math and science—neither of which came easily for me or my husband. We are fortunate to have marvelous teachers and mentors at our disposal to step into the areas where we cannot help our children.

Can you identify the attributes within yourself which you would categorize as genetic and those that are purely environmental? Take a moment to make a list:

Genetic   Environmental

_____   _____

_____   _____

_____   _____

Moses was not only a strange and wonderful combination of genetics and environment, but also a mix of two drastically different cultures.

In our previous week's study, we observed the increasing paranoia of the new Pharaoh as the Hebrew population increased across the land of Egypt. Exodus 1:7 says, *"But the children of Israel were _____ and _____ _____, _____ and grew exceeding mighty; and the land was _____ with them.* In an effort to control the increasing numbers, Pharaoh inflicted harsh conditions and grueling work schedules on the Israelites, making *their lives bitter with hard bondage—in mortar, in brick, and in all manner of service in the field.* (Ex. 1:14) Still, the Israelites multiplied, so the midwives, Shiphrah and Puah, were instructed to kill the male babies as they were born. Their non-compliance angered Pharaoh, but brought God-given blessings on their households with the births of their own children.

Review Exodus 1:22. What edict had just been given by Pharaoh prior to the birth of Moses?

_____

Although casting a child into the river is barbaric and merciless to our modern thinking, Pharaoh was following the ancient custom whereby babies were set adrift in baskets—they might sink and drown, die of exposure, or be rescued farther down river. He was ridding Egypt of male infants; not by actually killing them, but leaving their fate to the gods of the river. This was not viewed as infanticide but as a chance for life—*if* so desired by the river gods.

Based on Exodus 2:1-3, what was Moses' environment at this particular point in his life?

_____

_____

_____

_____

When Jochebed, Moses' mother, realized she could no longer keep her child quiet and hidden from the Egyptian soldiers, she was forced to make a difficult decision. I cannot imagine the ache in her heart as she wove the basket and smeared it with pitch making it as waterproof as possible. Although God knew all would be well for the baby, Jochebed's tears surely washed over his little face as she cradled him in her arms one last time before placing him in the basket. The hope in her heart that the basket would remain afloat until some kind person would mercifully pluck it from the river and rescue her child.

If Jochebed was still watching the basket, as the royal entourage approached, she must have quaked in horror, realizing the infant was about to be discovered by not just any Egyptian, but the Pharaoh's daughter! This was the first of many times when Moses would be in the right place at the right time—God's place at God's time. Although he was immediately recognized as a Hebrew child, the princess had compassion and chose to adopt him into the house of Pharaoh.

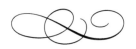

Many states have adopted what are commonly called "Baby Moses Laws" encouraging birth parents to bring infants to safe havens or emergency infant care providers rather than leaving them in a dangerous location. The parents are protected from criminal prosecution if they follow the guidelines of the Baby Moses Laws.

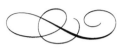

As a side note, have you noticed who thus far has been instrumental in thwarting Pharaoh's plan of suppressing the Israelites and in progressing God's plan to deliver them from bondage? The mid-wives blatantly disobeyed the edict; Jochebed gave birth to Moses, hid him three months, then trusted him to the river; Miriam watched over her brother and devised a babysitting plan for the Pharaoh's daughter; Pharaoh's daughter had compassion and adopted Moses. It is interesting in this period of male dominance and the rise of the patriarchs that God is using the women to raise up one of the greatest leaders of all time. As the adage says, "behind every great man is a great woman."

According to Exodus 2:9, Pharaoh's daughter did not keep Moses with her at this time. Miriam, the older sister of Moses, was watching from nearby and offered to find a nurse to care for the infant. Unbeknownst to the princess, Miriam ran straight to her own mother, and Jochebed (Ex. 6:20) was retained to care for Moses until "he grew up."

There is no other reference to the length of time Moses remained with his birth parents, so we are left with conjecture. Perhaps it was only until he was weaned at approximately three years of age, as fits with one traditional Jewish story. I believe a more accurate interpretation would have Moses returning to the Egyptian princess near the age of thirteen. Although the common Jewish tradition of Bar Mitzvah was not practiced in this period of history, a boy was still considered a man and responsible for his own actions at or around the age of thirteen.

Whether you believe Moses was with Amram and Jochebed (Ex. 6:20) for three months, three years, thirteen years, or something in-between, you can bet they were instilling as much of the Hebrew faith as humanly possible into his young heart and mind. Jochebed's heart must have ached on the day she brought him to the Pharaoh's palace to leave him with the princess. Although I am sure Moses had been told this was his fate, his mind was surely whirling with the contrast of his new home compared to his old.

Moses lived the next period of his life in the luxury of the palace. He undoubtedly sat under the tutelage of Egypt's finest and wisest minds. He learned Egyptian history, literature, art, music and the gods of his adoptive family. He became *"very great in the land of Egypt, in the sight of Pharaoh's servants and in the sight of the people"* (Ex. 11:3b).

And Moses was learned in all the wisdom of the Egyptians, and was mighty in words and deeds. Acts 7:22

What were the two events which caused Moses to flee from Egypt? (Ex. 2:11-15)

_____

_____

Exodus does not record Moses' age at this point in the story, but with a bit of research and a little subtraction we can come to an accurate deduction.

Deuteronomy 34:7: Moses was _____ years old when he died?

Numbers 32:13: The Israelites wandered in the wilderness for _____ years.

Exodus 7:7: Moses was _____ years old when he returned to speak to Pharaoh?

Acts 7:30: Moses had been in Midian _____ years at the time of the burning bush encounter?

Moses died at 120 years of age. By subtracting the 40 years in the wilderness we can deduce he was 80 years old when he returned to Egypt to confront Pharaoh. Timothy's sermon in Acts 7 tells us that Moses had been in Midian for 40 years at the time of the burning bush incident. Again, a little subtraction will help us surmise that he was approximately 40 when he killed the Egyptian taskmaster and fled his palace home.

Timothy confirms Moses' age in Acts 7:23 and also provides another bit of insight into the character of the man we are studying. *Now when he was forty years old, it _____ _____ _____ _____ to visit his brethren, the children of Israel.* It would be many years before God would speak directly to Moses and commission him to care for and lead the Israelites, but he already had a sensitive heart; a heart being molded by God for the people of God. That molding process would continue over the next 40 years as Moses became a resident in the land of Midian. Moses might have thought he was simply hiding from Pharaoh, when in actuality; he was being prepared for the most important job of his life.

Do you act when something "comes into your heart" even when it might lead to a major life change? If so, describe a specific situation.

_____

_____

_____

New influences now appear in Moses' life. He meets and is accepted into the household of Jethro, a fellow descendant of Abraham and high priest of Midian. Not only did Jethro (also known as Reuel) teach Moses how to care for his sheep, he exposed him to more of the traditions of his true ancestry. As we will see later in our study, Jethro is respected by Moses and looked to for direction and advice.

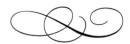

"*Long years must pass, during which God would drain away drop by drop his strength, his resolution, and his very desire to be an emancipator; that when he had become nothing, God through him might affect his almighty will.*"

F.B. Meyer, Theologian

Zipporah, the daughter of Jethro, becomes Moses' wife and the mother of his two sons, Gershom and Eliezer. She is only mentioned a few times in Exodus and later in Numbers, but each time she is depicted as a strong and opinionated help-mate (Ex. 4:24-26) and one not easily accepted by Moses' siblings (Num. 12:1).

As a review, list those we have specifically identified in today's study as people of influence in Moses' life prior to his return to Egypt:

_____   _____   _____

_____   _____   _____

_____   _____   _____

In today's study, what were the turning points in Moses life—specific events which set him on a new course?

_____

_____

_____

Regardless of your age, you can probably pinpoint a specific time when your life took a radically different course—perhaps, a move to a new city, a new career, a new school. Can you name the people of influence in your life up to that time? Take a moment to reflect and list those who come to mind.

_____   _____   _____

_____   _____   _____

_____   _____   _____

Just as Miriam watched over her baby brother from "afar off" as his little basket bobbed in the Nile River, do you know of someone who has watched you to know what would happen next in your life?

_____

_____

Whether Miriam watched her baby brother's basket bobbing in the river out of curiosity or concern for his safety, her actions helped set the stage for a future of diverse influences both genetically and environmentally.

◎⁀ Walking With Moses ⁀◎

Moses may not have been aware of the people of influence in his life, but they were making a huge impact on him nonetheless. From birth to death, God places those who can teach, guide, and support at each stage of life and learning.

◎⁀ Talking With God ⁀◎

God, thank You for the people of influence in my life.

_____

_____

_____

_____

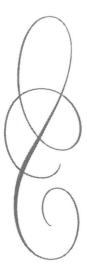

Day 2
The Burning Bush on Holy Ground

Text: Exodus 3:1-10

Focus: *Then Moses said, "I will now turn aside and see this great sight, why the bush does not burn."* Exodus 3:3

Several years ago, I helped lead the annual women's retreat at a lovely historic hotel in a quaint little college town. Although the site had wonderful character and much to offer in the way of hospitality and charm, the actual meeting space was a challenge. On the final day, we were crowded in a very small conference room, the sound system crackled off and on, dishes clanged in the nearby hotel kitchen, and it was miserably hot as the steam heat radiators hissed and rattled. Everything you could imagine was working against the plan for this to be a time of intense worship. Yet, as the music began and the ladies voices joined in song, it became obvious God had everything in control. Scripture was read, a prayer was offered and the retreat participants began to share. I sat to the side of the podium, knowing I would be bringing this worship experience and the weekend retreat to a close, as first one woman, and then another stood to tell of renewed commitment, new found friendships, release from snares, and restoration of body, mind and spirit. After quiet had enveloped the room again, I felt a pause in my spirit as I started to move toward the podium. In my soul I felt God leading me to remove my shoes, *"for the place on which you are standing is holy ground."* This room, cramped, hot, and noisy as it was, had been transformed through the power of the Spirit. I slipped my feet from my shoes and stood with the confidence a blessing had been bestowed on each of us in that room as we basked in the heat of our own burning bush experience.

Have you had a similar experience of standing on holy ground? If so, give a brief description.

_____

_____

_____

Were you surprised by the timing and power of the moment? Explain.

_____

_____

_____

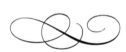

Draw nigh, shoes off thy feet, in silent awe and adoration. Draw nigh, as Moses drew near to the burning bush.

Two Listeners in *God Calling*

I can only imagine the blessing I would have missed if I had not removed my shoes acknowledging this strange encounter and the holiness of the moment.

Throughout my life, I may not remember the faces and names of those in the room on that day, but I will always remember how it felt to firmly plant my feet on Holy ground. In today's text, Moses was doing what he had done everyday since coming into the household of Jethro—tending sheep. On this particular day, however, perhaps in search of greener pastures, Moses ventured out of the desert and near to Horeb, the mountain of God. Although it was a new location, nothing was unusual until he noticed a strange light coming from a thicket at the foot of the mountain. Realizing it was a bush, wildly on fire yet without smoke or ashes, he cautiously approached to see *"this great sight."*

Blinking and rubbing his brow, Moses must have tried to make sense of what he was seeing. Finally, with courage and curiosity, he turned away from his doubts and walked closer to the bush. Moses not only witnessed a phenomenon that defied nature, but because of his obedience to the drawing power of the most Holy, he was invited to place his bare feet on holy ground and to ultimately embark on a remarkable journey with God.

As Moses approached the burning bush, God spoke, saying "Moses, Moses!" Throughout the Bible, a person's name, repeated twice, was characteristic of a divine call.

Who heard their name repeated in the following Scriptures, and how did each respond?

Genesis 22:11 _____

What was his response? _____

Genesis 46:2 _____

What was his response? _____

1 Samuel 3:4 _____

What was his response? _____

What was Moses' response in Exodus 3:4? _____

What two directives did God then give Moses in Exodus 3:5? "_____ _____
_____ _____ _____ _____! _____ the _____ off of
your feet, for the place on which you are standing is holy ground."

Frequently, when my children were younger I exclaimed, "Whoa! Don't move another step until you take off those muddy shoes." In some cultures the removal of shoes is

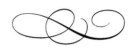

Throughout the Old Testament, fire symbolizes the manifestation of God. For additional examples, read Exodus 13:21, 19:18, Deuteronomy 4:12, & I Kings 18:24.

a sign of respect and humility; and in many Jewish synagogues, the rabbi removes his shoes before pronouncing the benediction. Based on his brief Hebrew upbringing in the house of Amram and Jochebed, Moses understood God's instruction. This was a significant moment. As Moses knelt to loosen the straps of his well-worn sandals, his mind must have raced in a jumbled confusion of curiosity, awe and fear.

Complete the following blanks with the anthropomorphic or human attributes found in Exodus 3:7. *And the Lord said: "I have surely _____ the oppression of My people who are in Egypt, and have _____ their cry because of their taskmasters, for I _____ their sorrows."*

Whether you believe God actually has physical eyes to see or ears to hear, we can be confident that God <u>does</u> see and <u>does</u> hear all that is going on in our lives.

Describe a time when you had a "burning bush" encounter with God.

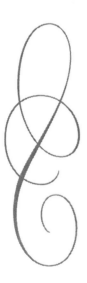

_____

_____

_____

_____

Did you argue and question or did you willingly agree to all God was asking of you?

_____

_____

_____

_____

In Week One, we heard the questions Moses asked God. What were the four that were asked at this particular encounter?

Exodus 3:11 _____

Exodus 3:13 _____

Exodus 4:1-2 _____

Exodus 4:13_____

Moses certainly had his questions and doubts, but ultimately, he obeyed. As he moved away from the burning bush and the ground declared holy, he stepped into the abyss of his future. A future where he would be called on to lead, teach, feed, organize, discipline, and ultimately die never tasting the milk and honey of the Promised Land. Moses never spoke again of the burning bush incident in any of recorded Scriptures, but I suspect he harkened back to that day when he needed assurance of his one-on-one encounter with God.

ᕼᕽ Walking With Moses ᕼᕽ

God may speak to you through an unusual circumstance or in an unusual setting, but ultimately, where God dwells is, by His very presence, deemed holy ground. Take off your shoes and step into your future.

ᕼᕽ Talking With God ᕼᕽ

God, help me not to turn away when I hear Your voice. I do not want to miss the blessing of placing my bare feet on holy ground.

_____

_____

_____

_____

Day 3
Hissing Snakes

Text: Exodus 7:2-13

Focus: *For every man threw down his rod, and they became serpents. But Aaron's rod swallowed up their rods.* Exodus 7:12

The Children's Minister at the church I attend is also a nationally recognized magician. He masterfully uses his gift of slight of hand and legerdemain to capture the attention of his audiences as he weaves his faith story throughout. Needless to say, even adults pay attention when he presents the children's sermon on Sunday morning, anticipating what he will pull out of his proverbial bag of tricks. On several occasions, I have been behind the scenes at this friend's magic shows and I still don't know how he does what he does. With a twinkle in his eye, he simply says, "It must be magic."

In the 2006 movie, *The Illusionist*, Eisenhiem the Magician tells the crowd that some things are not what they seem as he skillfully amazes the audience by producing something which in reality does not exist and is certainly not humanly possible. Such was the case in today's Scripture passage as the Pharaoh's magicians tried to outdo Moses and Aaron.

How long had it been since Moses fled from Egypt?

_____40 years

_____ 4 years

_____ 4 days

Based on Exodus 2:23, do you think Moses recognized this Pharaoh?

_____

Did Moses still have reason to think he might be arrested for murdering the overseer many years before? (See Ex. 4:19)

_____

With his older brother at his side, he made the ultimate demand, "Let my people go." The staff in his hand—the same one he had carried for 40 years and seen turn into a snake at the burning bush—was again to be an instrument of God's power. At Moses' instruction, Aaron threw the rod down and it became a snake. Not to be outdone, the magicians followed suit by casting their rods on the ground, and they became snakes.

Snake charmers have been a common street show entertainment for centuries and many county fairs include them in their side show tents. Old movies depict turban headed men sitting lotus style before a basket as a snake gracefully uncoils to the entrancing music played on the pungi, a flute-like instrument. Although it certainly appears the snakes are "charmed," they are in actuality simply exhibiting typical snake mannerisms. They slowly rise from the basket in response to the sudden rush of air and light when the cover is removed; they sway to detect the vibrations from the pungi and the tapping of the charmer's foot; and they do not strike the charmer based on their natural tendency to be defensive as opposed to offensive. The snake charmer makes his living by knowing his craft, his snakes, and his audiences.

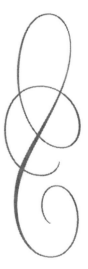

The magicians of Pharaoh's court were no less savvy to the gullibility of their audiences and the many ways snakes and other creatures could be controlled to make the impossible appear possible. There is evidence that when held by pressure points on either side at the base of the head, a snake can be rendered not only paralyzed, but straight and stiff until released. In this condition a snake would appear to be a rod or staff until it was thrown to the ground. The unknowing crowds believed in Pharaoh's ministers' magical abilities, until ruse met with reality as the snake created by God enjoyed the others for lunch.

Have you witnessed a magical illusion you could not explain? How did it make you feel? Give a brief description:

_____

_____

_____

Suppose the magician showed you how the illusion was performed. Would that change how you felt about his abilities?

_____

_____

Seated on his throne, snakes slithering at his feet, Pharaoh must have felt quite smug as his magicians matched wits with Aaron and Moses. I can almost hear him snarling "Tricks. Cheap parlor tricks. Is that the best your God can do?" His jaw, and those of his magicians, surely dropped when Aaron's rod-turned-snake began to eat all the others.

At this point in our study, several clichés come to mind relating to snakes and the attributes thereof. I'm also considering times when people and situations have reminded me of bromides such as: snake in the grass, speaks with a forked tongue, sheds his skin faster than a snake in the spring, or snake oil salesman. (If you are a fan of snakes, I offer my apologies.) Of course many of the circumstances where we might use the aforementioned figures of speech induce a smile or a chuckle, but there are certainly many situations where we have been hurt and maligned.

Several years ago, I was invited for a friendly lunch by a long time acquaintance. Light and mundane conversation ensued during the meal, yet by the time our dessert and coffee arrived I was being led down a much different path. Under the guise of sincere respect (*snake in the grass*) for my opinion, I soon found myself commenting on several very controversial topics. Assuming our conversation was between friends and would be held confidential, I freely spoke my mind. In the weeks following, I realized our conversation was not held in confidence and my words and opinions had been distorted to fit an agenda I wanted no part of (*forked tongue*). This person, whom I held in high regard, set a trap for me, betrayed my trust, and when confronted, denied the entire situation (*shed his skin*). Although to date our relationship is still strained, I am thankful God is powerful and willing to consume any illusion of deceit, ill-will, and trickery that I am faced with. Humorist Al Franken said, "Appreciate your mistakes for what they are: precious life lessons that can only be learned the hard way." Needless to say, I learned a very hard, but valuable lesson that day. Or back to the earlier reference to Eisenhiem the Magician, some things "are not as they seem."

Do you have a similar story to tell?

_____

_____

_____

Can you identify areas, situations, or relationships which "are not as they seem" in your life or areas of ministry? If so, give a brief description?

_____

_____

_____

_____

What are Christ's instructions to the disciples and ultimately to us in Matthew 24:4-14?

_____

_____

_____

_____

Ephesians 5:6: *Let no one* _____ *you with* _____ _____, *for because of these things the wrath of God comes upon the sons of disobedience.*

Colossians 2:8: *Beware lest anyone* _____ *you through philosophy and* _____ _____, *according to the tradition of men, according to the basic principles of the world, and not according to Christ.*

1 John 4:1: *Beloved, do not believe every spirit, but* _____ _____ _____, *whether they are of God; because many false prophets have gone out into the world.*

⤔ Walking With Moses ⤕

Only the truth as demonstrated by the loving hands of God can remove all illusion. Others may put on a good show and fool on-lookers into believing they hold power and abilities beyond human capacity, but only those imbued with the power of God can truly be effective in ministry.

∽⌒◯ **Talking With God** ◯⌒∽

God, please cleanse me of any deceit. Teach me to be an honest and forthright
instrument of Your grace and power.

_____

_____

_____

_____

Day 4
I AM Just Getting Started

Text: Exodus 7:14 - 8:15

Focus: *But when Pharaoh saw that there was a relief, he hardened his heart and did not
heed them, as the Lord had said.* Exodus 8:15

The summer before my son's tenth birthday, he attended several weeks at the local
YMCA day camp. His days were a healthy mix of group activities, sports, crafts,
and learning opportunities. Each afternoon I was anxious to hear of his adventures,
new experiences and budding friendships. Based on the condition of his clothes and
shoes, I could generally tell how involved he had been in the outdoor activities, often
spreading a towel over the car seat before allowing him to get in. He was always full of
stories and it was a rich time of sharing as we drove home.

One day in particular, he was unusually quiet as we made our way to the car and
I noticed he was carrying his backpack very carefully, instead of one strap slung
over his shoulder. With both hands outstretched, the backpack lay across his palms
much as pillow holding a crown at a coronation. Of course, when asked why, he
quickly answered, "I don't know," with nothing more than a sideways glance. Being
an experienced mom, I knew there had to be a reason for the kid glove treatment of
whatever he was protecting in his backpack. After a couple more inquiries and still

no clear picture of the contraband, I insisted he open the pack before we got into the car. As he slowly unzipped the main compartment, I was amazed to see, not a few, but dozens of tiny frogs meandering around his belongings. His group had spent the afternoon at the camp lake area and in his words, "Mom, it was awesome. When I went to the muddy places and jumped really hard, hundreds of baby frogs popped out. All I had to do was scoop them up. Cool, huh?" And then the words I dreaded hearing, "Can I keep 'em?" In a failed attempt to contain my astonishment, I shrieked, "Zip it up and keep it zipped until we get home; and, you may not bring those things into the house!"

That was the official onset of his fascination with frogs. Since then, we have had water frogs, tree frogs, toads of various sizes and colors, and even tadpoles on their way to becoming frogs. We have purchased special frog food, including live and freeze dried crickets, frog keeping equipment, and frog housing. We have argued over names, held funerals for the dearly departed and rescued escapees from our cats. You would think after such family involvement, I would have developed a mild affection for these critters, but the truth of the matter is, I still don't like frogs.

Although I admit I have used the "frogs in the backpack" story on several occasions to emphasize how you must jump into some activities with both feet to get to the "good stuff," in relation to today's Scripture lesson, I merely see a nightmare playing out.

The battle between Pharaoh and the God of the Hebrews was about to move to a new level, of nightmare proportions, for the Egyptians. Traditionally, Exodus 7:14 to 12:32 is described as the text outlining the ten "plagues" God brought upon Egypt.

In our previous day of study, Pharaoh was unmoved by the sight of Aaron's staff swallowing the snakes created by the magicians. Based on each word's definition, would you consider that particular event a plague, sign, wonder or miracle? Give a brief explanation of your choice.

_____

_____

_____

In today's Scripture, we find Moses and Aaron at the river's edge ready to follow the Lord's command to turn the water to blood. The same rod that had become a snake

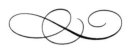

Plague: *1 anything that afflicts or troubles; calamity; scourge; 2 Bible any of various calamities sent down as divine punishment.*

Sign: *an act or happening regarded as a manifestation of divine will or power.*

Wonder: *a miraculous or apparently miraculous thing or act; miracle.*

Miracle: *an event or action that apparently contradicts known scientific laws and is hence thought to be due to supernatural causes, especially to an act of God.*

at the burning bush and again at Pharaoh's feet, would be the instrument used to turn not only the Nile River to blood, but also all the rivers, canals, and ponds in Egypt. The water soon became unfit to drink, the fish and vegetation died, and the whole land was a stinking mess. Yet, once again, the magicians were able to do the same feat and Pharaoh was unimpressed. He returned to his palace without giving a second thought to the plight of the Egyptians who were left without water for seven days.

Would you consider this event (water turning to blood) a plague, sign, wonder or miracle? Give a brief explanation of your choice.

_____
_____

Rods becoming snakes and rivers turning to blood did not sway Pharaoh, but God was just getting started with His plans: *"But if you refuse to let them go, behold, I will smite all your territory with frogs. So the river shall bring forth frogs abundantly, which shall go up and come into your house, into your bedroom, on your bed, into the houses of your servants, on your people, into your ovens, and into your kneading bowls. And the frogs shall come up on you, on your people, and on all your servants."* Exodus 8:2-5

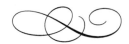

We are back to where we began in today's lesson—frogs, lots and lots of frogs. On the rare occasion that one of my son's frogs has actually jumped on me, I have been less than thrilled, so to imagine frogs all over me, in my bed and in my kitchenware, is more than I can comprehend. The Message *says "They'll be all over you, all over everyone—frogs everywhere, on and in everything!"* (Ex. 8:4) And to make matters worse, not only were the frogs produced by Moses and Aaron hopping around, but the magicians were able to do the same act "by their secret arts," thus adding to the number. Friends, that's a lot of frogs!

Would you consider this event (frogs everywhere) a plague, sign, wonder or miracle? Give a brief explanation of your choice.

_____
_____
_____

As a reassurance to myself and to those of you who appreciate my aversion to creepy crawly things, there's good news in Deuteronomy 28:5 "Blessed shall be your basket and your kneading bowl." I interpret that to mean no more frogs in the kitchen!

Finally Pharaoh realized Moses and Aaron, and the God they served, were forces to be

50

reckoned with. He called them back to the palace with the request they make the frogs go away. Moses seized the opportunity to show the power of God again by allowing Pharaoh to choose the exact time the frogs would die. *"So the Lord did according to the word of Moses. And the frogs died . . ."* (Ex. 8:13a) .

Would you consider this event (God acting on the day Pharaoh chose) a plague, sign, wonder or miracle? Give a brief explanation of your choice.

_____

_____

Barely aired out from the smelly aftermath of the rivers of blood, Egypt was left in an odoriferous state as the frogs were shoveled out of houses and courtyards and piled in the streets. Yet once again, Pharaoh, whose house was obviously upwind, hardened his heart and denied the request of Moses and Aaron.

Complete the following scriptures:

Exodus 7:3: *And I will _____ _____ _____,*
and multiply My signs and My wonders in the land of Egypt.

Exodus 7:13: *And _____ _____ _____ _____, and*
he did not heed them, as the LORD had said.

Exodus 7:14: *So the LORD said to Moses: "_____ _____ _____*
_____; he refuses to let the people go."

Exodus 7:22: *Then the magicians of Egypt did so with their enchantments; and*
_____ _____ _____ _____ and he
deed not heed them, as the LORD had said.

Exodus 8:15: *But when Pharaoh saw that there was relief, he _____*
_____ _____ and did not heed them, as the LORD had said."

Are you seeing a recurring theme? As we continue our study of the remaining days leading to the Israelites' departure from Egypt (Ex. 8:16 – 12:32) and beyond to the events at the Sea of Reeds (Ex.14), we will read a similar statement eleven additional times telling of Pharaoh's heart being hardened "just as the Lord had said." What does

Exodus 7:3 say the purpose will be for Pharaoh's heart being hardened?

_____

_____

_____

Pharaoh may have thought he was in control, but the plan of deliverance was perfectly orchestrated and would be carried out to demonstrate the power of the one true God.

∽◠ Walking With Moses ◠∼

Moses followed God's instructions regardless of the outcome: his best efforts matched by magicians, his environment became unpleasant and smelly, and the Israelites continued in captivity. Although you may be ready to jump to the end of your personal life story, allow God's glory to be revealed through the plan He has for each step of your life.

∽◠ Talking With God ◠∼

God, help me today to see beyond the snags and defeats of the day and rest in the assurance of Your plan for my life.

_____

_____

_____

_____

Day 5
I AM Means Business

Text: Exodus 8:16 - 12:51

Focus: *And the LORD said to Moses, "I will bring one more plague on Pharaoh and on Egypt. Afterwards he will let you go from here. When he lets you go, he will surely drive you out of here altogether. Exodus 11:1*

Today's Scripture reading is one of the longest of our entire study, but I encourage you to take the time to absorb each word. I cannot say it will be pleasant reading—plagues are usually anything but pleasant—but I suspect you will learn a few things along the way if you allow God to speak to your heart.

In our last day of study, you were asked to designate each event as a plague, sign, wonder or miracle. As we continue looking at the events leading up to the exodus from Egypt, keep those definitions in mind. Scholars and skeptics throughout history have attempted to downplay the significance of the events as nothing more that occurrences of natural phenomena and perhaps each could be so explained. What cannot be attributed to any power other than God are the timing, order, specific starts, abrupt stops, and the rapid succession of each. Who but God could orchestrate such a series of events?

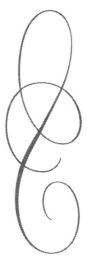

As you read Exodus 8:16 through Exodus 12:32, place a tally mark beside each of the following phrases each time you read it:

Then the Lord said to Moses	_____	(a word from God)
Stretch out your hand	_____	(a call to action)
Let my people go	_____	(a specific demand)
For if you do not let my people go	_____	(a consequence described)
He would not let the Israelites go	_____	(a decision made)
Go, worship/sacrifice to your God	_____	(a concession made)

In the midst of gnats (also translated stinging gnats or lice), flies, diseased livestock, boils, fire and hail, locusts, and total darkness, the same scenario played out again and again. A word would come from God calling Moses to action with a specific demand and a consequence described for Pharaoh's lack of compliance. Pharaoh's decision to deny the demand would unleash the consequence, causing him to temporarily concede. Each time, Pharaoh fell back into the same situation we discussed at length on Day 4 of this week's study; his heart was hardened.

In each of the events we have considered, who or what was affected?

	INDIVIDUALS	PERSONAL PROPERTY
1. Waters turned to blood	_____	_____
2. Frogs	_____	_____
3. Gnats (stinging gnats or lice)	_____	_____
4. Flies	_____	_____
5. Diseased livestock	_____	_____
6. Boils	_____	_____
7. Fire and hail	_____	_____
8. Locusts	_____	_____
9. Darkness	_____	_____
10. Death of firstborn	_____	_____

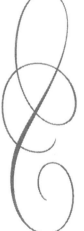

The events leading up to the Exodus of the Israelites can be further categorized into three specific delineations: individual discomfort (1-4 and 9), economic disaster (5-8), and finally, the loss of human life (10). Each development built on the one prior as Pharaoh's self-pronounced power was diminished.

The first four incidents were certainly annoying, uncomfortable, and sometimes smelly, but did not necessarily impact the livelihood or commerce of the Egyptians. The psychological implications began to mount as Pharaoh's advisors recognized the power of the God with whom they could not compete. The magicians used their incantations to call forth frogs, but only God could make the frogs die at a time specified by the seemingly unbelieving Pharaoh.

Did you notice I said "seemingly unbelieving"? If Pharaoh truly did not believe in the God of Moses, would he have said *"Entreat the Lord that he may take away the frogs from me and from my people"* (Ex. 8:8)? I wonder. What do you think was going on in Pharaoh's heart and mind?

_____

_____

_____

In Exodus 8:19a, how did the magicians explain the origin of the gnats which covered man and beast? *"This is the _____ _____ _____."* At this point, they admitted their powerlessness to Pharaoh, but, as previously noted, his heart remained hardened.

The distinguishing elements of each individual event continued to build. Frogs had been scooped into heaps and gnats had been on *every* human and animal throughout the *whole* land of Egypt; yet when the flies arrived, a clear and undeniable line was drawn. *And in that day I will _____ _____ the land of Goshen, in which my people dwell, that no swarms of flies shall be there, in order that you may know that I the Lord am in the midst of the land."* Exodus 8:22

It is important for us to pause in our study of Moses and remember the significance of this "land of Goshen". Although the book of Genesis is not formally a part of this particular study, the latter chapters, detailing the complex story of Joseph, give further insight into the extraordinary area in which the Israelites currently lived.

- Joseph was the son of Jacob and Rachel (Gen. 30:23-24); brother of Reuben, Simeon, Levi, Judah, Issachar, Zebulun, Dan, Naphtali, Gad, Asher, and Benjamin (Gen. 35:23-26).

- He was a shepherd by vocation (Gen. 37:2b); a dreamer by avocation (Gen. 27:5-10).

- He was the source of great jealousy for his brothers who considered killing him but sold him into slavery instead (Gen. 37:11-28); bought by the captain of the guard in the Egyptian Pharaoh's house (Gen. 39:1).

- He interpreted troublesome dreams for the Egyptian Pharaoh predicting seven years of plenty and seven years of famine for all the land (Gen. 41:1-36); rose to power over the land of Egypt and became a trusted advisor and overseer, ensuring that during the seven plentiful years enough grain was stored to last through the seven years of famine (Gen. 41:37-57).

- Jacob sent his sons to Egypt to buy grain from the governor (Joseph) whom they did not recognize (Gen. 42:1-8); Joseph ordered the brothers to return home and bring the youngest brother, Benjamin, back with them (Gen. 42:19-20). Joseph not only ordered their bags be filled with grain, but also secretly returned their payment to their bags, and gave them additional provisions for their return trip (Gen. 42:25).

- The brothers returned with Benjamin and were welcomed into Joseph's house (Gen. 43:16); after a meal together, Joseph sent them away, again hiding their money in their bags and his silver cup in Benjamin's bag (Gen. 44:1-2).

- The brothers were accused of theft and Benjamin was consigned to slavery because the silver cup was found in his bag (Gen. 44:6-17); Judah pleaded their case before Joseph (Gen. 44:18-34).

- Joseph finally revealed his true identity to the brothers and sent them to bring their father to Egypt (Gen. 45); the whole family returned to Egypt (Gen. 46:1-27); Joseph and his father enjoyed a tearful reunion (Gen. 46:29).

- Joseph requested land for his family from Pharaoh and was instructed to settle them in the best part of the land (Gen. 47:1-12).

Through that synopsis, we reach the significant aspect of the story as it pertains to our study of Moses. Re-read Genesis 47:11. Goshen was not just any part of Egypt; it was prime real estate. The Israelites of Exodus were still living in the best part of Egypt, the same land given to their forefathers by another Pharaoh four hundred and thirty years earlier (Ex. 12:40-41). Goshen—the best land for over four centuries and now a place of sanctuary. *"But against none of the children of Israel shall a dog move its tongue, against man or beast, that you may know that the Lord does make a difference between the Egyptians and Israel"* (Ex. 11:7). This place was so good, not even the dogs would growl.

Exodus 9 begins the second delineation—economic disaster. As the Israelites continued to be sheltered from the pestilence, the Egyptians pocketbooks were hit hard with the death of livestock by disease and boils, and the destruction of crops by hail and locusts. The economy felt the full impact of the unyielding acts of Pharaoh.

The ninth wonder is possibly the most intriguing to me. The Message translates Exodus 10:21 this way: *God said to Moses: "Stretch your hand to the skies. Let darkness descend on the land of Egypt—a darkness so dark you can touch it."* Have you participated in a cave tour? A standard element of every cave I have ventured into is the point where the guide instructs everyone to stand perfectly still while the lights are turned off. In absolute darkness the suggestions are made to raise your hand in front of your face, look to your left and right, look up and down. Of course, there is no light and all you see is darkness.

The original Hebrew word translated as "darkness" in Exodus 10:21 is *choshek*, also seen in Genesis 1:2a *The earth was without form, and void; and darkness was on the face of the deep.* Before God created any light whatsoever, there was only *choshek*—absolute darkness. This is the same darkness that engulfed Egypt in Exodus 10. For three long days, God withdrew the light created at the beginning of the world's existence, leaving only the land of Goshen in the light. The Egyptians were virtually paralyzed. *They did not see one another; nor did anyone rise from his place for three days* (Ex. 10:23b).

Has there been a time when an extreme or paralyzing darkness came over you? If so, give a brief description:

_____

_____

_____

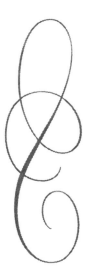

As the darkness lifted, Pharaoh's heart remained hardened and he continued to refuse Moses' demand, but he was obviously getting weary, saying to Moses, *"Get away from me! Take heed to yourself and see my face no more! For in the day you see my face you shall die"* (Ex. 10:28).

Exodus 11:1-12:30 details the final and most tragic event leading up to the Exodus. Moses passionately *("in hot anger"* Ex. 11:8b) delivered the warning to Pharaoh that all the firstborn in Egypt, both human beings and animals, would die. Specific instructions were given to the Israelites, and the first Passover was instituted and observed as *there was a great cry in Egypt, for there was not a house where there was not one dead* (Ex. 12:30b).

Then he [Pharaoh] called for Moses and Aaron by night, and said, "Rise, go out from among my people, both you and the children of Israel. And go, serve the Lord as you have said. Also, take your flocks and your herds, as you have said and be gone; and _____ _____ _____ *"* (Ex. 12:31-32). I find it curious, after everything that had transpired, that Pharaoh still would have the audacity to ask Moses for a blessing.

As we near the end of today's study and anticipate the triumphant departure from Egypt, take note of the following verses as you will see their significance on a later date.

Exodus 3:22a: *"But every woman shall ask of her neighbor, namely, of her who dwells near her house, articles of _____, articles of _____, and clothing;*

Exodus 11:2b: *"And let every man ask from his neighbor and every woman from her neighbor, articles of _____ and articles of _____."*

Exodus 12:35: *"Now the children of Israel had done according to the word of Moses, and they had asked from the Egyptians articles of _____, articles of _____, and clothing."*

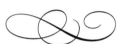

"A dispirited band of slaves, bound together only by their common plight, would never have become a people – a covenant community with a sense of historical vocation – had God not acted on their behalf when they were helpless and hopeless."

Bernard W. Anderson[1]

Moses' thoughts must have been reeling as he came to the full realization the journey was truly about to begin. His confidence was surely at an all-time high after seeing the faithfulness of God through each plague, sign, wonder, and miracle. The land of milk and honey seemed only a short distance away for Moses and this mixed multitude (Ex.12:38).

According to Exodus 12:40, how long had the Israelites been in Egypt?

_____

According to Exodus 12:41, when did all the companies depart Egypt?

_____

The New Revised Standard Version says, *That was for the Lord a night of vigil, to bring them out of the land of Egypt. That same night is a vigil to be kept for the Lord by all the Israelites throughout their generations* Exodus 12:42. According to that interpretation, what was God doing as the Israelites left Egypt?

_____

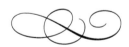

Vigil – a purposeful or watchful staying awake during the usual hours of sleep.

Not only did God set the Israelites free from the bondage of Egypt, God stayed up all night; keeping watch to make sure all was well.

As a parent there have been countless times I have kept vigil by the bedside of a feverish child. I watch the clock as I wait for my children to come home late at night from activities with friends. On those occasions when my husband is traveling, I rest easier once I know he has safely arrived at his destination. I keep watch until I am assured all is well.

Have you experienced a time of keeping vigil? If so, give a brief description.

_____

_____

_____

Describe a time when you knew God was keeping vigil over you?

_____

_____

Do you remember that significant event or time in a particular way? Is it something you will share with future generations as the Israelites were commanded to do? As we conclude today's study, consider God's faithfulness to deliver and watch over you.

ᏅᎾ **Walking With Moses** ᏅᎾ

Frequently, it takes very drastic measures for God to fully gain our attention so we will allow His perfect will and plan to unfold in our lives. Thankfully, under the new covenant, we are not plagued by disease and pestilence for disobedience or apathy, but God will ultimately prevail against the most hardened of hearts.

ᏅᎾ **Talking With God** ᏅᎾ

God, thank You for Your faithfulness to grab my attention when I stray from Your will.

_____

_____

_____

[1] Anderson, Bernard W., Darr, Katheryn Pfisterer, *Understanding the Old Testament,* Abridged and Updated, 4th Edition, © 1998, Pg. 49,73. Reprinted by permission of Pearson Education, Inc., Upper Saddle River, NJ.

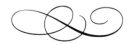

Week 3
GOD WILL PROVIDE – PART I

For the next two weeks we will be taking a look at the many ways God provided for Moses and the Israelites during their journey to the Promised Land. I hope you are not surprised there was more than could possibly be included in one week! This week we will look at the provisions of guidance, sustenance in the forms of food and water, patience, and wise counsel. Moses had his hands full with the crowd and God was faithful to provide.

This week, as you walk with Moses and talk with God, rest secure knowing God will provide as you strive to do His will.

Day 1
Pillars to Guide the Way

Text: Exodus 13:17-22

Focus: *He did not take away the pillar of cloud by day or the pillar of fire by night from before the people.* Exodus 13:22

Recently, my husband and I were forced, with great reluctance, to buy a new automobile. Although we had hoped his car would hang on for another year or two, a terrible noise deep within the engine revealed a problem creating a repair bill higher than the value of the vehicle itself. Neither of us was excited about looking at, or purchasing a new car, but after a bit of internet research, we narrowed our choices and ventured to the lots. I was dizzy with all the options—interiors, exteriors, motor size and horsepower, and of course the all important radio/CD/MP3 options. The days of simply choosing the make, model and color are long gone. Although we didn't come home with a new car that first day of looking, we did have a better idea of what we did and did not want or need in our next vehicle—most of which we agreed on.

One of the relatively new, and highly touted, features in many new cars is the GPS navigational system. There is an interactive map on the dash, a voice tells you when and where to turn, and it details the distance to your destination. These systems can be programmed to locate gas stations, restaurants, hotels and countless other services. It boggles my mind, and although I am confident it is frequently a valuable safety feature, it seems a bit intrusive to me. On my one test drive in a GPS equipped car, I was initially startled each time the voice piped up saying "turn left at the next stop sign, approximately 100 yards". Yet, after being on the road with my unseen companion for several miles and about fifteen minutes, I found myself blindly relying on the computerized directions instead of simply using my knowledge of the area to navigate my way back to the dealership. The entire experience was unnerving to say the least and was consequently deemed a feature I could do without. (I may regret that decision at some point, since I have been known to waste a good bit of time roaming instead of asking for directions—but that's a story for another day.)

Which of the following statements is true about you when you travel?

_____ I rely on a well-studied road map.
_____ I stop and ask for directions along the way.
_____ I rely on a GPS/satellite navigational system.
_____ I just keep going, making wrong turns along the way, until I eventually end up at my destination.
_____ I never go anywhere unfamiliar.

As a side note, I have read of several instances when the navigational guide was incorrect and vehicles have ended up on extremely narrow paths, driving off piers, and mired in construction sites. More reasons for me to stick with a map and common sense.

Verse 18 of today's Scripture passage holds the key to the navigational method of Moses and the Israelites; *So _____ _____ the people* ... (Ex. 13:18a). God held the well-studied map, gave the specific directions, was the only navigational system required, tolerated the Israelites' predisposition to make wrong turns, and encouraged them to venture into unfamiliar territory.

Complete the following Scriptures:

Genesis 24:27: *And he said, "Blessed be the Lord God of my master Abraham, who has not forsaken His mercy and His truth toward my master. As for me, being on the way, the _____ _____ me to the house of my master's brethren.* (This encounter led to the marriage of Isaac and Rebekah.)

Psalm 23:2-3: *He makes me lie down in green pastures; _____ _____ _____ beside the still waters. He restores my soul; _____ _____ _____ in the path of righteousness for His name's sake.* (David recognized the leading of God even in tough times.)

Luke 4:1a: *Then Jesus, being filled with the Holy Spirit, returned from the Jordon and was _____ _____ _____ _____ into the wilderness, being tempted for forty days by the devil.* (Jesus was led to overcome the temptations of Satan.)

Revelation 7:17: *". . . for the Lamb who is in the midst of the throne will shepherd them and _____ _____ to living fountains of water. And God will wipe away every tear from their eyes."* (In the final days God will lead.)

From the beginning, to the end of all time, God is in the business of leading His people.

Give a brief description of a time when you knew God was leading you.

_____

_____

_____

Often, when we think we have it all together and are ready for a particular endeavor, God will lead us down a much different path; sometimes, for our own protection. As the people left Egypt, in military fashion, company by company (Ex. 12:51), they were prepared for battle (Ex. 13:18b), but God knew what would happen if and when they came against a strong adversary . . . *God said, "Lest perhaps the people change their minds when they see war, and return to Egypt"* (Ex. 13:17b). Consequently, the Israelites were set on a serpentine path through the wilderness, guided by two distinctive navigational devices designed by the God of the universe.

And the LORD went before them by day in a pillar of cloud to lead the way, and by night in a pillar of fire to give them light, so as to go by day and night (Ex.13:21).

Do you have a pillar that gives direction to your life? If, so, give a brief description:

_____

_____

_____

_____

Do you believe others are guided by a similar pillar, or do you feel it is personal to your situation? Give a brief explanation:

_____

_____

_____

_____

How do you feel when you take your eyes off the pillar or it is obscured for some reason?

_____

_____

_____

_____

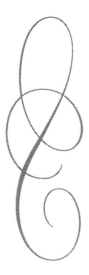

Some scholars have suggested the pillar was actually a burning brazier, or metal pan used to hold burning coals, affixed to a staff and carried at the front of the procession as was common in military tradition to indicate the path of the march. Regardless of the physical properties of the fire and cloud, God was leaving no doubt as to the path the Israelites were to take as they made their way out of Egypt and into the wilderness.

Nehemiah 9:12: *Moreover, you led them by day with a cloudy pillar, and by night with a*

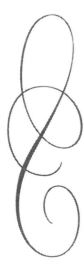

pillar of fire, to give them _____ on the _____ which they should travel.

Psalm 16:11a: *You will show me the _____ of _____.*

Psalm 78:14: *In the daytime also He led them with the cloud, and all the night with a light of fire.*

Psalm 119:105: *Your _____is a _____ to my feet and a _____ to my _____.*

Do you have any doubt God will lead you on your journey? Of course, the true pillar to which we should seek guidance is God alone, but thankfully He makes His will known through many avenues. I have wise and trusted friends that I consider pillars of faith; I look to them for counsel and example. Pastors, teachers, and gifted writers help to illuminate the right path for my days. And, ultimately, the study of God's Word is a true and accurate navigational guide.

Walking With Moses

Pillars of fire and cloud may not be in front of you, but God will be faithful to provide the pillars you need to guide you throughout your life.

Talking With God

God, thank You for the ways You lead me.

_____

_____

_____

_____

Day 2
Sweet Water to Drink

Text: Exodus 15:22-27

Focus: *So he cried out to the Lord, and the Lord showed him a tree. When he cast it into the waters, and the waters were made sweet.* Exodus 15:25

In the introduction to this study I warned you we would not always look at the events in chronological order and such is the case today. Next week we will take a good look at the events surrounding the crossing through the sea and the demise of the Egyptian army, but for today let's join Moses and the Israelites on the opposite bank, safe and sound. They turned to see Pharaoh and his charioteers swallowed as the water rushed over them and a joyous celebration broke out with Moses leading the song. As Moses completed his song, his sister Miriam took her tambourine and started the women in another round of *Sing to the Lord, for he has triumphed gloriously! The horse and its rider he has thrown into the sea!* (Ex. 15:21). Whether she repeated the entire song again, and it was simply not recorded in Exodus, or she was cut short by her younger brother, we abruptly see the Israelites on the move again.

They were now officially in the wilderness. As their provisions began to run out and their water jugs were found depleted, they cried to Moses for the solution. Three days passed before they came upon the waters at Marah. I can just imagine the hoard of people and livestock rushing to the waters edge expecting to find clear and refreshing water. Instead their jaws must have ached as the bitter taste puckered their mouths.

Can you relate to their expectation? Several years ago my husband and I ventured into an unusual ethnic restaurant in a distant city we were visiting. He is always braver than I when it comes to trying new things so he ordered one of the chef's specialties—I ordered the only recognizable item on the menu, a grilled cheese sandwich and fries. When his entrée arrived we both just stared, trying to discern what exactly he was getting ready to put in his mouth. Resolutely, he took the first bite and assured me it would probably be an acquired taste. He took the second and needed several big gulps before he was able to swallow. Before he even attempted a third bite, he covered his plate with his napkin and asked for one of my fries. Thankfully, there was a hotdog vendor on the corner as we traveled back to our hotel, so he did not go to bed hungry.

Can you remember a time when you had longed for a certain situation to come about and when it finally did, you were disappointed? Give a brief description.

_____

_____

_____

_____

The Israelites backed away from the bitter water and looked to Moses to provide for their needs saying "What shall we drink?" And once again, Moses turned to the true provider. Fill in the blanks from Exodus 15:25. So, he *cried out to the Lord; and the Lord showed him* _____ _____. *When he* _____ *it into the waters, the* _____ _____ _____ _____.

Have you looked to another person for a solution only God could provide? Did the person respond the way you expected? Did God provide for your need? Give a brief description of the situation and outcome.

_____

_____

_____

_____

Although Bible translations vary in what God showed Moses at the waters of Marah (NRSV & NIV each say a piece of wood). The New King James Version says in Exodus 15:25, "the Lord showed him a tree"—not a twig, not a branch, but a *tree*. Jewish tradition recounts the instruction for Moses to take a piece of a laurel tree with the name of God written on it and throw it into the bitter waters. After reading that in Louis Ginzberg's *Legend of the Jews*, I was intrigued by the specificity of the type of tree, which led to an interesting thought for me.

One of my fondest memories of growing up on the farm in rural Indiana is the many evenings my siblings and I would spend in the fields during planting season. Each day after school we would quickly pack a picnic supper and join our parents in the field.

Although there were a few activities we could help with, most of the time was left to our imaginations and creativity.

Of the many memories I have of those days, the ones that remain the strongest are the smells—freshly turned earth, chemically treated seed corn, honeysuckle in the fence rows, and frequently, pieces of sassafras root turned up by the disc. I loved the smell of those roots. Although sassafras is no longer considered healthful to ingest, in those days we would clean the roots and boil them for sassafras tea. It was a time honored tradition and a sweet and refreshing treat after a long day of work and play. I was surprised to read that sassafras is in the laurel wood family? Could it be the Israelites enjoyed a bit of sassafras tea at Marah.

The Israelites had seen amazing acts of God during their final days in Egypt, they had marched in mass out of their captivity; they had been delivered through the sea; they had survived three days in the desert without water; and they had seen God once again provide for their needs, even to the point of sweetening their water. Safely away from Egypt and with their thirsts temporarily quenched, it was time for God to make a few things clear before the journey continued.

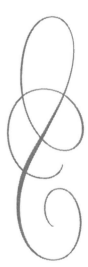

What does the latter part of Exodus 15:25 say? *There He made a _____ and an _____ for them, and there He _____ them.*

Webster's Dictionary defines these key words as:

> *Statute* - an established rule or formal regulation.
> *Ordinance* - a direction or command of an authoritative nature.
> *Test* - an examination, experiment, or trial, as to prove the value
> or ascertain the nature of something.

God proceeds to give them a very specific and clear directive—no flowery words, no beating around the bush—just plain and simple language. The rule (statute), the command (ordinance) to follow the rule, and the promise to hold them accountable (test). *"If you diligently heed the voice of the Lord your God and do what is right in His sight, give ear to His commandments and keep all His statues, I will put none of the diseases on you which I have brought on the Egyptians. For I am the Lord who heals you (Ex. 15:26).* Don't forget, there will be a test.

Complete the following Scriptures:

Exodus 16:4b: *That I may* _____ _____, *whether they will walk in My law or not.*

Exodus 20:20: *And Moses said to the people, "Do not fear; for God has come to* _____ _____ *and that His fear may be before you, so that you* _____ _____ _____.*"*

Deuteronomy 8:16: *"who fed you in the wilderness with manna, which your fathers did not know, that He might humble you and that He might* _____ _____, *to do you good in the end."*

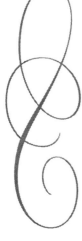

The Israelites heard the clear directions for their behavior and certainly understood the possible consequences of disobedience. They had seen, felt, heard, and smelled the results of Pharaoh's disobedience, yet as we continue our study we will see them err time and time again. Mercifully, God will not visit them with the plagues of Egypt, but they will keep on their walking shoes for a long, long time.

Perhaps the last eight words of Exodus 15:26 most clearly reveal God's truest affection for the Israelites—*for I am the Lord who heals you.* The Hebrew word for heal in this Scripture is *rapha*, which also means to repair. God not only wanted to keep the Israelites well, he wanted to repair the hurts and disappointments of their past, present and future. They had only to remain obedient to God's statutes and ordinances.

Describe a time when you, or someone you know, were *healed* by God.

_____

_____

_____

_____

Describe a time when you, or a situation, were *repaired* by God.

_____

_____

_____

_____

Fresh water to drink and a fresh word from God; all was well, so the journey continued to Elim, an oasis of seventy palm trees and twelve springs of water. As the Israelites looked ahead and saw the crown of green at the top of the palm trees, they were undoubtedly relieved, knowing they would have the provisions they needed. Palm trees provided food, fiber for ropes and baskets, and nectar easily made into wine. And please do not miss the significance of the twelve springs of water—one for each tribe. Further reading in Exodus 24:1, 9 and Numbers 11:16 will also reveal additional significance to the number seventy as Moses begins to give structure, under God's design, to the multitude.

What does the last part of Exodus 15:27 tell us the Israelites did when they arrived at Elim? . . . *so they* _____ _____ _____ _____

_____.

That sounds very familiar to me. When I arrive at a place of comfort in my faith, I am in no hurry to move on. I want to camp there for a while. I quickly realize however that the Christian walk is not about staying in one place—it is a journey.

Can you think of a time when you were tempted to camp by the water instead of moving to the next place on your journey? If so, give a brief description.

_____

_____

_____

Elim gave Moses a respite from the complaints of the Israelites, but as the journey continues we will see the same scenario play out time and again—times get tough and they run to Moses whining about their plight. In our next day of study we will take a closer look at the specific complaints and how Moses responded to each.

⌒ Walking With Moses ⌒

It is human nature to first seek a earthly solution to difficult situations we encounter along the way, when in actuality, seeking God's intervention first is always in our best interest. In God's best judgment, the answer might still come through human hands, but they will be God-ordained hands with a God-sent resolution to our dilemma.

⌒ Talking With God ⌒

God, help me to seek Your answers when I taste the bitter waters.

_____

_____

_____

_____

Day 3
Patience and Diplomacy

Text: Exodus 16:1-3, Numbers 12

Focus: *Then the whole congregation of the children of Israel complained against Moses and Aaron in the wilderness.* Exodus 16:2

For several years, I organized and prepared the Wednesday night dinners at my church. I took great pride in preparing well-balanced and appetizing meals for my fellow congregants and usually received compliments for my culinary endeavors. Complaints were few except for one particular person who had a negative comment about virtually every meal. I frequently saw this person return to the buffet line for a second plate, yet I knew to expect criticisms to be leveled before clean-up of the kitchen was complete. The comments were made with disdain of voice and scowl of face. I will admit, the first few times, my feelings were hurt and occasionally, it made me angry, but after a while I began to find it amusing. Silently, I imagined the terse responses I could make, but I held my tongue. This pattern of complaining went on for years until finally I was bold enough to ask, in my most respectful tone, the reason for the continued attendance if the meals were so terrible. The curmudgeon huffed out of the kitchen, continued coming for Wednesday evening dinners, yet never complained to me again. Have you been in my shoes? Do you know of someone who complains just for the sake of complaining? If so, without using names, give a brief description.

_____

_____

_____

How do you handle your encounters with this person?

_____

_____

_____

What were the complaints Moses heard in the following verses?

Exodus 15:22-24 _____
Exodus 16:2-3 _____
Exodus 17:2-7 _____
Numbers 11:4-6 _____
Numbers 12:1-2 _____
Numbers 14:2-3 _____
Numbers 16:12-14 _____
Numbers 20:2-13 _____
Numbers 21:4-5 _____

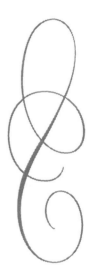

Moses had his hands full, didn't he? Deuteronomy 1:9-12 describes his despair at the magnitude of the problem. Who would have blamed him if he had thrown his hands in the air and said "Enough"? In most situations he cried out to the Lord for help (Ex. 15:25a and Ex. 17:4); other times he had to petition God not to obliterate the grumbling Israelites (Ps. 106:23). Whether asking for provision or pleading for mercy on behalf of the people, Moses was faithful to follow God's leadership and instruction.

Other than the fact that the people were actually hungry and thirsty, I suspect there were additional factors influencing their behavior. After all, they had left the only home most of them had ever known. While in Egypt, there was consistency and predictability to their days; even if unpleasant, they knew what to expect. Now, they were marching through a hostile land with no sight of the Promised Land.

When I was a high school senior, my parents informed me we were moving to another state. I complained and cried until they figured out a way for me to remain in Indiana and finish my senior year before I joined them at our new home. Regardless of the promising future offered by the move, I could not see anything except the few short months I had left with my high school buddies. After graduation, when I finally did make the move, I was still quick to point out how good things had been at our previous residence. Every little bump in the road resulted in a litany of complaints and murmurs from me. Looking back, I can see all was not as rosy as I thought at the place where I spent the first eighteen years of my life, but it was at least familiar. The fear of the unknown kept me from settling into my new surroundings for a very long time.

Everyday people choose to remain in unhealthy and dangerous situations including jobs, abusive relationships, and living arrangements because the fear of the unknown is more debilitating than staying in the familiar. The Israelites were no different from you and me. They were willing to give up the hope of the Promised Land and return to their old ways in Egypt.

Now, when the people _____, it _____ the Lord; for the Lord heard it, and His anger was aroused (Num. 11:1). In this particular verse, the translated word for complain is *anan* which literally means "to sigh habitually." I don't know about you, but I would much rather hear a clear and decisive complaint than constant and annoying sighs. No wonder God's anger was kindled; these Israelites were an exasperating lot.

American poet and United States Poet Laureate, Howard Nemerov, (1920-1991) penned the following verse testifying to the infamous complainers Moses was contending with:

> When Moses in Horeb struck the rock,
> And water came forth out of the rock,
> Some of the people were annoyed with Moses
> And said he should have used a fancier stick.
>
> *On Certain Wits* (1977)

Exodus 17:5 says Moses was told to use the same rod he had used to turn the water

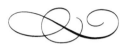

to blood in Egypt, but there is no doubt the Israelites found countless other things to complain about.

Write the following in your own words:

Jude 16: _____

_____

_____

_____

Philippians 2:14-15: _____

_____

_____

_____

Do you see yourself in either verse? If so, give a brief description:

_____

_____

_____

_____

While secluded in Goshen, the Israelites might not have fully understood all that was going on in Egypt during the plagues and negotiations with Pharaoh. They might have seen the river of blood and batted away the frogs and gnats, but the remaining plagues, signs, and wonders were not inflicted on those living in Goshen. Now, just a short time into their journey (the fifteenth day of the second month) as they witnessed the power of God first hand, they continued to succumb to the fear of the unknown and betray their trust in Moses' leadership and God's provision (Ex.16:3).

Then they despised the pleasant land; they did not believe His word, but complained in their tents, and did not heed the voice of the Lord (Ps. 106:24-25).

What does Psalm 103:7 reveal that might help explain the difficulty the Israelites were having in finding a level of trust? *He made known his _____ to Moses, his*

_____ *to the people.* They were seeing some unusual sights and wonders, but Moses understood what God was up to; he literally knew God's "ways". He could see the big picture, because he had personally met with the God who designed it. *So the Lord spoke to Moses _____ to_____, as a man speaks to a _____.* (Ex. 33:11a)

Jesus said to him, "Thomas, because you have seen Me, you have believed. Blessed are those who have not seen and yet have believed. (John 20:29)

The second section of text for today's study, Numbers 12, describes a dramatic scene between Moses and his siblings. What my mother called the "green eyed monster" had grabbed hold of Miriam and Aaron – jealousy had reared its ugly head. The incident began with harsh words against Moses' choice of spouse and quickly escalated to "you're not the only boss around here!" Doesn't that sound like classic sibling rivalry? I can picture countless scenes with my own brother and sister which played out in much the same way and culminated in my father's voice echoing up the steps, "All three of you get down here NOW!"

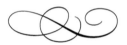

For additional New Testament reading see 2 Peter 2:4-11.

Numbers 12:4: *Suddenly the Lord said to Moses, Aaron, and Miriam, "_____ _____, you three, to the tabernacle of meeting!" So the three came out.*

Just as the Israelites suffered for the complaints they lobbied against Moses, Miriam in particular was punished for her jealousy and sin. Aaron did not suffer physically, but he felt mental and emotional anguish as he looked in horror to see his sister suddenly white with leprosy. He immediately turned to the brother he was berating only moments before and begged for mercy. Moses, true to his humble nature, true to his family loyalty, and true to his love of the Israelite people implored God to spare Miriam's life. True to His forgiving nature, God lessened the punishment to a time of banishment. I think this was a "time out" for Miriam. Yes, she still had to deal with the leprosy during the seven days while she sat outside the camp, but it also gave her time to think about her actions and words. I seriously doubt she or Aaron ever spoke against Moses again.

With that settled, the Israelites were once again on the move.

Whether in vocational ministry or lay ministry, difficult people will cross your path. How you choose to deal with them will set the stage for your effectiveness as a minister. Learning and demonstrating patience and diplomacy will serve you well.

∽⊚ **Talking With God** ⊚∽

God, continue to teach me to hold my tongue when I want to lash out at the complainers in my life. Help me to offer grace, patience, and forgiveness.

_____

_____

_____

_____

Day 4
Food from Heaven

Text: Exodus 16:4-36

Focus: *And the children of Israel ate manna forty years, until they came to an in habited land; they ate manna until they came to the border of the land of Canaan.* Exodus 16:35

In a report filed by the United States Department of Agriculture in 2007, "eighty-nine percent of American households were food *secure* throughout the entire year of 2006, meaning that they had access, at all times, to enough food for an active, healthy life for all household members." Based on the 2000 Census Bureau survey, 10.5 million households (approximately thirty-three million people) were considered food *insecure*. These numbers are staggering and remind me how blessed I am. Although I may occasionally declare in exaggeration that I am starving, the truth of the matter is I have never been truly hungry.

In today's text, the Israelites are just two months down the wilderness road and their provisions have been depleted. The unleavened bread they brought with them from

Egypt was consumed early in the journey, and their herds are dwindling. In the language of the Census Bureau, they are food *insecure*. Once again, they complain to Moses that it would have been better to die in Egypt, where they at least had meat and bread, than to die of starvation in the desert.

I wonder if Moses considered the magnitude of their demands or if he immediately turned to God for the solution. It has been estimated it would require approximately 1500 tons of food per day to feed the multitude in Moses' charge. As he gazed at the hungry and grumpy crowd, what else could he do but look heavenward?

Exodus 16:4: Then the LORD said to Moses, *"Behold, I will _____ _____ from heaven for you."* I can imagine Moses' puzzled face as he envisioned loaves of bread dropping from the sky. Mercifully, the bread was delivered in a far less dangerous form.

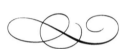

How is the bread described?

Exodus 16:14: _____
Exodus 16:31b:_____
Numbers 11:7: _____

I am the living bread which came down from heaven. If anyone eats of this bread, he will live forever; and the bread that I shall give is My flesh, which I shall give for the life of the world.

John 6:51

And they called it manna (*man-ha*)—which means "what is it?" Incredulously, they must have wondered how this "what is it" could truly be God's provision. Not only was it something never seen before, but after the Israelites arrival at *the border of Canaan* (Ex. 16:35b), it would never be seen again. So rare was this manna, and to commemorate its very existence, God instructed Moses and Aaron to fill a consecrated container and place it in the tabernacle *to be kept for all generations* (Ex. 16:33).

Economist Milton Friedman coined the phrase "there's no such thing as a free lunch" and such was the case with the delivery of the manna. This new form of heavenly sustenance still required effort, discipline, and self-control on the part of the Israelites.

When was the manna to be gathered? (Exodus 16:21)

_____

How much was each person to collect? (Exodus 16:16)

_____

How was the manna prepared? (Numbers 11:8)

_____

What did it taste like? (Exodus 16:31b, Numbers 11:8)

_____

What happened to the leftovers? (Exodus 16: 20)

_____

Only on the sixth day were the Israelites allowed to gather enough to last through the Sabbath and *it did not stink, nor were there any worms in it* (Ex. 16:24). *So the people rested on the seventh day* (Ex.16:30).

Matthew 6:11 says: _____

_____

The Israelites ate manna everyday for the next forty years!

Even a good thing can become tiresome after a while. My husband is never enthused about ordering pizza, saying he ate enough in college (over twenty-five years ago) to last him a lifetime. Such was the case with the Israelites and their appetites. Numbers 11:5 says they were thinking about fish, cucumbers, melons, leeks, onions and garlic— all foods with distinctive flavors and aromas. They were craving foods they could *taste*, but all they had was an abundance of bland manna.

Numbers 11:11-15 describes Moses' reaction to the complaints of the people. As my mother would say, he threw a little snit-fit. "Why me? What did I do wrong? What am I supposed to do? Why is this my problem? I can't handle this! Just kill me now!" (my paraphrase)

Again, God heard the complaints of the people and the cries of Moses. They soon had more quail than they knew what to do with, but this time, it was not out of benevolence God sent the provision, but to make a point and to punish the people for their complaints. Although the Exodus text alludes to the arrival of the quail in the evening, it is in Numbers 11:16-20 and 31-34 the intensity of the scene is revealed.

How many elders did God instruct Moses to bring to the tabernacle? _____

How were the elders to help Moses? _____

How many days did Moses say the people would eat the meat?

_____

Moses was obviously still having a difficult time getting his arms around exactly how God was going to provide meat for so many, assuming the only solution was in the slaughter of the herds and flocks.

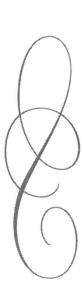

And the Lord said to Moses, "Has the Lord's arm been shortened? Now you shall see whether what I say will happen to you or not." (Numbers 11:23)

How do you think Moses responded when asked if God's power was limited? How would you answer that question?

_____

_____

_____

As God decreed, there would be so many quail, the Israelites would eat it until it was literally coming out their noses and they would become sick at the very thought of taking another bite (Num. 11:20). For two days the Israelites gathered the quail and spread the meat for drying on every spare inch of the camp. Those who had complained the loudest and *yielded to craving* as soon as the quail arrived were soon found dead because of their unbelieving and gluttonous behavior.

This event would not be forgotten. Read Psalm 78:23-32.

Time and again, God was expecting the children of Israel to trust in the divine plan and provision promised to them and their forefathers. Time and again, they failed to believe.

Deuteronomy 8:3: *So He humbled you, allowed you to _____, and fed you with _____ which you did not know nor did your fathers know, that*

He might make you know that man _____ _____ _____ *by*
_____ *alone; but man lives by every word that proceeds from the mouth of the Lord.*

Luke 11:3 _____

◌ **Walking With Moses** ◌

Each day of the journey Moses was faced with completely unmanageable situations, yet he trusted God to provide in all things. His life is a testament to the staying and preserving power of God in all matters. No need is beyond his supply.

◌ **Talking With God** ◌

God, on those days when my needs are great and the demands of life are looming, help me to trust You to provide.

_____

_____

_____

_____

Day 5
Good Counsel

Text: Exodus 18:1-23

Focus: *Both you and these people who are with you will surely wear yourselves out. For this thing is too much for you; you are not able to perform it by yourself.* Exodus 18:18

I frequently refer to my husband as one of the "good guys", even though as an attorney he is routinely the brunt of jokes involving sharks, high fees, and questionable admission to Heaven. In his daily legal practice he works very hard to mesh strong ethics, Christian values and pure kindness of heart as he deals with each person that comes through his door, whether client or colleague. Granted, the legal advice my husband offers his clients has been learned through years of experience in addition to law school and countless hours of continuing education; yet, other elements of his wise counsel have been fostered by countless individuals who have supported and encouraged him—his parents, pastor, mentor, and wife. His formula for good counsel is probably not found in the average text book, yet if such an inclusive book existed, every law school in the country would be prudent to add it to their required reading list. Those who seek his advice, or simply need a listening ear, are met with compassion, wisdom, and most important of all, an unhurried time of good counsel.

In Week 2, Day 1, we took notice of several people of influence in the life of Moses, and mentioned one man in particular who came in and out of Moses' life at specific and integral points. Jethro, also known as Reuel, was a respected priest and chief of the Midianite tribe. Shortly after fleeing into the desert, Moses encountered a group of sisters being harassed by some local ruffians at a well in the region of Midian. Naturally, he came to their rescue and a dinner invitation ensued from their father, Jethro. Not only did Jethro thank Moses for his gallant behavior with a nice meal, he gave his daughter Zipporah as a gift to be Moses' wife.

Exodus 2:21: *Then Moses was _____ _____ _____ with the man, and he gave Zipporah his daughter to Moses.* For the next forty years Moses was *content to live* with his father-in-law, tending his sheep and learning his ways. What a contrast from all he had known in Egypt—the finery and privilege of the palace exchanged for desert life and hard work.

Sometime during this same forty year period, the Egyptian king of Moses' childhood died and a new Pharaoh came into power instituting even harsher conditions for the Israelites.

So God heard their groaning and God remembered His covenant with Abraham, with Isaac, and with Jacob. And God looked upon the children of Israel, and God acknowledged them. (Ex. 2:24-25)

I am confident you remember this part of the story: God speaks to Moses through the burning bush, Moses argues, makes excuses, and asks lots of questions, but ultimately resigns himself to the task at hand.

Moses made an interesting decision as he returned to Jethro's camp that day. He had just experienced a remarkable and unbelievable sight at the burning bush; he heard the voice of God and learned of his destiny to be used by God to deliver the Israelites out of Egyptian bondage. Would anyone really believe his story? What should he tell Jethro? What should he tell his wife, Zipporah? Somewhere along the way, he obviously decided not to reveal all of the day's events—at least not just yet.

Exodus 4:18: *So Moses went and returned to Jethro his father-in-law, and said to him, "Please let me go and return to my brethren who are in Egypt, and see whether they are still alive." And Jethro said to Moses, "_____ _____ _____."* You know, in my book this is the ultimate gift of good counsel, *"Go in peace."* Anytime a friend, colleague or advisor can truthfully give me that admonishment, I know I am on solid ground. Such was the case with Moses—the sands of the desert would undoubtedly shift along the way, but his foundation was rock solid.

Time would pass and spectacular events would occur before the two men would meet again, but when Jethro heard *"that the Lord had brought Israel out of Egypt"* (Ex. 18:1b), he made haste to meet Moses at the encampment near the mountain of God.

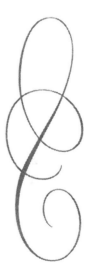

Recently we hosted a party celebrating our daughter's graduation from high school and one of the highlights of the day was visiting with friends we had not seen for a while. One couple in particular had been our dear neighbors for almost ten years and although we still reside in the same city, we had lost touch with one another due to the sheer busyness of life. On the afternoon of the party, I happened to be standing at my kitchen window as I saw them walking up the drive. I did not wait to greet them at the door, but just as Moses, I *"went out to meet"* them! We quickly caught up on each other's lives. We talked about the good things that were happening for each of us and shared some of the disheartening events of recent days. We reminisced about the days when we were neighbors; raising our children, working on our respective homes, establishing careers, and learning from one another. It was good to be with our dear friends again.

Exodus 18:7-12 reminds me of that visit with our friends.

Exodus 18:7a: *So Moses _____ _____ _____ _____ his father-in-law, bowed down, and kissed him.*

Exodus 18:7b: *And they asked each other _____ _____*

_____-_____, and they went into the tent.

Exodus 18:8: *And Moses* _____ *his father-in-law* _____ _____
_____ *Lord had done to Pharaoh and to the Egyptians for Israel's sake, and the hardship
that had come upon them on the way, and* _____ _____ _____
_____ _____ *them.*

Exodus 18:9: *Then Jethro* _____ _____ _____ _____
_____ *which the Lord had done for Israel, whom He had delivered out of the hand
of the Egyptians.*

Can you relate to a similar situation of re-establishing an old friendship? Were you able
to pick up where you left off years before? Did you hear one another's trials and rejoice
in victories? Give a brief description:

_____

_____

_____

_____

Jethro's response to Moses' stories of deliverance is significant. Although we would
like to assume, since Jethro is identified as a priest, he must surely worship the one
true God, we are never told that fact specifically in the Scripture. Historically, as a
Midianite priest, he might have worshiped many gods including Baal-peor (Num.
25) and Ashirah or Queen of Heaven (Jer. 7:17). Yet, after hearing Moses' account,
he declares *"Now I know that the Lord is greater than all the gods; for in the very thing in
which they behaved proudly, He was above them."* (Ex. 18:11)

For I know that the Lord is great, and our Lord is above all gods. Psalm 135:5

*O Lord of hosts, God of Israel, the One who dwells between the cherubim, You are God,
You alone, of all the kingdoms of the earth, You have made heaven and earth.* (Is. 37:16)

*The king answered Daniel, and said, "Truly your god is the God of gods, the Lord of kings,
and a revealer of secrets, since you could reveal this secret."* (Dan. 2:47)

Moses and Jethro have just moved to a new level in their relationship. They are no longer merely good friends and in-laws, but are now fellow believers—surely an added dimension to Moses' level of respect for his father-in-law—a dimension that would become very important in the coming days as Jethro observes Moses' management and leadership style.

What does Jethro see happening in Exodus 18: 13-14?

_____

_____

_____

_____

How does Moses explain his actions in Exodus 18:14-16?

_____

_____

_____

_____

The advice Jethro gives Moses is sound advice for all to hear. *"The thing that you do is not good. Both you and these people who are with you will surely wear yourselves out. For this thing is too much for you; you are not able to perform it by yourself."* (Ex. 18:17-18) I don't know about you, but I don't hear that kind of advice very easily. A former colleague once told me I had the "lone wolf" syndrome as for many years I preferred to work alone, without the counsel, aid or constraints of a committee or ministry team. Moses, obviously much less bull-headed than I, heeded his father-in-law's words and did just as he was counseled.

Advice #1 – Stand before God for the people.
Advice #2 – Teach them the statutes and laws.

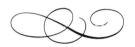

What a great favor God does to those He places in the company of good people!

St. Teresa of Avila

Advice #3 – Show them the ways they must walk and work they must do.

Advice #4 – Select able men who fear God, men of truth, who hate covetousness.

Advice #5 – Place the selected men as rulers over groups of thousands, hundreds, fifties, and tens.

Advice #6 – Let them judge the people and only bring the big matters to you.

Advice #7 – Let them bear the burden with you.

Every effective organization needs:

- God as the umbrella of divine inspiration over the organization (Ex. 18:23)

- Structure, guidelines, and a positive team mentality—the skeletal system to keep it standing strong (Ex. 18:21-22)

- A leader who understands the role as the head of the organization and is ready to see each and every task through to—this is where the proverbial buck stops (Ex. 40:33b).

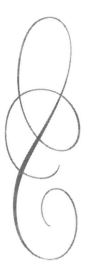

How does Jethro end his counsel in Exodus 18:23? *If you do this thing, and God so commands you, then you will be able to endure, and this entire people will also go to their place _____ _____*. With just a bit of variation in the phrasing, we again see those three wonderful words of counsel, *go in peace!*

Recently I advised a young friend assuming a new leadership role to surround herself with good people. Later in the day I thought again about those words and considered who I count in my circle of "good people" or those I look to, not just for friendship, but for good counsel. I call them my Council of Wise Counsel. I won't mention names, but I can easily assign very specific attributes and treasured qualities to each:

- smart, giving, feisty, and full of ideas
- always positive, wise, encouraging, clever, and fun
- sage, passionate, and steadfast
- solid, edgy, and always ready with a hug

- learned, mystical, and gentle
- protective, adoring, and loving
- supportive, sensitive and loyal
- eclectic, enlightened, and affirming

I encourage you to make your own list.

Council of Wise Counsel   Treasured Attributes and Qualities

_____   _____

_____   _____

_____   _____

_____   _____

_____   _____

Now take a few minutes to thank God for each person on your list and for the many ways they bring wise counsel to your life.

In any situation one of the wisest things we can do is to know where to seek good advise, to hear the words offered and then to seek the heart of God for ultimate counsel.

Isaiah 9:6b: *And His name will be called Wonderful, _____, Mighty God, Everlasting Father, Prince of Peace.*

Psalm 16:7: *I will bless the LORD who has given me_____; My heart also instructs me in the night seasons.*

Psalm 73:24-25: *You guide me with Your _____, and afterward You will receive me with honor. Whom have I in heaven but You? And there is nothing on earth that I desire other than You.*

〜 **Walking With Moses** 〜

It is human nature to attempt to handle many situations on our own. We think we can figure out the solution without asking for help; we want to appear strong and independent. In truth, it is only when we rely on others that we become strong. When our energies are depleted, so is our leadership effectiveness.

〜 **Talking With God** 〜

God, thank You for bringing wise and wonderful people into my life to help me navigate the path on which You have placed me. Help me to hear their words of advice and to sense their hearts of encouragement.

_____

_____

_____

_____

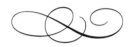

Week 4
GOD WILL PROVIDE – PART II

We continue our study of the many ways God provided for Moses and the Israelites after their hasty departure from Egypt. From the dramatic rescue at the Sea of Reeds to the support of friends and need for quiet time away from the masses, God continued to be faithful to His people. Specifically, we will see God provide protection, safe passage, stamina, support, and rest. (I don't know about you, but the promise and provision of rest is at the top of my list.)

This week, as you walk with Moses and talk with God, rest secure knowing God is your provider and protector during days of calm and days of tumult.

Day 1
Rumble of Chariots

Text: Exodus 12:33 - 14:15a

Focus: *And when Pharaoh drew near, the children of Israel lifted their eyes, and behold, the Egyptians marched after them. So they were very afraid, and the children of Israel cried out to the Lord.* Exodus 14:10

One of my favorite places to read, write, and think is outside under the awning on my deck. My house backs up to dense woods, so there is no shortage of wildlife or the sounds of nature. Other than an occasional airplane overhead, all I hear are birds, tree frogs, and the wind moving through the trees. Today, as I write, I hear a rumbling in the distance as a thunderstorm slowly moves into my area. Although the sun is still shining, I see clouds forming, smell the rain in the air, and hear the frequent low rumble of the thunder. I've always loved thunderstorms so I am in no hurry to head inside. The power of a summer storm can be exhilarating. And, why should I pack up my notes and laptop when the wind might shift causing the storm to move past without a single drop of rain or streak of lightning. Surely I can stay a while longer— it's a chance I'm willing to take.

In today's study, we hear a distant, yet approaching storm, as Pharaoh once again changes his mind regarding the future of the Israelites. Just days earlier, after tolerating all the plagues he could handle, he told Moses and the Israelites to go, saying *"Rise, go out from among my people, both you and the children of Israel."* (Ex. 12:31b) Great rejoicing resounded as the enslaved nation began their journey to the land of milk and honey—a land that was only a hope the day before is now a reality in the making.

The Israelites wound their way through streets paved with bricks laced with their ancestors' blood. Their spirits surely soared as the reality of their freedom began to settle in; four hundred and thirty years of captivity finally over.

How does Exodus 12:33 describe the Egyptians' feelings regarding the departure of the Israelites?

_____

_____

_____

_____

What do the following Scriptures tell us the Israelites took with them as they left Egypt? What do you suppose the significance of each will be in the future?

Exodus 12:34 _____

_____

Exodus 12:35 (Exodus 3:22a; Exodus 11:2) _____

_____

Exodus 12:38 _____

_____

Exodus 13:19 _____

_____

Led by the pillars of fire and cloud, the Israelites skirted the main highway, camping for a short time at Etham, and then at Pi-hahiroth near the Sea of Reeds (traditionally believed to be the Red Sea). Still riding high on the excitement of their successful departure from the rule of Pharaoh, I doubt many even considered this location as less than ideal. Imagine for a moment what the activity and mood in the seaside camp might have been at this point in the story. Give a brief description.

_____

_____

_____

_____

How do you suppose the scene changed when the Israelites began to hear the rumble of Pharaoh's chariots coming across the desert? Could they see the dust of the chariots and feel the ground shake as the horses pounded the dry earth? Were they assuming Pharaoh would keep his word and let them continue their journey, or remembering how many times he had changed his mind before? Briefly describe how you envision the scene.

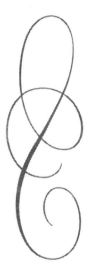

_____

_____

_____

_____

I suspect they were scurrying like mice as they attempted to fold their tents and gather their meager belongings, all the while, turning their fear and wrath on Moses as they questioned his leadership.

Fill in the blanks from Exodus 14:11-12. *Then they said to Moses, "Because there were no _____ in Egypt, have you taken us away to die in the _____?*

Why have you so dealt with us, to bring us up out of Egypt? Is this not the word _____ _____ _____ in Egypt, 'Let us alone that we might _____ the Egyptians'? For it would have been better for us to serve the Egyptians than that we should die in the wilderness."

Have you responded in the same manner as the Israelites when your back was against the wall (or a proverbial sea)? Did you blame those who had given you counsel or led you to the place of your distress? Give a brief description.

_____

_____

_____

_____

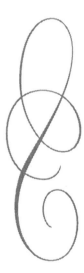

Moses easily could have joined the panic as it permeated the camp. The potential for disaster was obvious and he knew how ruthless Pharaoh could be, but he also was privy to God's plan to bring glory to Himself (Ex. 14:4). What did God tell Moses He wanted the Egyptians to know in Exodus 14:4b? *"_____ am the _____."*

With *apparent* confidence, Moses commanded the masses to stand still and wait for the Lord to deliver them, *"The Lord will fight for you, and you shall hold your peace."* (Ex. 14:14). Their necks must have ached as they craned to see the chariots through the cloud of dust, and then turned to see the expanse of sea barring their escape.

Did you notice in the previous paragraph the emphasis placed on the word *apparent* when referring the Moses' confidence. What does verse 15 say Moses is doing? *And the Lord said to Moses, "Why do you _____ to me?"* Just for fun, use your imagination to write a brief (modern day) dialogue between God and Moses at this point in the story.

Moses said, "God, do you see what I see?"
God said, _____ "
Moses said, "_____ "
God said, "_____ "
Moses said, "_____ "
God said, "_____."

This all sounds so familiar to me. I continue hoping for a particular thing or situation even when it seems it will never come to fruition. I fuss and fume, arguing and bargaining with God. Then, one day, when it seems the way is made clear and the future is bright, I hit another wall.

Years after I acknowledged God was leading in a particular area of ministry, it seemed things were finally falling into place. I, along with many others, had witnessed plagues of disinterest and disillusionment, but it appeared the way had been made clear and it would be smooth sailing. Similar to Moses and the Israelites, there was a group of people who needed leadership; there was a cohesive and committed circle of advisors and helpers; the necessary resources were in place to insure a quality program, and there was a promised land ahead. Yet, with every step forward, it seemed we were forced to take two steps back. Personally, as I grew into the leadership role, I frequently heard the chariots of jealousy and power rumbling behind me, and on more than one occasion, found myself backed to the sea with no means of resolution except by the mighty hand of God. Oh friends, I can tell you, He was always faithful.

Where are you today? Are you making your way along in a blissful state of freedom? Are you hearing ominous thunder in the distance? Are you trapped against a seemingly insurmountable obstacle? Are you standing still? Are you listening for God's next instruction for your life?

⤸⟋⟍ Walking With Moses ⟍⟋⤸

In spite of evidence to the contrary, Moses' confidence was based on his past experiences with God. He had witnessed the faithfulness of God time and time again, and could resolutely say *"the Egyptians whom you see today you shall never see again."* Each battle won, with the loving help and guidance of God will build confidence as you face the next challenge on down the road.

God, when my back is against the wall, help me to rest in the confidence that You can and will make a way for me.

_____

_____

_____

_____

Day 2
Crossing Through the Deep Water

Text: Exodus 14:15 – 15:19

Focus: *Then Moses stretched out his hand over the sea; and the Lord caused the sea to go back by a strong east wind all that night, and made the sea into dry land, and the waters were divided.* Exodus 14:21

In our previous day of study, we saw Moses speaking to the Israelites with great authority as they watched the Egyptian army getting closer and closer. Perfectly composed and confident, at least on the outside, Moses proclaimed the saving power of God. Yet, as soon as the Israelites faces turned back toward the approaching chariots, Moses was crying to God for help.

What did Moses tell the people to do? (Ex. 14:13) _____ _____!

What did God tell the people to do? (Ex.14:15b) _____ _____!

Obviously, the manner of deliverance God had in mind was very different from what Moses expected. Moses must have thought God would simply blow in a sand storm to blind the Egyptians, or perhaps a swarm of hornets to distract them. After all, God had issued some very effective plagues just a few days earlier. Surely he could just repeat one of those until the Israelites made their escape around the sea.

When you call on God for help do you have a pre-conceived notion of how He will respond?

_____

_____

_____

_____

God gives Moses three very specific orders:

1. Use the tool I have given you—*Lift up your rod.*
2. Look directly at the obstacle in your way—*and stretch out your hand over the sea.*
3. Take action—*and divide it.*

It was a God-style version of *ready, set, go!*

As a reminder, look back at Week 3, Day 1. What were the two specific navigational aids God provided for the Israelites? _____

_____

Describe the change that took place in Exodus 14:19-20: _____

_____

_____

_____

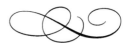

yam = sea
suph = reeds, flags, weeds,

*** Suph is also translated as to be consumed, to have an end, and to perish utterly.

The cloud and the fire came together to become a double barrier between the Egyptian army and the Israelites. Pharaoh and his men were once again in a cloud of darkness, while there was plenty of fire light for Moses and his people.

Do you think Moses felt a sense of familiarity as the water lapped at his feet. Many historians, scholars and theologians interpret the body of water blocking the Israelite's escape, as *Yam Suph,* the Sea of Reeds. Although Moses was certainly too young at the time to remember, he had been rescued once before in the midst of reeds (Ex. 2:3). And, as he raised his rod over the sea, his memory must have raced back to a few days before when Aaron stretched the same rod *over the waters of Egypt, over their streams, over their rivers, over their ponds, and over all their pools of water* and they became blood (Ex. 7:19). Once again the rod would be used to exact justice on the Egyptians as they came to *suph*, to perish utterly (see additional translation in inset on page 93).

The image I have in my mind right now is probably not much different from yours if you too have seen the Cecil B. DeMilles epic movie, *The Ten Commandments*. Right or wrong, I picture actor Charlton Heston, standing on a rock at the edge of the sea with his staff raised high in the air. Martin Noth, in the *Pentateuchal Traditions*, describes this scene as "the bedrock of an historical occurrence" an event "so unique and extraordinary that it came to constitute the essence of the primary Israelite confessions and was regarded as the real beginning of Israel's history and the act of God fundamental for Israel."[1] This would be a day to remember.

Moses obeyed God's instructions. He raised the rod in the air and the waters began to pull back.

What caused the waters to divide? (Ex. 14:21) _____

Or, as Moses sang after the event, "*And with the blast of his nostrils the waters were gathered together; the floods stood upright like a heap; the depths congealed in the heart of the sea.*" (Ex. 15:8) Yes, you read that right, God blew His holy nose and the waters divided.

How long did it take? (Ex.14:21) _____

What did the Israelites walk on? (Ex. 14:22) _____

Come and see the works of God; He is awesome in His doing toward the sons of men. He turned the sea into dry land; they went through the river on foot. (Psalm 66:5-6)

He divided the sea and caused them to pass through; and He made the waters stand up like a heap. (Psalm 78:13)

Moreover, brethren, I do not want you to be unaware that all our fathers were under the cloud, all passed through the sea. (I Corinthians 10:1)

In the darkness, the Egyptian army pursued the Israelites, evidently not realizing where they were. What a scene this must have been!

Approximately how many Israelites left Egypt? (Ex. 12:37) _____

_____

How many Egyptians were in pursuit? (Ex. 14:6-7) _____

_____

Exodus 14:24 is another one of those verses which tells me of the ever abiding nature of God. *Now it came to pass, in the morning watch, that the LORD looked down . . .* Just as in Exodus 12:42 when God kept vigil as the Israelites left Egypt, He was keeping the morning watch as they made their way through the sea.

But the children of Israel had walked on dry land in the midst of the sea, and the waters were a wall to them on their right hand and on their left. (Exodus 14:29)

Have you experienced a time when you felt God keeping watch? If so, give a brief description.

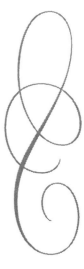

_____

_____

_____

_____

Frequently, as I read the Scriptures, I come across a verse that I have never noticed before. Such is the case with Exodus 14:25. *And He took off their chariot wheels, so that they drove them with difficulty. "* Although at first I was amused by the image of this scene, I then considered the dire consequences for the Egyptian army, and again realized the "creative" ways God was choosing to deliver his people. Other translations say God *clogged their wheels* (NRSV) or *made the wheels of their chariots come off* (NIV), but regardless which version you are reading, those chariots were going no where.

Hebrews 11:29 *By faith they passed through the [Red] Sea, as by dry land, whereas the Egyptians attempting to do so, were drowned.*

Nehemiah 9:11: *And You divided the sea before them, so that they went through the midst of the sea on the dry land; and their persecutors You threw into the deep, as a stone into the mighty waters.*

Psalm 106:11-12: *The waters covered their enemies; there was not one of them left, then they _____ His _____; they _____ His_____.*

Exodus 14:31: *Thus Israel saw the great work which the Lord had done in Egypt; so the people feared the Lord, and believed the Lord and His servant Moses.*

Take a few minutes to read Exodus 15:1-19 aloud. Is there any doubt this was a group of very happy people singing a song of praise to a mighty God? No doubt whatsoever. Yet, in the coming days we will continue to see how fickle the Israelites are in their trust in God's promise to deliver them. The next verse of Psalm 106 attests to this, *They soon forgot His works; they did not wait for His counsel* (vs.13).

Walking With Moses

Moses might have given the wrong order initially when he told the Israelites to stand still, but once he heard God's voice saying to move through the middle of the waters, there was no doubt God was preparing to show His might in a big way as He provided safe passage for the Israelites. Stepping out in faith, is just that, a step. God will be faithful to direct and redirect your steps.

Talking With God

God, thank You for being a God of wonders, mighty enough to part the waters and offer safe passage.

_____

_____

_____

_____

---

[1] Anderson, Bernard W., Darr, Katheryn Pfisterer, *Understanding the Old Testament, Abridged and Updated,* 4th Edition, © 1998, Pg. 73. Reprinted by permission of Pearson Education, Inc., Upper Saddle River, NJ.

Day 3
Days in the Wilderness

Text: Exodus 20:1 - 23:33

Focus: *Behold, I send an angel before you to keep you in the way and to bring you into the place which I have prepared.* Exodus 23:20

Today is another occasion where I have asked you to read a rather lengthy passage of Scripture. And, though each verse is chock-full of merit and meaning, we will devote most of today's discussion to a very limited section of the reading. In an effort to be good stewards of our time, let's do a quick recap of those areas even though I will rely on other writers to expound on them:

- Exodus 20:1-17: Moses meets God on the mountain and receives the first set of tablets containing the Ten Commandments:

  You shall have no _____ _____ before Me.
  You shall not make for yourself a _____ _____.
  You shall not take the name of the _____ _____ _____ in vain.
  Remember the _____ day, to keep it _____.
  Honor your _____ and your _____.
  You shall not _____.
  You shall not _____ _____.
  You shall not _____.
  You shall not _____ _____ _____ against your neighbor.
  You shall not _____.

- Exodus 20:18-23:19: Moses receives specific instructions for the people concerning the construction and use of the altar; the observance of the Sabbath and annual feasts; and domestic, civil, commercial, and corporal laws.

Exodus 23:20 is our focus Scripture for today's study: *Behold, I send an Angel before you **to keep you in the way** and to bring you into the place which I have prepared.* Did you notice the highlighted words? God knows Moses and the Israelites are on a prolonged journey through the wilderness and He will care for them regardless how long it takes for them to reach the Promised Land.

What comes to your mind when you think of a wilderness?

_____

_____

_____

_____

A few years ago my husband and I took a very wrong turn while traveling in the southwest. We realized first hand what our definition of "wilderness" might be. We drove for several hours without seeing a living being (human or animal); a dwelling of any kind; a living plant—green or otherwise; or any other indication that we were crossing through a habitable land. Luckily, we had a full tank of gas, several bottles of water, snacks, and a healthy dose of good humor to see us through. The road we were traveling changed several times from pavement to gravel to sun-baked dirt; yet, each time we began to fear the road might disappear completely; it mercifully began edging back toward pavement again. Without a cell phone signal, we wondered what we would do if our rental car broke down or if our adventure lasted longer than our tank of gas. Several interesting and comical scenarios came to mind resulting in stimulating fodder for conversation. We were reminded of the importance of being prepared for the unknown and always having a good road map. We laugh about our day in the desert now, but at the time, we were not sure it was a good place to be.

Comparatively speaking, my husband and I spent a mere fraction of time in our wilderness experience. Moses, on the other hand, lived 80 of his 120 years in desert or wilderness regions—40 years prior and 40 years after the Exodus. As I consider those days, I wonder which were harder or more challenging for him, the 40 years he lived in the desert before returning to Egypt or the 40 years required to lead the Israelites to the Promise Land?

During Moses' first wilderness experience, he was a fugitive from justice after killing the Egyptian taskmaster. The Scriptures do not tell how long he wandered before he eventually came upon the well near the family compound of Jethro, but I suspect those first few days afforded quite an education as he adjusted to life on the outside of the palace walls. The necessities and amenities at his beck and call as a member of the royal family were no longer available and he was forced to find his own food, clothing and shelter. Under his father-in-law's tutelage, he learned to shepherd, manage a family compound, navigate unfamiliar areas, and how to be a good husband and father. The skills he acquired before returning to Egypt would serve him well when the time came to lead the Israelites to the Promised Land—those years would teach him to see, hear, feel, and believe. The following are just a few comparative thoughts:

40 YEARS BEFORE	–	EXODUS	–	40 YEARS AFTER
Alone				With a crowd
Brooding				Eager
Searching				Leading
Learning				Teaching
Scared				Empowered
Running from justice				Delivering justice
2 way conversations between God and Moses				3 way conversations between God, Moses and people

It has humorously been observed that the shortest route is usually under construction, and so it was for Moses and the Israelites. God had a huge amount to teach Moses about leadership in the 40 years before he returned to Egypt; and in the 40 years after the Exodus, God had even more to teach the Israelites of how to live successfully in the Promised Land.

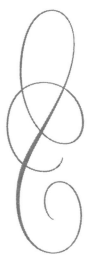

I can identify wilderness times in my own life when I, like Moses, have been alone, brooding, searching, learning, and engaging in constant one on one conversations with God. At other times, I can be just as deep in the wilderness but surrounded by people who are expecting me to lead them through a particular situation or event. Those times of "construction" can be confusing for even the most qualified and confident leader, let alone people such as me. There are many times I feel as though I am slogging through the mud with my wheels removed like the Egyptians, surely heading for total disaster. Other days I wander in a land of questions about decisions made, hoping I have made the best choices. And, thankfully, on some days I think I can see past the last "under construction" sign to the smooth road ahead—those are really good days.

What are your "under construction" days like? Give a brief description:

_____

_____

_____

It was shaping up to be a bumpy ride for Moses and the Israelites. God was certainly giving them every possible tool to help them arrive at their destination as expeditiously as possible, but the Israelites would spend 40 years trying, failing, and trying again to get it right.

What a merciful God to send an Angel to keep them on the way—and not just any old angel at that. What does the latter part of Exodus 23:21 say sets this angel apart from any other? _____

The Angel, a messenger of guidance, authority, and righteousness, would go before them to clear the way of obstacles and adversaries. All the Israelites had to do was obey the commandments and statutes set out by God and everything would go as planned.

Exodus 23:22: *But if you indeed obey His voice and do all that I speak, then I will be an enemy to your enemies and an adversary to your adversaries.*

The following verses give further details of exactly how the Israelites are to behave with four "you shall" statements and several "I will" statements. So as not to miss their significance or impact, list them below:

You shall: Not bow down to their gods

                      _____

                      _____

                      _____

I shall/will: Bless your bread and your water

                      _____

                      _____

                      _____

                      _____

                      _____

                      _____

❧ Walking With Moses ❧

God will be faithful to see your construction and instruction through to His satisfaction while you *are on the way* to the place He has prepared for you; *a land for which the Lord your God cares; the eyes of the Lord your God are always on it, from the beginning of the year to the end of the year.* (Deut. 11:12)

❧ Talking With God ❧

God, help me to realize You are with me, even in the wilderness valley, teaching and preparing me for Your will.

_____

_____

_____

_____

Day 4
Arms Held High

Text: Exodus 17:8-16

Focus: *But Moses' hands became heavy; so they took a stone and put it under him, and he sat on it. And Aaron and Hur supported his hands, one on one side and the other on the other side; and his hands were steady until the going down of the sun.* Exodus 17:12

A few years ago, while attending a women's conference in Memphis, Tennessee, I witnessed a sight that left a lasting impression on me. At the conclusion of a full day of conference sessions, I was sitting in the hotel lobby, enjoying a cup of coffee with friends, when I saw the speaker and her staff come in. I was concerned as I watched a gentleman on either side of this well-known leader literally holding her up as they passed through to the elevator. Another person carried the speaker's shoes—her bare feet hardly touching the floor as she leaned into her aides. I assumed she was ill and the conversation with my friends turned to skepticism as to whether she would be well enough to teach the following morning. I was relieved to see her bound onto the stage the next morning with energy restored.

Have you witnessed a similar scene? A minister, speaker, or leader exhausted and "carried" along by others? If so, give a brief description.

_____

_____

_____

_____

One of the duties I enjoyed most while on church staff was event planning. Whether a concert, conference, church-wide dinner, or a weekend retreat just for the women, I would invest all of my energies attending to the details. Most of the time, I was successful and proud as the endeavor came together. Anyone who looked at me in those final moments before an event or at its conclusion would surmise that I was tireless and unflappable.

In truth, I was only as strong as those around me—precious friends and colleagues who held me up when I was too exhausted to stand any longer. One friend brought my soft drink of choice, another delivered favorite snacks, and yet another simply reminded me to breathe. Others on the sidelines faithfully prayed for my stamina and for the success of the event. Seemingly small offerings that provided just the support needed at a tiring time.

Can you think of a time when someone held you up when you were physically and/or emotionally exhausted and too tired to carry on? If so, give a brief description.

_____

_____

_____

In the following passages, who was being held up, and who were the friends at their sides?

	ONE IN NEED	FRIENDS
Ruth 1:11-17	_____	_____
Matthew 8:5-13	_____	_____
Mark 2:1-5	_____	_____
Acts 14:19-20	_____	_____

As the Israelites camped in the valley of Rephidim, Moses was surely thinking he would have a moment to rest. He had successfully negotiated the release of the Israelites from Egypt and choreographed their exit; he had marched them through the sea, and petitioned God to provide food and water for the journey. Just as he removed his sandals, propped up his feet, and settled for an afternoon nap, the army of Amalek showed up. Moses did not engage in the battle but sent Joshua to lead the troops.

Where did Moses station himself? _____

From this lofty post, Moses could watch the ensuing battle in the valley below.

Who did he take with him? _____ and _____

What did he take with him? _____

Take a moment to return to Week 1, Day 3 as a reminder of the awesome power God had infused into the staff Moses carried.

Briefly describe the ways we have seen the staff used in our study to this point.
Exodus 4:2-4 _____
Exodus 7:9-12 _____
Exodus 7:20-21 _____
Exodus 8:5-6 _____
Exodus 8:16-17 _____
Exodus 9:22-23 _____
Exodus 10:12-13 _____
Exodus 14:15-16 _____
Exodus 17:5-6 _____

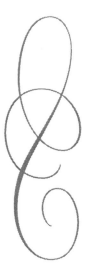

Once again, this common shepherd's tool became a mighty conduit of God's power. As long as Moses held his hands and the staff in the air, the Israelites prevailed, but as soon as he would lower his arms to rest, Amalek moved ahead. Needless to say, as the battle waged on, Moses' arms became tired and he was no longer able to hold them aloft. Just as the earlier mentioned conference speaker had aides to hold her up, and as my friends have supported me on countless occasions, Moses was fortunate to have Aaron and Hur nearby. They settled their weary leader on a rock, moved to either side of him, and held his arms high in the air until the battle was won.

At the end of this scene chronicled in Exodus 17, it is interesting to note that Moses built an altar and called it *"The Lord is my Banner"* (Ex. 17:15). *Webster's Dictionary* describes a banner as "a piece of cloth bearing a design, motto, slogan, etc., sometimes attached to a staff and used as a battle standard." It was surely Moses' aching arms that prompted the naming of this particular altar. The children of Israel were victorious through the power of a sign held high with the mighty *"rod of God"* (Ex. 17:9)— a victory won with the help of a friend on the left and another on the right.

✍ Walking With Moses ✍

Moses was given the authority and tools to lead the Israelites, but his physical limitations found him at the edge of exhaustion on countless occasions. God was faithful to provide others to step alongside this great leader to help, support, and carry the load when necessary. You are not alone in your ministry.

✍ Talking With God ✍

God, thank You for those who walk alongside me as I seek to do Your will.

_____

_____

_____

_____

Day 5
Retreat

Text: Exodus 33:7-11

Focus: *Moses took his tent and pitched it outside the camp, far from the camp, and called it the tabernacle of meeting. And it came to pass that everyone who sought the Lord went out to the tabernacle of meeting which was outside the camp.* Exodus 33:7

What do you think of when you hear the word *retreat*? If you have served in the military you may think of the bugle call when the flag is lowered at the end of the day.

A student of history might consider great army commanders ordering their troops to move away from battle. I instantly think of quiet and rest, a time away from the daily demands of life.

I am a huge proponent of a regular time of retreat. Whether alone or with friends, for a day or a week, silent or interactive; a designated time away from regular routine can be restorative and is worthy of consideration on a regular basis. I consider it a time for my soul to catch up with my racing mind and heart.

One of my favorite responsibilities while on church staff was coordinating the annual spring women's retreat. Each year I would encourage, and attempt to empower, women of all ages to embrace the value of taking time away to consider their relationship with God and one another. It was always a rich time of rest and renewal for those who attended.

When was the last time you had a time of personal retreat? Briefly describe the setting. Were you alone or with a group? How long did you stay? Was their a particular theme or format? What did you take with you?

_____

_____

_____

_____

List four unique characteristics of your retreat:

_____   _____

_____   _____

What were the benefits of the retreat described in Psalm 23:1-3?

_____

_____

_____

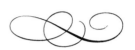

retreat >verb
1 (of an army) withdraw from confrontation with enemy forces.
2 move back from a difficult situation.
3 withdraw to a quiet or secluded place.
>noun 1 an act of retreating.
2 a quiet or secluded place.
3 a period or place of seclusion for the purposes of prayer and meditation.
4 a military musical ceremony carried out at sunset.
-ORIGIN Latin retrahere 'draw back'.

What was the purpose of Jesus' retreat into the wilderness in Matthew 4:1-10?

_____

_____

_____

_____

Matthew 4:11: *Then the devil left Him and behold, angels came and ministered to Him.* Have you experienced the ministry of angels while on retreat?

Who joined Jesus on the mountain in Matthew 17: 1-8 and what was their experience?

_____

_____

_____

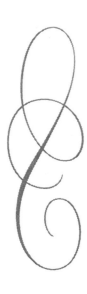

Jesus sought times of retreat at other times for other reasons including the evening after He fed the five thousand when He needed rest, and in the Garden of Gethsemane when He asked God to *"take this cup away"* (Mark 14:36).

Moses had been with the Israelites for a long time. Day in and day out he had led, instructed, and basically been in charge of every detail of their journey. He was undoubtedly physically tired and probably tired of dealing with a frequently ungrateful crowd. It was time for a retreat.

In today's focus Scripture, where did Moses go? _____

Was it near or far? _____

What did he take with him? _____

It is significant to note the "tabernacle" spoken of in Exodus 33:7 is *ohel,* which literally means a tent of habitation and not the structure *mishkan* described in Exodus 26 and 40 containing *"the holy place and the Most Holy Place."*

What was his retreat called? _____

Why and when did others join him? _____

Exodus 33:9: Was Moses inside or outside this tabernacle? _____
            Was God inside or outside this tabernacle? _____

Exodus 40:34-35: Was Moses inside or outside this tabernacle? _____
                Was God inside or outside this tabernacle? _____

Why do you think it was important for Moses, as the leader of the Israelites, to have a place of retreat? _____

_____

Consider for a moment the answer to the earlier question. Was Moses' tent near or far? Why do you suppose Moses specifically recorded that the tent was set up "far off from the camp"?

_____

_____

_____

_____

On occasion, I have attempted to have a day of retreat in my own home, but I have yet to make this a successful venture. I can turn off the phones, hide the TV remote controls, ignore the doorbell and the stack of correspondence awaiting my attention, but I am still surrounded by the daily-ness of life. It is only when I physically move myself away from the norm that I am able to settle into a level of relaxation that allows me to hear God in a fresh way.

Reread Exodus 33:9. What covered the door of the tent after Moses entered?

_____

Earlier in our study, we explored the significance of the pillar of cloud that was with the Israelites as they journeyed through the wilderness. It is interesting that this cloud of leadership stayed very near to Moses, just outside the door as he spoke with God.

Fill in the blanks of Exodus 33:11a. *"So the LORD* _____ *to Moses* _____ *to* _____, *as a man speaks to his* _____.*"*

When was the last time you heard God speaking to you as a friend? When did you last speak to God as a friend speaks to a friend? If it has been a while, I encourage you to take whatever steps necessary to move your tent away from camp for while, allow the cloud to cover the door, and listen for the voice of God.

❧ Walking With Moses ❧

Moses recognized the value of a time of retreat. Of course he had few significant "mountain top" experiences with God, but he also took deliberate measures to ensure times to be alone with God in the daily-ness of his life. You can be confident your efforts to step away from your daily routine as you seek to hear God's voice will be honored.

❧ Talking With God ❧

God, thank You that You are faithful to meet me when I enter into a time of retreat.

_____

_____

_____

_____

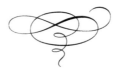

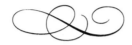

Week 5
MILE MARKERS

This week we will focus on several specific events which help to define the rich history of Moses and the Israelites' journey through the wilderness. Each mile marker, good, bad, and even horrific, became a learning experience for Moses and gave clarity to his calling as a leader of this fickle people.

This week, as you walk with Moses and talk with God, rest secure knowing you too have significant mile markers to remind you of God's faithfulness in all things.

Day 1
Altars Along the Way

Text: Exodus 24:1 -18

Focus: *And Moses wrote all the words of the Lord. And he rose early in the morning and built an altar at the foot of the mountain.* Exodus 24:4a

One of my preferred places to visit for quiet and solitude is a monastery in rural, southern Indiana. As often as my busy family's schedule will allow, I try to break from my regular routine of work and home life to escape to this haven of quiet. Times of silence and contemplation are not only suggested, but are expected of all who come to visit this tranquil environment.

The traditions of this particular order and denomination are far removed from my own religious background, but I have come to appreciate their call and respect for the Holy. Whether attending evening vespers, walking the Stations of the Cross, enjoying

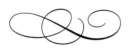

Lectio Divina – Latin for divine reading - a method of prayer and scriptural reading which calls one to study, ponder, listen, and pray from God's Word. The Monk's Ladder, written in 1150 A.D by Guigo II describes four rungs: reading, meditation, prayer and contemplation.

As a side note, Numbers 3:4 details how Nadab and Abihu died after disobeying God's command to use only holy fire, taken from the altar of God, in their censers or personal fire/incense trays. Although we will not delve into that particular story in this study, you can see the ramifications of their disobedience in Leviticus 10:1-11.

the beautiful flower gardens, or sitting in reverent silence in the Chapel, it is in this place I often hear God speak to me, giving me direction, assurance, and comfort. A gentle breeze reminds me of God's ever abiding presence and unfailing love, and the rhythmic Lectio Divina prayers offered by the Benedictine sisters deepens my meditation, allowing me to hear God's voice speaking to my heart.

Today's Scripture finds us at a critical point in the Exodus story as Moses prepares for another one-on-one meeting with God to receive direction and affirmation of the covenant.

What is God's invitation to Moses in Exodus 24:1? *Now He said to Moses,* " _____ _____ _____ _____ _____ ."

Who does God say should accompany Moses to the base of the mountain? _____, _____, _____, and _____ of the elders of Israel.

What is the relationship between Nadab, Abihu, and Moses? (Exodus 6:23)

_____

Why do you think they were chosen to join Moses and Aaron at the base of the mountain? (Exodus 28:1, Numbers 3:3) _____

_____

_____

Who were the seventy that accompanied Moses, Aaron, Nadab and Abihu and why do you think they were chosen? (Numbers 11:16) _____

_____

Which other two men are named in Exodus 24:13-14, suggesting that they are included in the seventy? _____ and _____

Joshua is identified as Moses' assistant and will play a major role as the Israelites finally arrive at the Promised Land. Hur, you will recall, was one of the men who held up Moses' arms during the battle with Amalek (Week 5, Day 1). (Jewish tradition also suggests Hur was the husband of Miriam, Moses' sister).

Now that we have established the players in this particular scene: Moses, Aaron, Nadab, Abihu, Joshua, Hur and sixty-eight additional unnamed elders, let's look at the actual events chronicled in this short chapter.

After hearing the invitation from God, Moses turned to the Israelites to prepare them for his departure. Before he leaves, he not only reminds them of the rules, but he actually writes them down—lest they forget during his absence. In unison, they twice declared their intentions:

Exodus 24:3c: *"All the _____ which the LORD has said _____ _____ _____."*

Exodus 24:7b: *And they said, "All that the LORD has said _____ _____ _____, and be _____."*

In an effort to seal their commitment, Moses built an altar of stone. It is interesting to note this particular type of altar or *mizbeach* is for a particular purpose and is mentioned in Scripture only a few times prior to this event.

Who before Moses had constructed a mizbeach—an altar of blood sacrifice?

Genesis 8:20: _____
Genesis 12:7; 13:18; 22:9: _____
Genesis 26:25; 33:18-20: _____

It is impossible to know what the altars of blood sacrifice built by Noah, Abram/Abraham, and Jacob might have looked like, but Moses had been given detailed building specifications (Ex. 20:24-26). After the oxen were slain, the blood was collected before they were burned on the altar. Although, it seems quite grisly in our culture, the Israelites understood the solemn oath of obedience they had made when Moses sprinkled, or dashed (NRSV), the blood on them. It gave visual, and I suspect visceral, impact to help them remember their covenant with God.

What did Moses say as the oxen blood covered the upturned faces of the crowd?
Exodus 24:8b: *This is the _____ of the _____ which the*

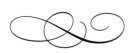

*Mizbeach –
miz-bay'-akh –
slaughter place; altar
of blood sacrifice;
altar of burnt
offerings.*

111

Lord has made with you according to all these _____.

Does that verse sound familiar to you? Record the following New Testament Scriptures:

Matthew 26:28: _____

_____

Mark 14:24: _____

_____

Luke 22:20: _____

_____

1 Corinthians 11:25b: _____

_____

COVENANT	=	a need to remember
ALTAR	=	a place to remember
BLOOD SACRIFICE	=	a sign to remember

Many years ago, my husband and I were part of a marvelous Sunday School class with a devoted teacher. Each week, Ken would hand out little strips of yellow paper with the Scripture references for the day's lesson. I still occasionally find those strips of paper tucked away in my Bible and I am reminded of lessons learned and covenants made.

My friend Anita has given me countless bookmarks, each lovingly chosen and included with a card of encouragement or concern. Those markers are scattered throughout my Bible as well, marking the verses that have brought me comfort and assurance throughout the years. The pages seem to naturally fall open to Jeremiah 29:11 and Psalm 139, with specific events associated to each.

I have pictures of my children and precious friends clipped to pages throughout my Bible with dates and names written near significant Scriptures. Each time I see those faces and read the verses associated with each, I am reminded of special times of love and friendship.

Perhaps little strips of paper, inspirational bookmarks and pictures are not ordinarily considered altars, but they nevertheless serve to remind me of the need to remember, they direct me to a specific place to remember; by keeping them in significant and meaningful places, they are signs that help me remember.

What "altars" help you remember your covenants with God? Give a brief description.

_____

_____

The remaining verses of today's lesson describe the assent up the mountain. Moses, Aaron, Nadab, Abihu and the seventy elders progressed to the base of the mountain where they saw God standing on a *"paved work of sapphire stone"* (Ex. 24:10). Can you imagine being able to eat after seeing such an amazing sight? But, that is exactly what happened; they enjoyed a meal together, then Moses and Joshua started up the mountain, leaving Aaron and Hur as the "deputies in charge" with the elders. (My natural curiosity makes me wonder how Aaron felt when Moses chose Joshua to accompany him and not his own brother.) We are not told when or why Joshua stopped the climb, but by the seventh day, it was only Moses who was called into the cloud at the apex of the mountain. There he remained forty days and forty nights receiving the *"tablets of stone, and the law and commandments* _____

_____ _____ _____, *that you may teach them"*
(Ex. 24:12b).

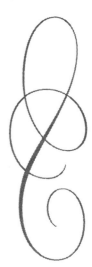

◦⁄◦ **Walking With Moses** ◦⁄◦

Moses was faithful to acknowledge situations and times that should be remembered by himself and the Israelites by building altars of remembrance and of sacrifice. It may not be necessary for me to build actual altars, but any device which can help me remember the faithfulness of God is a worthwhile endeavor.

◦⁄◦ **Talking With God** ◦⁄◦

God, thank You for the many ways You remind me of Your faithfulness through the gifts and treasures from family and friends.

_____

_____

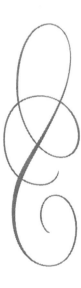

Day 2
Lowest Valleys and Highest Mountains

Text: Exodus 19:1-25. Deuteronomy 2:1-37

Focus: *For the LORD your God has blessed you in all the work of your hand. He knows your trudging through this great wilderness. These forty years the LORD your God has been with you; you have lacked nothing. Deuteronomy 2:7*

Whoever said the Christian walk would meander down an easy road must have had a very different travel guide than the one I have. I don't know about you, but I am daily faced with hairpin turns, potholes, and washed out bridges. Speed limits and no passing zones keep me inching along, and road construction is a constant nuisance. I endure long expanses of deserted highway and lonely hours of solitude due to poor judgment and wrong turns along the way. And, just as some of my valleys have been despairingly deep, I have also enjoyed the view from many mountaintop overlooks.

How would describe the path you are traveling at this particular time in your life?

    _____ Smooth and easy going
    _____ Serpentine with no clear view around the next corner
    _____ At a dead end
    _____ Stranded in the desert
    _____ Over crowded and bumper to bumper
    _____ Dark and lonely
    _____ A little bumpy
    _____ Inching along at a snail's pace
    _____ Narrow and clearly defined
    _____ Enjoying the view from the mountaintop
    _____ Other _____

Countless biblical figures shared similar experiences, but none so extravagantly or clearly detailed as Moses. From the day he fled the splendor of Pharaoh's palace to his final conversation with God on Mount Nebo, his life adventure was replete with desert valleys and mountaintop experiences.

Exodus 2:15b: *But Moses fled from the face of Pharaoh and dwelt in the land of Midian; and he _____ _____ by a _____.*

As we established earlier in our study, there is no way for us to know how long Moses had been in Median before he met his future wife and father-in-law, but we do know he was on the run. His crime of murder against the Egyptian taskmaster had been witnessed and Pharaoh was seeking vengeance. Tired, hungry, confused, and lost, he came to a well in an unfamiliar land. The Hebrew word used here is "yashab" which means to sit down and be still. It was time for Moses to stop running—to sit down and be still so he could be prepared to take the next slow steps into his future. As a follow-up to our previous week's last day of study, this was perhaps Moses' first retreat experience.

Have you considered a time in a valley as a time to sit down and be still? If so, give a brief description.

_____

_____

_____

_____

For Moses, the next forty years in the desert lands of Midian, helped prepare him as a leader to lead the Israelites to the Promised Land. What are some of the basic lessons he learned while living in Midian?

Exodus 2:21a _____
Exodus 3:1   _____
Exodus 3:12   _____
Exodus 3:13   _____
Exodus 4:17   _____

Contentment, leadership skills (of sheep and people), the assurance of God's presence, the name of the one true God, and God given tools to do the job, all good things for any leader to have and to know. While shepherding Jethro's sheep, he learned to read the stars for direction, understand the unpredictable weather of the desert, and to be ever watchful for predators. In addition to the skills already mentioned, he learned:

• To recognize God's voice (Ex. 3:4)
• How it felt to stand on holy ground (Ex. 3:5)
• He could be in the presence of God without being consumed (Ex. 3:6)

- God is a God of compassion and deliverance (Ex. 3:7-8)
- God is a God of miracles and wonders (Ex. 4:1-9)
- To be honest with God (Ex. 3:10)
- God could only be pushed so far (Ex. 4:14)

Midian may not have been Moses' first choice of places to spend forty years of his life, but it was valuable valley time as God prepared him for the forty years he would wander in the desert with the Israelites.

As Moses led the Israelites out of Egypt, his expectations must have been very high as they headed to the Promised Land. Each day as the desert continued to stretch before them, I can imagine his mood becoming more and more somber, but there were still many lessons to be learned.

Exodus 13:19: *And Moses took the _____ _____ _____ with him, for he had placed the children of Israel under solemn oath, saying, "God will surely visit you, and you shall carry up my bones from here with you."*

Moses fulfilled a promise made many years earlier (Gen. 50:25) that Joseph's bones would not be left behind when God finally delivered the Israelites from the bondage of Egypt. Moses carried these literal "old bones" on the journey, but I suspect he carried some figurative "old bones" as well – resentment, jealousy, fear, despair, loneliness, distrust. He would have ample time in the wilderness valley to consider each.

What "old bones" have you carried with you in the valley?

_____

_____

_____

_____

Exodus 14:3: *For Pharaoh will say of the children of Israel, "They are _____ by the land; the _____ has _____ _____ in."*

As we saw in Week 4, Pharaoh did indeed believe the Israelites were confused and closed in at the Sea of Reeds. To the Egyptians, it seemed Moses was leading his band of refugees aimlessly and to ultimate ruin. Appearances are not always what they seem, are they? God had not for one moment lost sight of His children, even in the valley, regardless of how it looked to Pharaoh.

Job knew how it felt to have others define his condition. His friends certainly were of little help or support as they considered his suffering brought on by personal sin. Even his wife questioned his integrity and faith. In his deepest, darkest valley Job was still able to say, *"But He knows the way that I take; When He has tested me, I shall come forth as gold."* (Job 23:10)

During David's days in the valley he wrote, *"Where can I go from Your Spirit? Or where can I flee from Your presence? If I ascend into heaven, You are there; If I make my bed in hell, behold, You are there. If I take the wings of the morning, and dwell in the uttermost parts of the sea, even there Your hand shall lead me, and Your right hand shall hold me.* (Ps. 139:7-10)

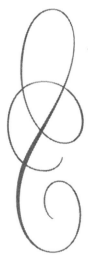

With full knowledge of God's faithfulness, Moses admonished the Israelites by saying, *"He knows your trudging through this great wilderness. These forty years the Lord your God has been with you; you have lacked nothing."* (Deut. 2:7b)

Consider the following Scriptures and the possible lessons Moses gleaned from each. Time in the valley can:

- Exodus 17:7 - lend itself to grumpiness and questioning
- Exodus 18 – be a good place to hear valuable advice and counsel
- Exodus 33:12-19 – be a time of grappling with the hard questions
- Deuteronomy 8:2-5 – be a time to be humbled and tested
- Deuteronomy 32:10-14 – be a time to simply be cared for by God.

One final valley experience and lesson is possibly my favorite—our desert and wilderness valleys prepare us for our mountaintops. *And the Lord said, "Here is a place by Me, and you shall stand on the rock."* (Ex. 33:21) It is a monumental comfort to know God will only allow me to dwell in the valley for a while. Just as the Israelites, I need to be ready when it is time to approach the mountain.

Read Exodus 19:10-20.

What were the Israelites told to do in preparation? (vs. 10) _____

_____

What would happen on the third day? (vs. 11) _____

_____

What were they not allowed to do? (vs. 12) _____

_____

What was the signal for them to approach the mountain? (vs. 13) _____

_____

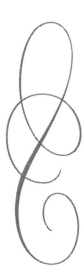

What were the conditions on the mountain on the third day? (vs. 16) _____

_____

What did God invite Moses to do? (vs. 20) _____

_____

Fulfilling the promise He made in Exodus 3:12, God invited Moses to meet Him on the mountaintop. Moses was not only ready, he was prepared. He had done everything God had required of him to this point, even the tasks that fell far outside his comfort zone. The responsibility of leading the Israelites had weighed heavy on his shoulders and the days in the wilderness had been harsh and difficult. If ever a man was due a mountaintop experience, it was Moses.

Earlier in today's study we listed the experiences which prepared Moses to lead the Israelites. Which of those also might have prepared him for the unknowns of this first trip up the mountain?

_____

_____

_____

_____

Can you identify specific events which set the stage for a significant mountaintop experience in your life?

_____

_____

_____

Exodus 34:29: *Now it was so, when Moses came down from Mount Sinai (and the two tablets of Testimony were in Moses' hand when he came down from the mountain), that Moses did not know that the skin of his face shone while he talked with Him.*

Moses' very countenance had changed. His face glowed because of his encounter with God. Have you had a mountaintop experience which changed you? Could others see the change in you?

_____

_____

_____

_____

Of course, Moses was called to meet with God on other occasions on the mountain and each time he returned full of power and wisdom for the people. Although he probably became less intimidated by the fire and smoke, thunder and lighting, and pure awesomeness of the presence of God, I feel confident he never took his times alone on the mountain with God for granted.

What was Moses' final mountaintop experience, as recorded in Deuteronomy 34?

_____

_____

_____

_____

As we conclude today's study, there is one final distinction for us to consider in regards to lowest valleys and highest mountains.

Who was with Moses in the wilderness valley? _____

Who was with Moses on the mountain? _____

Days in the valley certainly can be lonely, but usually, there are those who are more than willing to commiserate with me with I am down. Whether it is truly their desire to boost my spirits, or simply a need to share their own tale of woe, the adage "misery loves company" seems to prove true. Perhaps it is a gift to know we need not walk alone in hard times.

On the other side of the coin, my most meaningful mountaintop experiences have been just between me and God—one on one, face to face, heart to heart. I might have been worshiping alone or with a crowd, but the actual encounter was extremely personal and could not be added to or lessened by anyone else's experience.

As I continue to walk with God, on a road fraught with trials and concerns, I want to be ready when God calls me out of the valley saying, *"Here is a place by Me, and you shall stand on the rock."* (Ex. 33:21)

⌒⌒ Walking With Moses ⌒⌒

Moses knew what it was to walk the unpredictable road of life, and although it seems his days in the valley far exceeded his mountaintop experiences, the latter were significant enough to carry him through the difficult days. As much as he might have wanted to live on the mountaintop, he understood his calling was walking the dusty road through the wilderness "on the way" to the Promised Land.

⌒⌒ Talking With God ⌒⌒

God, thank You for the mountaintop experiences and for the valleys in-between.

_____

_____

_____

Day 3
Written by the Finger of God

Text: Exodus 25:1 – 31:18

Focus: *And when He had made an end of speaking with him on Mount Sinai, He gave Moses two tablets of the Testimony, tablets of stone, written with the finger of God.* Exodus 31:18

The six chapters prior to today's focus are devoted to the words spoken to Moses while on the mountain with God. I realize today's text was a lengthy task, and although this study will not focus on the specifics of the tabernacle and accouterments thereof, I encourage you not to skip over it. If nothing else, the detailed instruction will convince you God is indeed in the details. As a quick summary before we get to the heart of today's study, record the instructions given by God in the following Scriptures:

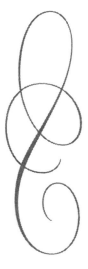

Exodus 25:2: *". . . bring Me an _____."*
Exodus 25:8: *"And let them make Me a _____ . . ."*
Exodus 25:10: *"And they shall make an _____ . . ."*
Exodus 25:17: *"You shall make a _____ _____ . . ."*
Exodus 25:23: *"You shall also make a _____ . . ."*
Exodus 25:31: *"You shall also make a _____ . . ."*

Exodus 26–31:11 give further details for the construction and design of the temple, the ordination and attire of the priests, and the types of offerings to be accepted in the sanctuary. Exodus 31:12-17 reminds the people to keep the Sabbath as a day of rest in the midst of all the work God has given them to do. No doubt an entire study could be created around each of these particular subjects, but for our purposes today, let's focus our attention on Exodus 31:18. Please, take a moment to reread that Scripture now.

Do you like to finger paint? There is a freedom that comes when creating something colorful, albeit messy, with our fingers. Many years ago, we allowed a dozen three year olds to paint our basement walls. Although we provided neat little cups of primary paint and foam brushes, they quickly abandoned the brushes and instead used pudgy little fingers to create their masterpieces. Surprisingly, as their parents realized the joy in their abandon, they joined in the fun. It was with a genuine sense of regret several years later, as we updated the area to suit our pre-teens that we painted over the artwork.

Finger paints are just the tip of the iceberg when it comes to the creativity and artistic endeavors of our fingers. I am always amused by what is written on dusty car windows such as "wash me," "Joe ♥ Sue," and "I'm not dirty, I have true grit." Tiny fingers rake across the side of birthday cakes positioned perilously close to the counter edge. And my all time favorite, freshly poured concrete. As a child, along with my brother and sister, I was encouraged to write my name in the freshly poured foundation of the new grain bin before the metal walls were erected. I remember considering then who might someday see those names and wonder about the lives of Rose Ann, Bobby, and Cindy. A few years ago, after having some much needed work done in our leaky basement, my husband, children, and I wrote our names in the wet concrete before the carpet was replaced. One day in the future, after my husband and I have moved into our retirement home, some young family will pull back the carpet in the basement of the gray house on Fox Hill and know that this place was loved by a family of four humans and two cats. (Yes, we pressed their little paws in the wet concrete too.)

Have you had a similar experience of leaving your personal mark on something that will be discovered at a later time? If so, give a brief description.

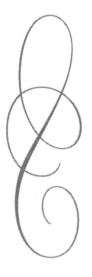

_____

_____

_____

_____

There is such great value in writing things down. My husband writes his goals for the future. Motivational speakers recommend posting your main life goal on the wall so you see it everyday. Habakkuk 2:2 says, *Write the vision and make it plain on tablets, that he may run who reads it.* An American proverb says, *the pen is mightier than the sword.* As a writer, I choose words carefully to convey specific meanings—and when I want the sentiments to be as personal as I feel them in my heart, I move away from the keyboard and pick up a pen. A handwritten note is a gift all unto itself.

I suppose it is because of those experiences and the personal attention required when creating anything with my fingers that I am intrigued when Moses records the Ten Commandments were *written by the finger of God.* The attachment of anthropomorphic (human) attributes to God can be troubling to some, but it helps me better understand the God who created and understands mankind. I can imagine Moses peeking out from the cleft in the rock and seeing the words being inscribed on stones perfectly chiseled by God. The personal touch of that Holy hand gave each word power and life to last for all eternity.

Exodus 24:12b: *". . . I will give you tablets of stone, and the law and commandments _____ _____ _____ _____, that you may teach them."*

Before we go any further, let's refresh our knowledge of the Decalogue or Ten Commandments (Ex. 20:3-17; Deut. 5:7-21).

- You shall have no other gods before me.
- You shall not make for yourself a carved image.
- You shall not take the name of the Lord your God in vain.
- Remember the Sabbath day, to keep it holy.
- Honor your father and your mother.
- You shall not murder.
- You shall not commit adultery.
- You shall not steal.
- You shall not bear false witness against your neighbor.
- You shall not covet.

Exodus 32:15-16 – *And Moses turned and went down from the mountain, and the two tablets of the Testimony were in his hand. The tablets were written on both sides; on the one side and on the other they were written. Now the tablets were the _____ _____ _____, and the writing was the _____ _____ _____ engraved on the tablets.*

Earlier in our walk with Moses (Week 2, Day 5), we saw another event attributed to the finger of God. It seems the Egyptian magicians in Exodus 8:16-19 were equally intrigued. What did they attribute to the finger of God?

_____

Tablets of stone and a plague of gnats are surpassed by the beauty of Psalm 8:3, *When I consider Your heavens, the work of Your fingers. The moon and the stars, which You have ordained.*

And, 2 Corinthians 3:2-3 moves us from the old covenant to the new—*You are our epistle written in our hearts, know and read by all me; clearly you are an epistle of Christ, ministered by us, written not with ink but by the Spirit of the living God, not on tablets of stone but on the tablets of flesh, that is, of the heart.*

Have you considered the finger of God writing on your heart? What does that mean to you?

_____

_____

_____

Matthew 22:37-39: *Jesus said to him, "You shall love the L<small>ORD</small> your God with all your heart, with all your soul, and with all your mind. This is the first and great commandment. And the second is like it: You shall love your neighbor as yourself. On these two commandments hang all the Law and the Prophets."*

Deuteronomy 6:4-9: *Hear, O Israel: The L<small>ORD</small> our God, the L<small>ORD</small> is one! You shall love the L<small>ORD</small> your God with all your heart, with all your soul, and with all your strength. And these words which I command you today shall be in your heart. You shall _____ _____ diligently to your children, and shall talk of them when you _____ in your house, when you _____ by the way, when you_____ _____, and when you _____ _____. You shall bind them as a sign on your hand, and they shall be as frontlets between your eyes. You shall _____ them on the doorposts of your house and on your gates.*

Would you pass the test? How would you answer the following questions?

Do you love God with all your heart, soul, mind, and strength? How does that effect how you live your life?

_____

_____

_____

Are His words in your heart? How does that help you during the course of the day?

_____

_____

Have you taught His words to others? If so, give an example of whom, when, and how.

_____

_____

_____

Do you talk about God's Word in your house?

_____

_____

_____

Do you talk about God's Word in your workplace?

_____

_____

_____

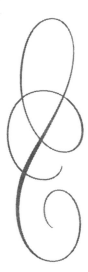

Are God's words the last on your mind and in your heart at the end of the day and the first at the beginning of the day?

_____

_____

_____

Are God's words displayed anywhere in your home or workplace as a witness to others?

_____

_____

_____

Psalm 119:105: _Your word is a lamp to my feet and a light to my path._

Moses had no doubt he was the custodian of the handwritten words of God and he was faithful to impart their significance to the Israelites. The words and history recorded by Moses have eternal merit and help to light the way for each of us on our individual journeys as we seek to love God with our entire beings.

⚬⚬ Talking With God ⚬⚬

God, help me to love You with all my heart, soul, mind, and strength.

_____

_____

_____

_____

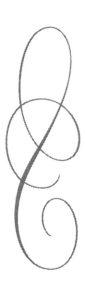

Day 4
Idols Consumed by Fire

Text: Exodus 32:1-20

Focus: *The he took the calf which they had made, burned it in the fire, and ground it to powder; and he scattered it on the water and made the children of Israel drink it.* Exodus 32:20

As a parent of school aged children, one phone call I always dreaded receiving was from the principal or school counselor, not reporting illness, but a discipline problem. Knowing you are about to hear the words, "Please come to the school to pick up your child because he/she has been involved in an incident" is enough to cause any parent to invest in caller ID and not pick up the phone.

Forty days Moses had resided on the mountain listening to God's voice give instruction and details for the tabernacle. Imagine . . . forty days on a mountain, in a cloud, alone with God . . . sweet communion. And then, the dreaded call arrived.

Exodus 32:7: *And the LORD said to Moses, "_____, _____*

_____! For your people whom you brought out of the land of Egypt have _____ themselves."_

Moses had been gone too long and the people were getting restless. The mountain continued to rumble and was covered by the cloud of smoke, but there was no word from Moses, or even from Joshua who was waiting halfway up the hillside. In fear and absolute lack of faith in the God who had delivered them to this point, the people went to Aaron asking for leadership. They wanted new gods to lead them and Aaron did exactly what they asked. He took their gold earrings and baubles, created a golden calf, and they declared, _"This is your god, O Israel, that brought you out of the land of Egypt!"_ (Ex.32:4b) Not simply the god that would lead them forward, but the god that had led them thus far. What were they thinking!

Where do you think they got the gold that was used to make the calf? Look back at Week 2, Day 5 for a possible answer.

_____

There has been much speculation as to Aaron's motivation for responding in the manner in which he did, but personally, I think the sudden power and attention simply went to his head.

- The people gathered around Aaron (Ex. 32:1)
- And brought them (gold earrings) to Aaron (Ex. 32:3)
- He received the gold from their hand (Ex. 32:4)
- He fashioned it and made a calf (Ex. 32:4)
- They said, "This is your god" (Ex. 32:4)
- Aaron saw it and built an altar before it (Ex. 32:5)
- Aaron proclaimed, "Tomorrow is a feast to the Lord." (Ex. 32:5)

Have you ever suddenly been thrown into a position of authority or leadership and then been expected to make snap decisions on behalf of the group? Did you find it an easy or daunting task?

_____

_____

_____

_____

Aaron had been second in command from the day Moses had returned to Egypt. To this point, Moses had been the one in charge and Aaron was simply the mouthpiece. *So he [Aaron] shall be your spokesman to the people. And he himself shall be as a mouth for you, and you shall be to him as God.* (Ex. 4:16) Even the most loyal brother might have been a little jealous when considering the good fortune of his younger sibling to this point. After all, Moses had been:

- Spared Pharaoh's edict that all baby boys should be cast in the river.
- Rescued from the river by Pharaoh's daughter.
- Raised in the house of Pharaoh with the privileges and splendor thereof.
- Chosen by God to lead the Israelites out of bondage.

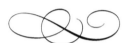

Nearly all men can stand adversity, but if you want to test a man's character, give him power.
Abraham Lincoln

When you add the element that Moses had obviously chosen Joshua to become his apprentice and aide-de-camp, it is no wonder Aaron saw this as his moment to shine. Moses and Joshua were both gone and the people were calling out to *him,* not to his brother. Faith and experience should have helped him process his actions more wisely, but some other force took over and he created an idol which he was obviously quite proud of. *So when Aaron saw it, he built an altar before it.* (Ex. 32:5)

I remember the pride I felt when my first article was published in a magazine and I actually got paid for it. I was convinced I had *arrived* as a writer. My husband had the article matted and framed; it still hangs on my kitchen wall. I didn't build an altar in front of it, but every time I walk past it, I still remember that feeling of pride. Of course, as every writer learns, one published article does not a writer make, so my ego was quickly put in check as future rejection notices arrived, but it was a brief ego boost nonetheless.

Aaron is certainly the man of the hour. He provided the Israelites the god they clamored for, declared a feast day, and is reveling in his acclaim with the people. They sat down to eat and drink, and rose up to play, all the while having no idea while they were partying at the base of the mountain, Moses was getting a full report from a very angry God. *"Now therefore, let Me alone, that My wrath may burn hot against them and I may consume them."* (Ex. 32:10)

How did Moses respond to God's anger toward the Israelites? (Ex. 32:11-13)

_____

_____

How did God respond? (Ex. 32:14)

_____

What is Moses' reaction when he witnesses the spectacle as he reenters the camp?
(Ex. 32:19) _____

When God first told Moses what the people were up to and expressed His wrathful desire to obliterate them, Moses was very quick to come to their defense. Perhaps until he saw with his own eyes the uncontrolled behavior in the camp he could not believe Aaron would have allowed such a situation to occur. After convincing God to calm His anger, Moses turned around and completely lost his own temper. He cast down the tablets he had just been entrusted with—*the work of God* and *the writing of God*—symbolically demonstrating the broken covenant. He then turned his rage toward the golden calf and destroyed it in the fire.

Two specific memories came to mind as I read Exodus 32:20. The first recollection was of a class I participated in several years ago while working at an historic home/ living history museum. This particular class demonstrated the old-fashioned method for making soap. One of the key ingredients, lye, in colonial days was acquired by leaching water through ashes. The ash substance was added to animal fat, cooked over an open fire and then poured into molds. It was the lye from the ashes that provided the lathering and cleansing aspect of the soap. The other memory was of a childhood friend frequently getting his mouth washed out with soap for saying a curse word. Read that verse again: *Then he took the calf which they had made, burned it in the fire, and ground it to powder; and he scattered it on the water and made the children of Israel drink it.* It occurs to me Moses literally washed the Israelites' mouths out with soap for offering their worship to another god.

While the people spit and sputtered, Moses turned his attention to his brother as he tried to get his arms around the situation. He could not imagine Aaron would have created the idol without being coerced or forced by the people.

What was Aaron's response?

_____

_____

_____

It was obvious he was not going to take responsibility for his actions; he blamed Moses for being gone too long and the people for being evil. He even had the audacity to say, "I just threw the gold in the fire and out popped the calf." (Ex. 32:24) Although the absurdity of that statement makes me chuckle, it was no laughing matter to Moses as he positioned himself at the entrance of the camp and called forth all those with true allegiance to God. Exodus 32:25-29 details a gruesome scene as approximately three thousand men are slain by the swords of the Levites—at Moses' command. This sacrificial purging was a necessary atonement for the sin of the golden calf.

Aaron did not receive a specific and personal punishment for creating the calf, but he did have to stand by and watch as thousands of his countrymen were massacred, knowing full well he had a hand in the retribution they were paying. In spite of Aaron's failing and caving to the wishes and demands of the people, he is forgiven and is raised to the priesthood in the tabernacle of meeting. The witness of his life gives me hope that even when I allow a sin as grievous as the worship of an idol or other god to creep into my life, I can be forgiven and restored to a right relationship with God.

Earlier Moses pleaded with God to let the Israelites live (Ex. 32:11-14), now he was prepared to ask God to forgive them.

Exodus 32:32: *Yet now, if You will _____ _____ _____ – but if not, I pray, _____ _____ _____ of Your book which You have written.*

If God would not forgive the Israelites, Moses was willing to take the same or worse punishment. He was a true team player and the quintessential leader. Perhaps because the Israelites had not had the opportunity to see the first commandment on the stones (since Moses broke them in his fit of anger), God decided not to end the journey. What is the first commandment? (Ex. 20:3)

_____

_____

Instead, God simply told Moses to keep leading the people toward the Promised Land and this particular situation would be dealt with on another day. However, to the sadness and dismay of the people, God's anger is not completely assuaged.
And I will send My Angel before you . . . for I will not go up in your midst, lest I consume you on the way, for you are a stiff-necked people. (Ex. 33:2-3)

Before we leave today's study, I want us to focus for a few more moments on the concept of idols. Martin Luther, in The Book of Concord, expounds on the first commandment by saying "Whatever your heart clings to and confides in, that is really your God." [1]

What is your definition of an idol?

_____

Some days my idols take the physical form of a person or thing, but often, my heart is clinging to idols that cannot be seen or touched such as worry, fear, or jealousy. On those sleepless nights when my mind swirls with "what if" scenarios, I am dancing at the altar of a foreign god; an idol of my own making and needing to be consumed by a holy fire.

I will bless the LORD who has given me counsel; My heart also instructs me in the night seasons. I have set the LORD always before me; because He is at my right hand I shall not be moved. Therefore my heart is glad, and my glory rejoices; my flesh also rest in hope. (Psalm 16:7-9)

What are the idols of your own making? _____

_____

_____

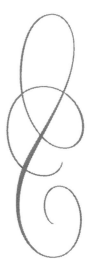

While visiting the Mayan ruins in Mexico several years ago, I was intrigued by one particular bit of folklore. The Mayans worshiped countless gods, including gods of the heavens, gods of the underworlds, and gods of all things in-between. During the Spanish conquest and influence of European beliefs, the Mayan religion and traditions were oppressed. Christian icons replaced Mayan icons in the temples and the people were expected to convert and bow before these new symbols of faith. In desperation, the Mayan artisans devised a clever plan to appear submissive to the new rule, while remaining true to their own beliefs. They conceded to fashion the new statues and symbols for the temple according to the Christian mandate, yet secretly enclosed statues of their own gods inside. They could, in this way, continue to bow before their own gods while appearing to submit to the new religion of their conquerors.

What are the idols you have cleverly disguised? _____

_____

_____

Moses had lived his first forty years in a palace full of lifeless and powerless idols. The second forty years he lived with the many gods of the Midianites, while encountering the one true God. As he entered his final forty years of life, he acknowledged no other God but the great I AM. Is it any wonder his rage burned so intently at the sight of the golden calf? He understood the folly of false gods.

∽⌒◌ Walking With Moses ◌⌒∽

Idols, seen and unseen, keep us from true fellowship and communion with God. Only by casting them into Holy fire are we able to totally be released from the hold they can have on our hearts and minds.

∽⌒◌ Talking With God ◌⌒∽

God, You are the One true God. Help me to see the idols I have erected and pay homage to. Consume them with Your holy fire.

_____

_____

_____

_____

[1] Martin Luther, *Book of Concord, Large Catechism* (1529) "The First Commandment."

Day 5
Replacement Tables

Text: Exodus 34:1-35

Focus: *And the LORD said to Moses, "Cut two tablets of stone like the first ones, and I will write on these tablets the words that were on the first tablets which you broke."* Exodus 34:1

My mother was a remarkable and gifted woman. She could turn a meal planned for a family of five into a feast for unexpected company simply by "throwing another potato in the pot." She could sew, drive a tractor, decorate elaborate cakes for celebrations, and keep complicated farm records. For years she rocked babies in the church nursery, organized banquets and receptions, and probably made hundreds of gallons of ice cream for the youth groups that would converge on our home during the 70s.

I don't remember any challenge that my mother ever shied away from with the exception of one—housekeeping. It might have been in rebellion against her own upbringing by my grandmother who was fanatical about the tidiness and cleanliness of her home, but I suspect it was more a case of priorities. Mother had many other things to do, so cleaning could wait. If the pastor stopped by and had to move the unfolded laundry before he sat on the couch, she jokingly suggested he fold towels while they chatted. Her home was always warm and welcoming, regardless of the disarray.

If my mother's questionable housekeeping methods were in rebellion to her own upbringing, perhaps my penchant for neatness is a similar yet opposite rebellion. Many times, during my growing up years, I would wage war on a particular room, scrubbing, dusting, organizing and throwing away anything that didn't seem important to me.

Occasionally, my zeal for my grandmother's way of housekeeping got me into trouble. One year our church was preparing to do a new pictorial directory and as usual, my mother was asked to take charge. The directory company sent the forms and specific instructions of how to contact each member, set appointments, check and cross check so no one was left out. Mother meticulously followed the guidelines and as the photo dates approached, she was very proud of the organizational time she invested in the project. The entire congregation had been contacted. Needless to say, as this was in the

133

early seventies, she did not have a computer, but her record keeping rivaled the best spreadsheet program. She held the only copy and she guarded it dutifully.

The week before the directory representative was scheduled to begin taking the long awaited photos, I went into one of my cleaning frenzies and not only tossed the entire file into the trash; I carried it to the burn pile behind the barn and set it ablaze. I will never forget the sight of my mother sitting on the porch steps sobbing when she realized what had happened. I had destroyed records she had been entrusted with, a project she had taken great pride in doing well for her fellow church members, and the fruit of countless hours of phone calls and visits. After vowing never to clean again, I joined her at the burn pile to see if there were any charred remains that might be salvageable. Not so much as a paper clip was found. We returned to the house and both sat on the porch steps and cried. After dinner, she closed her bedroom door and did not come out for the rest of the evening.

Can you think of a similar situation when good intentions ended up being disastrous? If so, give a brief description.

_____

_____

_____

_____

Did those involved respond with anger or mourning? What was your own reaction?

_____

_____

_____

_____

The morning after I destroyed the church directory file, I found my mother sitting at the kitchen table with the church roster, calendar, phone book and a stack of carefully hand-drawn scheduling charts. She was resolutely piecing together the mess I had made. Although I think she was embarrassed when the company photographer arrived and she handed him the homemade forms, the appointments went off with few problems and the directory became a well-used resource for the good people of Elberfeld First Baptist Church.

Moses had a similar situation to deal with. He had been entrusted with some very specific instructions on tablets formed and written by God. Clutching them tightly to his chest, he made his way down the mountain, knowing the stones contained information not easily replicated, details he could never remember on his own, in a format created by a higher power. The destruction of the tablets was not at the hand of a well-meaning adolescent, but by the rage surging within him as he witnessed the Israelites worshiping around the golden calf. In a moment, the stones were broken at the foot of the mountain and the handwriting of God was gone. With intense, yet mixed emotions, Moses surely knelt to see if there was a recognizable word amid the shards.

Describe how you think Moses' must have felt as he looked at the broken tablets?

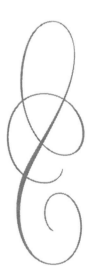

_____

_____

_____

_____

Can you think of a time when you responded in anger to a situation that ultimately caused an even bigger mess? If so, give a brief description.

_____

_____

_____

_____

As the days passed, Moses' anger turned to mourning over the fickle and sinful behavior of the Israelites. He moved his tent away from the camp so he could continue his intense conversations with God. Moses must have felt great relief when God finally said, *"Cut two tablets of stone like the first ones, and I will write on these tablets the words that were on the first tablets which you broke. So be ready in the morning . . ."* (Ex. 34:1-2a).

Recently my husband and son made a pilgrimage to a remote area in Utah to experience for themselves a place called U-Dig Fossils, one of the world's richest deposits of trilobites. My son had seen the location featured on the Discover Channel and had been pestering us for two years to take him. With goggles, picks, hammers, and buckets in hand, they set out for a day of digging. Several hours (and a few skinned knuckles) later they loaded up their treasures—a bucket full of rocks that upon closer examination would reveal nickel to quarter size fossils. Although they deemed it an adventure, neither was inclined to devote more time or energy to the grueling work of hammering and breaking rocks.

God had chiseled the first set of tablets; Moses would chisel the second. After hours of hearing iron on stone, the Israelites emerged from their tents to see Moses, with homemade tablets in hand, heading back up the mountain to piece together the mess that had been made days earlier.

Reread Exodus 34:27. The first tablets had been cut by God and written by the finger of God; the second tablets were cut by Moses (vs. 4) and written by the hand of Moses. Did this make the commandments and instruction any less legitimate or God-spoken?

_____

_____

_____

_____

Write Exodus 34:6-7 in your own words.

_____

_____

_____

_____

Can you think of a time when you were given a second chance to make a bungled situation right? If so, give a brief description.

_____

_____

_____

_____

My mother, as Moses, had a deep and abiding affection for the people she served. She took her responsibilities seriously and although my actions in her absence had created a significant problem, she did what was necessary to keep moving forward. A little time behind a closed bedroom door, a few more tears, a plea for direction, and ultimate resolve. Perhaps King Solomon had Moses, my mother, and you and me in mind as he pinned the words found in Ecclesiastes: *a time to break down, and a time to build up; a time to weep, and a time to laugh; a time to mourn, and a time to dance; a time to cast away stones, and a time to gather stones.* (Eccl. 3:3b-5a)

✎ Walking With Moses ✎

God has always been the God of second chances. He understands our human tendencies to make mistakes (even with good intentions), to respond in anger or frustration, and to make a mess of His best plans for us. He will always make a way for the situation to be reconciled.

✎ Talking With God ✎

God, thank You for showing me how to fix the messes I've made as I have tried to do Your will.

_____

_____

_____

_____

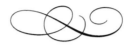

Week 6
TOMORROW IS ANOTHER DAY

Our final week of study brings us to the final days of Moses' life. The journey we have endured for six short weeks spanned 120 years for this unlikely leader. His ultimate fate was decided much earlier, yet this week we will witness first hand the disappointment he felt when his steps were stopped just a short distance from the Promised Land. During these final days we will learn by example how this leader of questionable background, qualification, and talent managed to end his duties with dignity while empowering and encouraging the one stepping into his well-worn sandals.

This week, as you walk with Moses and talk with God, rest secure knowing God will continue to lead you into your best future.

Day 1
Hope of a New Beginning

Text: Deuteronomy 10:1 - 11:32

Focus: *And now, Israel, what does the LORD your God require of you, but to fear the LORD your God, to walk in all His ways and to love Him, to serve the LORD your God will all your heart and with all your soul.* Deuteronomy 10:12

My children have been fortunate to attend very good public schools in our city, and although both have teachers they consider their favorites and others who might not make the list, they have received a good education and excellent instruction in matters far beyond *reading, writing, and 'rithmetic.* When my daughter returns home for visits from college, I feel certain she will drop in on one or two of her high school teachers to say hello. My son, still in middle school, has yet to move beyond a student/teacher relationship to the level of friendship often fostered in high school, but I feel certain his experience will be much the same when he reaches that stage.

Along the way, as my children have learned from their teachers, so have my husband and I. One of my son's teachers sent notes home many days detailing the antics which kept him from getting a reward or requiring additional homework. She ended each and every note with the words "Tomorrow is a new day and we will start anew." Those became key parenting words for us for several years. Everyday offered a clean slate, a new start, a second chance.

Describe a time when you were given a second chance by a friend, colleague, or family member?

_____

_____

_____

Describe a time when you were given a second chance by God?

_____

_____

_____

_____

I could list countless examples of second chance stories, including those of sports stars, television and movie celebrities, religious leaders and, of course, my own story. Even a recent *Veggie Tales* movie chronicles the story of Jonah and his second chance. In one way or another, we have all been given a second chance at some point in our lives and that is exactly where we find the Israelites today. The fiasco with the golden calf is yesterday's news, the second set of tablets are complete and safely stored in the ark of the covenant under the watchful eye of the Levites, and Moses has been instructed to set out again on the journey toward the Promised Land. It was time for them to begin again, or as Deuteronomy 10:12 begins *"And now, Israel . . . "* It was time to stop talking about the problems of the past and look to the future.

Do you begin each day with a sense of expectancy and a hope for a new beginning? As a personal month long commitment and experiment, I began my morning journal entries by personalizing the words of Deuteronomy 10:12, beginning each day with *"And now, Cinda . . ."* I was astounded by the freedom which welled up within me to truly release yesterday's failures and to move forward into the challenges and ultimate successes of the new day. Needless to say, it was not a practice I was willing to forfeit at the end of my original commitment time and it has consequently become part of my daily routine to include those words in my morning prayers. I encourage you to give it a try.

And now, (your name) _____ . . .

_____

_____

By the time Moses finished speaking the words recorded in today's text, the Israelites should have had no doubt about God's expectations. If you have not yet read Deuteronomy 10 & 11, please do so now; otherwise, glance back through your reading and note each time you read a variation of the words "keep the commandments of the Lord." Your translation may differ slightly, but in the NKJV, I found six (10:13; 11:1, 8, 13, 22, & 27). Minister and author, Norman Vincent Peale described how easily a thought or action can become a habit and automatic reflex if repeated often enough. Moses must have been working on the same principle.

In Deuteronomy 10:12-13, what are the five requirements God is looking for?

1. _____
2. _____
3. _____
4. _____
5. _____

Micah 6:8: *He has shown you, O man, what is good; and what does the Lord require of you but to do* _____ *, to love* _____ *, and to walk* _____ *with your God.*

Matthew 22:37-40: *Jesus said to him, "'You shall love the Lord your God with all your* _____ *, with all your* _____ *, and with all your* _____ *.' This is the first and great commandment. And the second is like it: 'You shall love your*

_____ _as_ _____.' On these two commandments hang all the Law and the Prophets."

I must tell you; today's text was a surprise to me—a really good surprise. Various phrases within our reading are found elsewhere in the Bible, so those Scriptures seemed familiar, but until this study, I had never taken an intense look at these two particular chapters of Deuteronomy. Tucked amidst God's admonishments and instructions are countless words of tender compassion and affection for the Israelites; in spite of their behavior to this point. _The Lord delighted only in your fathers, to love them; and He chose their descendants after them, you above all peoples, as it is this day._ (Deut. 10:15) Or, as _The Message_ says, _but it was your ancestors that God fell in love with; he picked their children—that's you!—out of all the other peoples._ On this new day, God reminded the Israelites He was in love with them before they were born and would be long after they were gone. This was a good day for the Israelites.

Deuteronomy 10:16: _Therefore_ _____ _the_ _____ _of your heart, and be stiff necked no longer._ For a gentler translation of this particular verse, _The Message_ says, _so cut away the thick calluses from your heart and stop being hard headed._

What does it mean to be hardhearted? _____

_____

What does it mean to be hardheaded? _____

_____

How do you think the Israelites had demonstrated these two characteristics to this point in their journey?

_____

_____

_____

Would you describe yourself as hardhearted and/or hardheaded? If so, give a brief description.

_____

_____

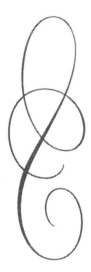

I mentioned earlier how this text was a pleasant surprise for me; the next passage is a perfect example. In the middle of a speech about keeping commandments and doing away with hard hearts and heads, Moses stops dead in his tracks and has a little praise session: *For the Lord your god is God of gods and Lord of lords, the great God, mighty and awesome, who shows no partiality nor takes a bribe. He administers justice for the fatherless and the widow, and loves the stranger, giving him food and clothing.* (Deut. 10:17-19) I can just imagine him ending with a resounding "Ain't God good!?!" or as we like to say at my church, "Amen, with Joy!"

Are there times during the normal course of your day when you stop to simply praise the goodness of God? How does that act and acknowledgement change your mood or outlook?

_____

_____

Deuteronomy 10 ends with a "therefore clause." *Webster's Dictionary* defines the word *therefore—as a result of this or that; for this or that reason; consequently.* In other words, since Moses has already established God is a good God who is just, compassionate and giving, the Israelites are to emulate those characteristics.

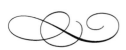

As a clarification before we leave chapter 10, the seventy persons noted in verse 22 refer to the descendants of Jacob who originally came to Egypt. Read Exodus 1:1-7.

Therefore _____ the _____, for you were strangers in the land of Egypt. You shall _____ the Lord your God; you shall _____ Him, and to Him you shall _____ _____, and take _____ in His name. **He is your praise**, *and* **He is your God**, *who has done for you these great and awesome things which your eyes have seen.* (Deut. 10:19-21)

The eleventh chapter of Deuteronomy outlines an "if—then" scenario with the bottom line being, obey God's commandments and good things will happen. Moses first identifies his audience specifically and ensures he has their attention.
Who is he NOT speaking to? (Deut. 11:2) _____

Why does Moses say he is not speaking to the children? (Deut. 11:2b-6)

_____

_____

Deuteronomy 11:7: *But _____ eyes have seen every great act of the Lord which He did.*

IF you keep every commandment;
>   THEN (vs. 8) _____
>   (vs. 9) _____

IF you earnestly obey my commandments;
>   THEN (vs. 14) _____
>   (vs. 15) _____

IF you carefully keep all these commandments;
>   THEN (vs. 23) _____
>   (vs. 25) _____

Bottom line, the Israelites had a choice to make; a choice for a blessing or a curse; a choice that needed to be made before they would step into the Promised Land.

Obviously, Moses had faith in them to make the right decision and gave instructions of the best way to keep his words and God's commandments at the forefront of their thoughts and actions. As we discussed in Week 5, Day 3, the Israelites were expected to know the commandments by heart, to carry them on their hands and foreheads, write them on their doorposts and gates, and talk about them all the time. *You shall teach them to your children, speaking of them when you sit in your house, when you walk by the way, when you lie down, and when you rise up.* (Deut. 11:19)

◌◌ Walking With Moses ◌◌

Moses lived the "and now . . ." scenario day after day with the Israelites. He understood disobedience carried consequences, and obedience carried blessings. His diligence to teach the "if/then" wisdom of God's laws and instruction was seemingly unflappable. So too should ours be.

◌◌ Talking With God ◌◌

God, help me begin each day with "and now . . ." always expectant of Your guidance and grace.

_____

_____

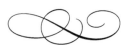

Proclaim liberty throughout all the land, unto all the inhabitants thereof.

Leviticus 25:10

Inscribed on the Liberty Bell, Philadelphia, PA

Day 2
Is There Someone Else? – Part II

Text: Deuteronomy 31:1-29

Focus: *Then Moses called Joshua and said to him in the sight of all Israel, "Be strong and of good courage, for you must go with this people to the land which the Lord has sworn to their fathers to give them, and you shall cause them to inherit it."* Deuteronomy 31:7

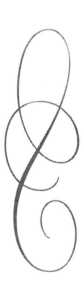

I will confess, today's topic is for me personally the most intimate of our entire study in terms of preparation and openness. Of the many lessons and challenges I have encountered along the way, none have been as difficult as letting go of leadership roles and ministry responsibilities. Perhaps it is my ego, or simply my sincere belief in the particular ministries and hope for their continued growth. Regardless of my motivation, I admit to having a very difficult time trusting anyone else to take over the leadership roles I have held in the past.

Can you relate to my dis-ease? How do you handle similar situations when it is time to step down from a leadership role? Are you able to release the reins, trusting the new leader to carry on?

_____

_____

_____

_____

Are you convinced no one can do the job as well as you?

_____

_____

_____

_____

How does it make you feel when you see changes being made?

_____

_____

_____

_____

Do you feel threatened by the new leadership?

_____

_____

_____

_____

If you are still an active member of the organization, do you think the new leadership feels threatened by you?

_____

_____

_____

_____

These are questions I grapple with daily.

From the text of today's Scripture, Moses apparently accepted the lesson, at this point in the story, with a heightened level of dignity. A forty-year journey full of trials, hardships, miracles, victories, and a prolonged one on one conversation with God was coming to an end. His days of leadership were over and someone else had been chosen to take over.

I found the manner in which Moses prepared the Israelites for his departure very true to human nature and comical. Please indulge my very loose paraphrase of Deuteronomy 31:1-2, "I won't be the one leading you into the Promised Land. The truth of the matter is, I'm old and my gitty-up has got up and gone. Oh yeah, and did I mention God said I can't go?" That sounds so familiar to me. First I try to explain with excuses and human reasoning; then, almost as an after thought I disclose the reality of God's intervention and plan.

Obviously assuming the Israelites were going to panic when he announced the change in leadership, he expounded on the faithfulness of God to go into the land before them to vanquish all their foes. So, regardless who was leading them, all would be well because God would be in control. What does Moses say God will do for them specifically?

Deuteronomy 31: 3: *The LORD your God Himself* _____ _____ *before you. He will* _____ *these nations from before you, and you shall dispossess them.*

Deuteronomy 31:5: *The LORD will* _____ _____ *over to you, that you may do to them according to every commandment which I have commanded you.*

He then proclaimed what I think is one of the most remarkable encouragements in the entire Old Testament: *Be strong and of good courage, do not fear nor be afraid of them; for the LORD your God, He is the One who goes with you. He will not leave you nor forsake you.* (Deut. 31:6)

Many years later, David would use similar words speaking to his son Solomon: *Be strong and of good courage, and do it; do not fear nor be dismayed, for the Lord God—my God—will be with you. He will not leave you nor forsake you, until you have finished all the work for the service of the house of the Lord. (I Chr. 28:20)*

Christ Himself spoke of the coming of the Holy Spirit saying *I will not leave you orphans. (John 14:18).* Some versions of the Bible say orphans and others say comfortless, but the meaning is the same, *for the LORD will not forsake His people, for His great name's sake, because it has pleased the LORD to make you His people. (I Sam. 12:22)* Before we go any further in today's study, let's take a look back at one of the questions Moses asked as he stood before the burning bush. *But he said, "O my Lord, please send by the hand of whomever else you shall say." (Ex. 4:13).* The NIV says *"O Lord, please send someone else to do it."* Now, forty years later and many miles away from Egypt, Moses is getting what he requested at his original encounter with God. Someone else would indeed be leading the Israelites into the Promised Land. You've heard the adage, "Be careful what you ask for, you just might get it." So it was for Moses, at least for these last few steps of the journey.

Have you had an experience of praying for a particular outcome and then being surprised when your prayer is answered many years later? If so, give a brief description.

_____

_____

_____

_____

Then Moses called Joshua. (Deut. 31:7a) American Journalist, Walter Lippman said, "The final test of a leader is that he leaves behind him in other men the conviction and the will to carry on." [1] Moses proved, once again, his aptitude for effective leadership by doing exactly that. He had been training and mentoring Joshua for more than forty years and was confident of his conviction to finish the task at hand.

So, who is Joshua and what qualifies him to take over? What three things are revealed about Joshua in Exodus 33:11?

- He was Moses' _____
- He was the son of _____
- He was a _____ _____

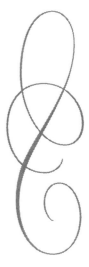

Joshua was born during the years of captivity in Egypt. He was the son of Nun of the tribe of Ephraim. Ephraim was one of the sons of Joseph, and Joseph was one of the twelve sons of Jacob—the original Israelites to come to Egypt. Read Exodus 1:1-7. *But the children of Israel were fruitful and increased abundantly, multiplied and grew exceedingly mighty; and the land was filled with them.* (vs.7) Thus, Joshua was a child of Israel and a slave under the reign of a cruel and unrelenting Pharaoh.

The Scripture does not detail whether Moses' true heritage was common knowledge among the Israelites during the years he lived in Pharaoh's palace, but obviously his immediate family knew the story, so I believe others must have known his identity as well. If you remember, from an earlier lesson, Exodus 11:3b says, … *the man Moses himself was very great in the land of Egypt, in the sight of Pharaoh's servants and in the sight of the people.* (Although it cannot be known for sure, it is surmised that Joshua was approximately forty years younger than Moses.) As a small child Joshua probably heard stories about Moses and wondered about this Hebrew child adopted into royalty; as a teen he probably admired the bravery of the man who rejected his adopted family to rescue one of his own; and as a young man he perhaps had a foreboding their paths would one day cross in a significant way.

Who is someone you knew of by reputation and then were honored to meet and/or work with?

_____

_____

_____

What responsibility did Moses entrust to Joshua in Exodus 17:8-13?

_____

_____

Numbers 11:28 says Joshua was one of Moses' _____ men.

What additional job was Joshua given in Numbers 13?

_____

_____

_____

_____

After the twelve spies returned from Canaan, all agreed it was a good land that "flows with milk and honey" (Num. 13:27), but dissension arose as to whether the Israelites were strong enough to overtake the Amalekites, Hittites, Jebusites, Amorites, and Canaanites who dwelt there. Only Caleb and Joshua spoke out favorably, saying, *"If the Lord delights in us, then He will bring us into this land and give it to us, 'a land which flows with milk and honey.'"* (Num. 14:8)

From this additional scene in Joshua's life would you describe him as a man who sees the glass as half empty or half full? _____

Moses surely recognized this positive outlook and the impact such an attitude could have on the well-being of the Israelites in the future.
Scholars and theologians have long debated Joshua's age at the time of his

commissioning by Moses to lead the Israelites into the Promised Land, but the general consensus is approximately 80 years of age—the same age Moses was when the journey out of Egypt began.

How long was Moses in the wilderness before returning to Egypt? _____

How long was Joshua in the wilderness with Moses before reaching the Promised Land? _____

Forty years in the wilderness learning to see, hear, feel, and believe. Forty years learning to lead an unruly and fickle people. Forty years learning to worship the one true God and to trust Him for all things. Moses had taught Joshua all he could and it was time to pass the proverbial torch.

Numbers 27:20: *And you shall _____ some of your _____ to him, that all the congregation of the children of Israel may be obedient.*

Numbers 27:22: *So Moses did as the Lord commanded him. He took Joshua and set him before Eleazar the priest and before all the congregation. And he _____ _____ _____ on him and inaugurated him, just as the Lord commanded by the hand of Moses.*

Deuteronomy 3:28: *But _____ Joshua, and _____ him and _____ him; for he shall go over before this people, and he shall cause them to inherit the land which you will see.*

Based on this instruction given to Moses, what are our responsibilities as we pass on leadership responsibilities to others?

_____

_____

_____

_____

How should we do this? _____

Deuteronomy 34:9: *Now Joshua the son of Nun was full of the spirit of wisdom, for Moses had _____ _____ _____on him; so the children of Israel heeded him, and did as the Lord had commanded Moses.*

✏ **Walking With Moses** ✏

Moses knew his job was almost complete. He faithfully set the stage for Joshua to step into the role as leader of the Israelites, showing his own strength of character and love for the people. He wanted the best for them, even after his departure from their midst. His example of passing the torch, is a challenge, but an action to be emulated.

✏ **Talking With God** ✏

God, teach me to step down from leadership roles with grace and dignity while encouraging the one stepping in.

_____

_____

_____

_____

[1] Walter Lippman, American Journalist 1889-1974 in NY Tribune, April 14, 1945.

Day 3
Look, but Don't Touch

Text: Deuteronomy 31 - 32

Focus: *Yet you shall see the land before you, though you shall not go there, into the land which I am giving to the children of Israel.* Deuteronomy 32:52

Frequently when shopping, I will hear a mother say to her youngster, "Look with your eyes, not with your hands." Of course, it is every parent's fear that their child will accidentally send a piece of merchandise crashing to the floor, resulting in a purchase they never intended to make, for an item that is broken and useless. Other places we see and hear this admonition to look but not touch include the animal cages at the zoo, newly painted surfaces, and freshly planted grass. For several years I worked at an historic home in my city. When I needed to handle an artifact or antique item in the house, I knew to wear gloves to protect the surfaces from the natural oils and dirt that might be on my hands; and, guests were always instructed to stay behind the cord barriers. In each of these scenarios, the warning serves to protect from a harmful, unpleasant or dangerous outcome. We may not enjoy hearing the cautionary phrase, but we know it is ultimately for our own good.

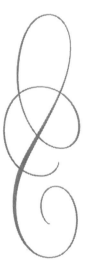

In today's lesson, we see a much different situation for Moses as he hears God say he will only be allowed to look into the Promised Land. His weary feet will never touch it.

There are variations in the interpretations of what happened at Massah and Meribah in Exodus and Numbers, when Moses *not so gently* coaxed water from the rock, but regardless of the details, or the actual chain of events, it is clear God exacted a disappointing judgment on Moses for his disobedience and lack of faith.

At the beginning of today's text, and as a bit of repetition from our earlier study involving the choosing and blessing of Joshua, we see Moses knew his death was near and was working at a fevered pitch to get his affairs in order.

Deuteronomy 31:2: *And he said to them: "I am _____ years old today. I can no long go out and come in. Also the LORD has said to me, 'You shall _____ _____ _____ this Jordan.'"*

Deuteronomy 31:9: *So Moses _____ this law and _____ it*

to the priests, the sons of Levi, who bore the ark of the covenant of the LORD, and to all the elders of Israel.

Deuteronomy 31:14b: *So Moses and Joshua _____ and _____ themselves in the tabernacle of meeting.*

Do you think Moses was prepared for the message he would hear from God when he entered the tabernacle of meeting? Re-read Deuteronomy 31:16-18. Can't you just imagine Moses saying, "Okay God, I get the part about me dying, but these people are going to do WHAT, with WHOM, WHERE, and WHEN? WHY would they do such a thing?" And God replied as He has frequently replied throughout history when the hard questions are asked. He said, *"Now therefore, write down this song for yourselves, and teach it to the children . . ."* (Deut. 31:19a). The Song of Moses recorded in Deuteronomy 32 is one of praise, warning and redemption.

Read Psalm 23 and consider the questions on David's mind as he penned those words or Luke 1:46-55 as Mary tried to understand her future.

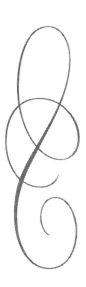

In 1870, Horatio Spafford wrote "It Is Well With My Soul" after his four beloved daughters were lost in the sinking of the S.S. Ville Du Havre.

> *When peace, like a river, attendeth my way,*
> *When sorrows like sea billows roll;*
> *Whatever my lot, thou has taught me to say,*
> *It is well, it is well , with my soul.*

"What A Friend We Have In Jesus" was written in 1857 by Joseph Scriven out of his deep need to understand his lonely existence after losing two fiancées, one to drowning and one to illness, and then suffering estrangement from his family after his Christian conversion.

> *Are we weak and heavy laden,*
> *Cumbered with a load of care?*
> *Precious Savior, still our refuge;*
> *Take it to the Lord in prayer.*

For contemporary Christian artist Tammy Trent, the words to "Rescue Me" came as she cried out to God following the drowning death of her husband off the coast of Jamaica on September 10, 2001.

I need you to rescue me
From this feeling I won't breathe again
Need you to rescue me
And make my spirit strong within.

Deuteronomy 31:22: *Therefore Moses _____ this song the same day, and _____ it to the children of Israel.*

Deuteronomy 31:30: *Then Moses _____ in the hearing of all the assembly of Israel the words of this song until they were ended.*

Deuteronomy 32:45 : *Moses _____ _____ all these words to all Israel, and he said to them: "Set your hearts on all the words which I testify among you today, which you shall command your children to be careful to observe – all the words of this law. For it is not a futile thing for you, because it is your life, and by this word you shall prolong your days in the land which you cross over the Jordan to possess."*

Write a song, learn a song, sing a song, memorize a song, teach a song. *Set your hearts on all the words. . .* (Deut. 32:46a)

Is there a song that has carried you through a difficult period or helped you make sense of a seemingly senseless situation?

_____

_____

_____

_____

In the days after the September 11 attacks I, along with many others in our nation, found great comfort in the song "You Raise Me Up," written by Brendan Graham and Rolf Lovland. Since that time it has been recorded over 400 times by artists from around the world.

The song Moses sang to the Israelites told of troubles past and troubles yet to come, but in the end, God would look with favor on His people.

Deuteronomy 32:48-52 brings us to the climax of today's lesson—*you may look, but you may not touch.*

Although I cannot fathom the disappointment Moses must have felt, I can imagine other modern day scenarios that seem as grim. Consider with me the following:

- A young wife is unable to join her husband in another country because of immigration restrictions.
- New parents are not allowed to touch their critically ill newborn as it struggles to survive in the neonatal intensive care unit.
- A rescue worker can see the victim in distress, but cannot reach him in time to save him from the burning building.

Several years ago my husband and I toured Ellis Island while attending a conference in New York City. I was astounded by the number of people who passed through those buildings leaving behind all things familiar in search of a new life in a new country. I was equally astounded by the numbers who, after surviving the arduous journey, were separated from their traveling companions and turned away because of lack of identification or a medical condition which had often developed aboard the overcrowded ships. They stood on Ellis Island and looked across the bay to what they considered their Promised Land, but they were not allowed to cross over into it. Frustration, disappointment, heartbreak, and despair—all words inadequate to describe the feelings that accompany such situations.

My son just turned fourteen and he is a typical teenager. He would rather play video games than read a book; torment his sister than get along with her; and sleep until noon than get an early start to the day. He can be infuriating one minute and hilarious the next, yet usually by the end of the day, I am still glad he is my son (Moms, you know what I mean.) On those days when he is on my last nerve, I need only recall the beginning of his story to remember what a blessing he is to me and my family.

Samuel was born in El Salvador. We began working toward his adoption five months before he was born, yet he was eighteen months old when we were finally able to bring him home. Two years of red tape, mishandled documents, and political under-workings by two diverse governments stole precious time from us and from Samuel.

The whole saga is a story for another day, but during that time, I felt the despair of being able to look but not touch. We heard our son over the phone and saw many pictures of him, but we could not get our hands on him. Of course, we finally were able to bring him home, but it was not until we made our way through the customs gates of the Miami airport, that we felt confident he was safely and irrevocably ours.

Do you have your own story of "look but don't touch"? If so, give a brief description:

_____

_____

_____

_____

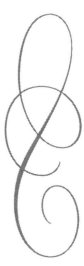

During those many months as we waited for Samuel, I prayed for God to intervene and change the situation. The truth is, I begged. I could not understand how the delay could possibly be God's best plan for our lives or for Samuel's.

How did you handle your situation? Did you petition God to change it?

_____

_____

_____

Well, friends, you will be glad to know, we are in good company. Read Deuteronomy 3:23-25. Moses not only pleaded with God to allow him to enter the Promised Land, he even tried to do a little "buttering up" by extolling God's great works and mighty deeds. I must admit, I can relate to that tactic as well.

Based on your previous study this week, you know how things progressed. As a reminder, read Deuteronomy 3:26-28. God held firm to His judgment. Joshua was installed as the new leader, blessings were given to the children of Israel, and Moses resigned himself to his fate.

In the introduction to this study, I explained how my walk with Moses began. As a quick reminder, I was reading the books of Exodus, Leviticus, Numbers and Deuteronomy out of curiosity to know more about the man Moses. During that time, I was also trying to decide whether I should resign from my fourteen-year position on church staff. Ultimately, I did resign and it has been an interesting adjustment, especially as my husband and I are still active members of the congregation. Many of the ministries I was involved with are not only continuing, but are flourishing under their new leadership; others are working hard to find their balance. Yet, even now, more than a year since my departure, I occasionally catch myself feeling uneasy when I see others doing jobs that were my responsibilities for many years—sitting at *my* desk, answering *my* phone, organizing *my* programs, and planning *my* events. Amazing how territorial we can become, even in ministry, isn't it? With a heavy heart, I find myself standing atop my own Mt. Nebo—able to look, but not touch.

Hebrews 11:1a: *Now faith is the substance of things hoped for . . .*

Moses' job was done. He would have the opportunity to look into the Promised Land before he died and that would have to be enough. His faith had carried him to this point and now his hope was in the leadership mantle placed around Joshua's broad shoulders.

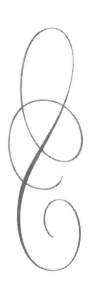

Walking With Moses

Moses was a leader who began well and was preparing to end well. He looked into the Promised Land with faith and hope for the Israelites; faith in the God who would continue to guide them and hope for their new beginning. Looking into a future that does not include our leadership or participation can be extremely difficult, but Moses led the way for us.

Talking With God

God, thank You for all that has been and for all that will be.

_____

_____

_____

_____

Day 4
Blessings to One and All

Text: Deuteronomy 28:1-14, Deuteronomy 33

Focus: *Now this is the blessing with which Moses, the man of God, blessed the children of Israel before his death.* Deuteronomy 33:1

Almost every Monday, while on the church staff, I was expected to attend the weekly staff meeting. After my resignation, I attended the last staff meeting, with a bit of trepidation, but also with a quiet knowing that the right decision had been made. In typical "play it to the end" fashion, the pastor had asked me to provide the devotion at the start of the meeting and I willingly agreed, knowing it would be one more chance to share the discernment process I had been engaged in over the past several months. After chronicling my experiences of walking with Moses and talking with God, I requested the opportunity to do one of the things Moses had done before he left the people for the last time.

Forty years they had wondered together in the wilderness. Forty years trusting God, following Moses as their leader, and not knowing if the next morning would find them in the Promised Land or still on desert sand. And now, at the edge of the Jordan, the long awaited day was finally upon them. There was no longer a cloud before them, only the expanse of the river and the land of milk and honey on the horizon. As they expectantly looked to Moses for the command to cross over, they must have stood in stunned amazement as he stood, called Joshua forth, laid his hands upon him and recognized him as their new leader. He sang a song reminding the people of the importance of the Law and the words of the Lord. And, as a final act, he prayed a blessing over the people with a specific word for each tribal leader. He brought closure to his unlikely life of leadership.

Reread Deuteronomy 33:6-25. List those who received a specific blessing by Moses.

_____

_____

_____

These are the same names listed in Jacob's farewell words in Genesis 49:3-27. Do you see any particular differences in what Jacob and Moses each had to say? Of particular interest is the charge to Levi. From Jacob we see condemnation and a curse; whereas Moses acknowledges Levi's commitment to the covenant. F. B. Meyer said, "If ever there was an illustration of the power we have to turn a curse into a blessing, it is here."

Read Numbers 1:5-16. List those who are commissioned to stand with Moses.

_____

_____

_____

"These were the chosen from the congregation, leaders of their fathers' tribes, heads of the divisions of Israel." (vs.16), now receiving a final and far reaching blessing from Moses. If time allows and you want to see the magnitude of the blessing offered by Moses in Deuteronomy 33:6-25, read Numbers 1:17-49.   Verse 46 reveals the total number as six hundred three thousand five hundred fifty men *"twenty years old and upward, everyone able to go to war in Israel."* Add in the women, children and men unable to go to war, and you end up with quite a crowd receiving this final blessing of Moses.

Did Moses receive a blessing himself as he spoke the words over the people of Israel? If so, explain how and why.

_____

_____

_____

_____

At the final staff meeting with my colleagues of fourteen years, all eyes were on me as I stood at the head of the conference table, each of them wondering if I would be so bold as to name my successor and sing a song reminding them of the importance of God's word. Mercifully, I refrained from delivering either. I did, however, ask to say a blessing. As I began making my way around the table, I'll admit I felt that familiar "I can't speak in public" knot in my stomach. Thoughts of inadequacy raced through my mind. What if I lisp and someone chuckles? Most of my fellow staff members have considerably more education, they've been to seminary for heaven's sake! Who am I to invoke a blessing on them? What if they think I'm being melodramatic? Gently, God calmed my fears reminding me that He had called me to this place, He had allowed me to be blessed by these people, and though I had not been ordained by the rites of man, He had ordained this moment.

So it was, with many tears and precious words of love and blessing I made my way around the room, laying my hands on the shoulders of those I had ministered with for so many years. It was good, it was right, and it helped each of us to move on.

How did the Israelites know they were being blessed even during their enslavement in Egypt? (Ex. 1:7)

_____

Proverbs 28:20a: *A* _____ *man will abound with blessings.*

How do you define the word *blessing*? _____

_____

_____

_____

How would differentiate between being a blessing to someone and bestowing a blessing upon someone?

_____

_____

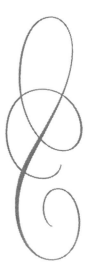

Webster's New World College Dictionary defines "blessing" as "the act or prayer of one who blesses with an invocation or benediction; a grace said before or after eating; the gift of divine favor; good wishes or approval." The Hebrew translation of the word "blessing" is *berakah* and is the same word used for "present."

Describe a time when you invoked a blessing on a person or group. How did you feel as you spoke the words? Did you sense that you were giving them a present?

_____

_____

_____

Do you think the blessing went beyond the person or group you called by name, just as Moses' blessing reached beyond the leaders of each tribe? If so, explain.

_____

_____

_____

_____

Who is God leading you to deliver a blessing to? Do you think that blessing will have a ripple effect to others?

_____

_____

_____

_____

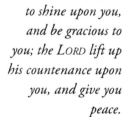

The LORD bless you and keep you; the LORD make his face to shine upon you, and be gracious to you; the LORD lift up his countenance upon you, and give you peace.

Numbers 6:24-26

✧ Walking With Moses ✧

You are called not only to lead, but to bless those you come in contact with throughout your ministry. Whether as a final act before moving on to a new leadership role or as a daily practice, the blessing from God you deliver to those around you has a ripple effect that reaches far beyond the one standing before you.

✧ Talking With God ✧

God, show me who I might bless through my words and actions today.

_____

_____

_____

_____

Day 5
My Presence Will Go With You

Text: Exodus 33:14, Deuteronomy 34:1-12

Focus: *He said, "My presence will go with you, and I will give you rest."* Exodus 33:14

Don't you love today's focus Scripture? I know I do. As we come to the end of our six weeks of study, there is such assurance knowing the very presence of God will go with us into all our tomorrows. Take a moment to re-read Exodus 33:12-23 and envision Moses asking for God's active involvement in the journey the Israelites have embarked upon. Keep in mind, this particular conversation occurred after:

- the plagues, miracles and wonders leading up to the departure from Egypt
- the exodus from Egypt
- the appearance of the cloud by day and the fire by night
- the trip through the Red Sea
- the bitter water of Marah turned sweet
- food fell from heaven
- water flowed from the rock
- the first tablets were *"written with the finger of God."*

Glory! That's quite a list as proof of God's favor and provision, isn't it? Yet still Moses implores "show me your ways." God continues by:

- dictating a new set of tablets
- designing the tabernacle and ark of the covenant
- detailing worship practices
- and affording countless other manifestations of His goodness.

Just as the Israelites lingered at the wells of Elim, I want to camp out on Exodus 33:14 for a few moments lest we miss the eternal significance of this promise as we look at Moses' final moments on this earth. Each step of the journey, God's patient reply was the assurance of His presence with Moses and the Israelites. The most frequently used Hebrew translation of the word *presence* is *panim*, literally meaning *face*. However, in this particular case, and based on verse 20 saying Moses cannot see God's face, we can be confident the word *panim* in verse 14 is the lesser used translation meaning a *presence* or *countenance*. (Countenance is defined as showing one's nature or feelings.)

Think about the last time you were in a darkened room with friends or loved ones. Perhaps you could not see their face, but you knew they were there—you could simply feel their presence? Many years ago, I heard a story about a man and his young daughter who were grieving the sudden death of wife and mother. As they settled into bed on their first night alone, the little girl asked her father to sleep in her room. Shortly after the lights were turned out, she whispered "Sure is dark, isn't it daddy?" "Yes, honey it sure is." "Isn't this the darkest night ever, Daddy?" "Yes, honey I think it is." "Daddy, is your face turned toward me?" "Yes, honey it is." And then she slept. It must have been very similar for Moses and the Israelites. Although they could not see the face of God, they knew God's holy presence was turned toward them. Moses had secured this promise for the Israelites before he ascended Mount Sinai for the second time.

Exodus 33:15-17: *Then he said to Him, "If Your Presence does not go with us, do not bring us up from here. For how then will it be known that Your people and I have found grace in Your sight, except You go with us? . . . So the LORD said to Moses, "I will also do this thing that you have spoken; for you have found grace in My sight and I know you by name. "*

How does God manifest His presence to you? Do you feel the face of God turned toward you?

_____

_____

_____

_____

Exodus 40:34-38 recounts God's presence within the tabernacle. As long as God's presence, in the form of a cloud, filled the tabernacle or tent of meeting, the Israelites would not move forward. When the cloud was taken up, they would set out on their trek once again. The NRSV says, *For the cloud of the LORD was on the tabernacle by day, and fire was in the cloud by night, before the eyes of all the house of Israel at _____ _____ of their _____.* (Ex.40:38) A childhood friend of mine frequently said, "a promise is a promise, and you can't break a promise." And so it was with the promise of God's presence.

The other part of verse 14 that I appreciate is the promise of rest. Not just rest at the end of the day, or a respite on the journey, but divine rest given by the God of deliverance, miracles, provision, and eternity. In Hebrew, the word *nuach* means "to cause to rest". Don't we all need to hear God saying, "I am not only going to give you rest, but I am telling you to take a nap, take a time out, take a selah. I am telling you it is time to be finished with your task."

Have you heard and heeded God's instruction to rest?

_____

_____

_____

_____

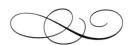

selah (Hebrew) to weigh, measure, pause, stop and reflect, observe, think, rest.

Throughout Moses' life he had received the promise of Exodus 33:14. God's presence had been with him from the very beginning as his tiny body was cradled in a watertight basket lovingly woven by his Hebrew mother.

In the past six weeks we have seen countless times when the promise of God's presence and rest were manifested. Take a few moments now to glance back through our previous days of study and consider anew the many steps that brought us to our final day with Moses.

Read Exodus 3:7-9. The job entrusted to Moses as he stood before the burning bush so many years before has been completed and we find ourselves at the end of Moses' life. And, what a life it was! The Israelites were preparing to cross into the Promised Land; Joshua was ready to lead, Moses had bestowed final blessings and instructions; all that remained was for Moses to gaze upon the long awaited destination.

A few years ago, my husband and I decided it was time to visit a tourist attraction we had driven past countless times on our way to and from Florida. If you have traveled north or south of Chattanooga, on I-75, you have no doubt seen the "See Rock City" signs advertising the attractions on top of Lookout Mountain. Although I chose not to ride the Incline Railway and our schedule did not allow time for Ruby Falls, we did take in the massive rock formations (and the occasional gnome sighting) of Rock City. Another significant draw to this particular site (other than the gnome statues, of course) is the observation point where you experience the panoramic view from 1700 feet above sea level, seeing seven states while standing in one spot. It is quite impressive if you happen to visit on a clear day—you truly can see forever.

What do you think were the "signs" along the way for Moses and the Israelites?

_____

_____

_____

_____

What are the signs you can identify in your own life, which have assured you that you were on the right road to your destination?

_____

_____

_____

_____

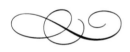

Mount Nebo is an elevated ridge that is approximately 2680 feet above sea level, in what is now western Jordan.

High atop Mt. Nebo, God provided Moses with the panoramic view of *"the whole land"*, saying *"This is the land of which I swore to Abraham, to Isaac, and to Jacob, saying 'I will give it to your descendants."* (Deut. 34:4a). Even on the clearest day, it is doubtful Moses could have truly seen to the farthest boundaries of the Promised Land, but with spiritual eyes, he could see the glorious borders of the promise itself. His heart was surely pounding with excitement as he realized the culmination of his life's work. And then God spoke the words Moses undoubtedly hoped he would not hear, *"I have caused you to see it with your eyes, but you shall not cross over there."* (Deut. 34:4b) I can imagine the sigh that must have escaped Moses' lips as he realized God had not changed His mind. The Israelites would continue across the Jordan under the qualified leadership of Joshua, but Moses would take his last breath on Mount Nebo. His job was done.

My thoughts are tender as I consider this final conversation between Moses and God. I have heard countless stories of remarkable scenes witnessed by family and friends as dying loved ones began their face to face dialogue with God, yet I have experienced only one.

In August, 2004, my mother suffered a massive stroke and never regained consciousness. At one point, on the day mother died, I wiped tears from her feverish cheeks. Although the doctors assured us there was no discomfort or brain activity, I was troubled that she might have been in pain or frightened. Some days later, I mentioned my concern to a dear friend who reminded me my mother was getting her first glimpse of the riches in Glory (Phil. 4:19), being welcomed into the arms of God, and hearing His voice speaking words directly to her ears. When I remembered how she always cried at happy occasions such as the sight of new babies, weddings, family reunions, and unexpected company, her tears on that day in August made perfect sense to me.

No one knows what went on between Moses and God in those final moments, but I suspect Moses heard words similar to those recorded much later in Biblical history, *well done, good and faithful servant.* (Matt. 25:23)

Exodus 33:11: *So the Lord spoke to Moses _____ to _____, as a man speaks to his friend.*

 Still face to face, Moses died; joining his spirit with the God of Abraham, Isaac, and Jacob; the God of Moses.

But since then there has not arisen in Israel a prophet like Moses, whom the Lord knew face to face, in all the signs and wonders which the Lord sent him to do in the land of Egypt, before Pharaoh, before all his servants, and in all his land, and by all that mighty power and all the great terror which Moses performed in the sigh of all Israel. Deuteronomy 34:10-12

⤙⤚ **Walking With Moses** ⤙⤚

Of all the lessons that are gleaned from the life of Moses, today's holds the most eternal significance. God's promise of presence and rest are foundational to our walk in this life and into the next.

Talking With God

God, thank You for the promise of Your presence and rest.

_____

_____

_____

_____

Conclusion

Friends, it has been a pleasure walking with you. And, though you have arrived at the end of this study, you have in no way reached the end of your journey. There are still many lessons to be learned and many words to be spoken by God to your heart. Don't stop now. Keep going through every valley and to the top of every mountain. Trust God for protection and provision. Be on the lookout for God's active presence in your life and build altars of remembrance along the way. Step boldly into each tomorrow until you reach your final Promised Land and hear God say "well done good and faithful servant."

BIBLIOGRAPHY

Anderson, Bernard W.; Darr, Katheryn Pfisterer, *Understanding the Old Testament,* Abridged and Updated, 4th Edition. (Pearson Education Inc., 1998, Upper Saddle River, NJlewood Cliffs, NJ)

Berlin, Adele and Marc Zvi Brettler, eds., *The Jewish Study Bible* (Oxford University Press, 2004, New York)

Ginzberg, Louis, *The Legends of the Jews,* Vol. III, Moses in the Wilderness, translated by Paul Radin (Johns Hopkins University Press, 1998, Baltimore, MD)

Knowles, Elizabeth, ed., *The Oxford Dictionary of Quotations* 6th Ed. (Oxford University Press, 2004, New York, NY)

Laymon, Charles M., ed., *The Interpreter's One-Volume Commentary of the Bible* (Abingdon Press, 1971, Nashville, TN)

Lazareth, William H., ed., *Reading the Bible in Faith: Theological Voices from the Pastorate* (Wm.B. Eerdmans Publishing Co., 2001, Grand Rapids, MI)

Meyer, F.B., *Great Verses Through the Bible* (Marshall, Morgan & Scott, Ltd., The Zondervan Ed., Zondervan Publishing House, 1972, Grand Rapids, MI)

Nemerov, Howard, *The Collected Poems of Howard Nemerov* (University of Chicago Press, 1977, Chicago, IL)

Peterson, Eugene H., *The Message* (NavPress, 2002, Colorado Springs, CO)

Russell, A.J., ed., *God Calling: by Two Listeners* (Jove Books, The Berkley Publishing Group, 1986, New York, NY)

Troccoli, Kathy, *My Life Is in Your Hands* (Careers – BMG Music Publishing, Inc. and Floating Note Music, 1994)

Young, Robert, LL.D, *Young's Analytical Concordance to the Bible* (Wm.B. Eerdmans

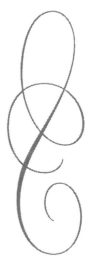

Publishing Co. 1977, Grand Rapids, MI)

www.jewfaz.org/moshe.htm   Judaism 101 Moses, Aaron and Miriam

www.jhom.com/topics/fire/bush.html

www.net.bible.org/illustration/php?topic-3 Quartermaster General's Report

www.net.bible.org/illustration/php?topic=1025 Unmasking Egypt's Magicians

www.religion.ucumberlands.edu/hebrewsbible/hbnotes/mosnotes.htm

www.religion.ucumberlands.edu/hebrewsbible/hbnotes/plaguenotes.htm

www.rrfb.org/media/food_security.htm

Note to Leaders

Visit www.randallhouse.com and receive a free Leader's Guide for *Walking With Moses—Talking With God*.
.

Discover tools to aid you in leading your church or small study group through a six-week journey that will cultivate a deeper walk with God. In this on-line resource you will find teacher suggestions, discussion springboard questions, lists of additional resources, and several handouts for the group. You will also find a personal note from Cinda King.

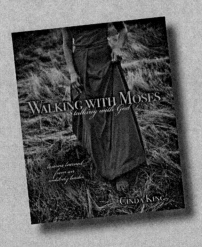

To order additional copies of
Walking With Moses—Talking With God
call **1-800-877-7030** or
log onto **www.randallhouse.com**.

Call for quantity discounts.

Experience

the Power Behind the Passages You've Known for Years

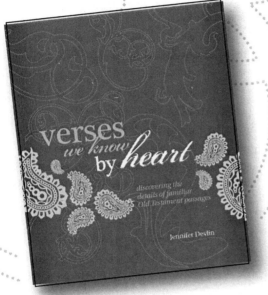

Verses We Know By Heart
Jennifer Devlin

$10.99- Group Discounts Available!
ISBN: 9780892655656

Verses We Know By Heart is a six-week study of familiar Old Testament passages. Throughout this study, you will gain a more insightful look into the background, context, and meaning of each passage. The variety of topics applies to various stages of life and will ignite you with a passion to search the Word of God for truths needed to overcome all of life's obstacles.

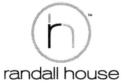

randall house

**To order call 1-800-877-7030
or visit www.randallhouse.com**

The Verses We Know By Heart study covers these following passages:

- *Genesis 1:1—2:3*
- *Exodus 20:1-17*
- *Proverbs 3:5-6*
- *Psalm 23*
- *Ecclesiastes 3:1-14*
- *Isaiah 40:10-31*

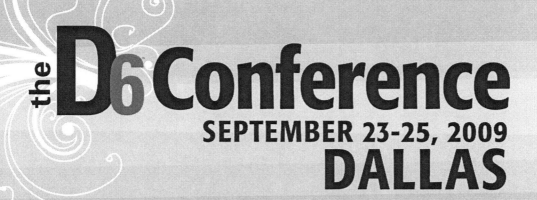
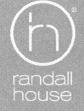

CPSIA information can be obtained at www.ICGtesting.com
Printed in the USA
LVOW121432310512

284057LV00002B/6/P